12/17/12
#131.95

PAIN

Psychological Perspectives

PAIN

Psychological Perspectives

Edited by

Thomas Hadjistavropoulos
University of Regina

Kenneth D. Craig
University of British Columbia

LAWRENCE ERLBAUM ASSOCIATES, PUBLISHERS
2004   Mahwah, New Jersey   London

BF
515
P29
2004

Lawrence Erlbaum Associates, Inc., Publishers
10 Industrial Avenue
Mahwah, New Jersey 07430

Cover design by Sean Sciarrone

Library of Congress Cataloging-in-Publication Data

Pain : psychological perspectives / edited by Thomas Hadjistavropoulos, Kenneth D. Craig.
    p. cm.
Includes bibliographical references and index.
ISBN 0-8058-4299-3 (alk. paper)
    1. Pain—Psychological aspects. I. Hadjistavropoulos, Thomas. II. Craig, Kenneth D.,
    1937–

BF515.P29   2003
152.1'824—dc21   2003052862
                                                                                   CIP

Books published by Lawrence Erlbaum Associates are printed on acid-free paper,
and their bindings are chosen for strength and durability.

Printed in the United States of America
10 9 8 7 6 5 4 3 2 1

We dedicate this volume to those who mean the most to us:

Heather, Nicholas, and Dimitri
—T. H.

Sydney, Kenneth, Alexandra, and Jamie
—K. D. C.

Contents

Contributors

Gordon J. G. Asmundson   Faculty of Kinesiology and Health Studies, University of Regina, Regina, Saskatchewan, Canada

Stephen Bruehl   Department of Anesthesiology, Vanderbilt University School of Medicine, Nashville, Tennessee

Christine T. Chambers   Department of Pediatrics, University of British Columbia, Centre for Community Child Health Research, Vancouver, British Columbia, Canada

C. Richard Chapman   Pain Research Centre, Department of Anesthesiology, University of Utah, Salt Lake City, Utah

Ok Yung Chung   Department of Anesthesiology, Vanderbilt University School of Medicine, Nashville, Tennessee

Kenneth D. Craig   Department of Psychology, University of British Columbia, Vancouver, British Columbia, Canada

Amanda C. de C. Williams   INPUT Pain Management Unit, St. Thomas' Hospital, London, United Kingdom

Shannon Fuchs-Lacelle   Department of Psychology, University of Regina, Regina, Saskatchewan, Canada

Steven J. Gibson   National Ageing Research Institute, Parkville, Victoria, Australia

Heather D. Hadjistavropoulos   Department of Psychology, University of Regina, Regina, Saskatchewan, Canada

Thomas Hadjistavropoulos   Department of Psychology, University of Regina, Regina, Saskatchewan, Canada

Joel Katz   Department of Psychology, York University, Toronto, Ontario, Canada

Victoria L. Mason   Department of Psychology, University of Bath, Bath, United Kingdom

Ronald Melzack   Department of Psychology, McGill University, Montreal, Qeubec, Canada

Elena S. Monarch   Department of Anesthesiology, University of Washington, Seattle, Washington

Gary B. Rollman   Department of Psychology, University of Western Ontario, London, Ontario, Canada

Suzanne M. Skevington   Department of Psychology, University of Bath, Bath, United Kingdom

Dennis C. Turk   Department of Anesthesiology, University of Washington, Seattle, Washington

Arthur D. Williams   Department of Anesthesiology, University of Washington, Seattle, Washington

Kristi D. Wright   Dalhousie University, Halifax, Nova Scotia, Canada

Preface

This volume offers a state-of-the-art, comprehensive account of the psychology of pain that encompasses clinical perspectives but also basic social and behavioral science as well as biopsychological contributions to the field. The relatively recent focus on pain as a subjective experience has led to dramatic improvements in our understanding of the complex psychological processes that represent and control pain. There has also been an enhanced understanding of the ontogenetic, socialization, and contextual determinants of pain. Mechanisms responsible for the complex synthesis of sensations, feelings, and thoughts underlying pain behavior have been the target of concerted research and clinical investigation. This volume explicates our current understanding of the current theory, research, and practice on these complex psychological processes. We are proud of our list of contributors that includes some of the most influential and productive pain researchers in the world.

Although the book is primarily intended for psychologists (practitioners, researchers, and students) managing, investigating, and studying pain, it would also be of interest to a variety of other professionals working in this area (e.g., physicians, nurses, physiotherapists). The book is also suitable as a textbook for graduate and advanced undergraduate courses on the psychology of pain.

We owe a debt of gratitude to the many sources of support made available to us. In the first instance, we are most appreciative of the commitment, inspiration, and hard work of the people who work with us in the common cause of developing a better understanding of pain and pain control. Our graduate students and project staff continuously offer fresh perspectives, ideas, and boundless energy, giving us a great hope for the future and confidence in our work today. We also acknowledge many outstanding colleagues who generously exchange ideas with us about important issues relating to the psychology of pain. These ideas are a source of inspiration and make us proud of the many scientific and clinical advances our field has achieved.

Work on this project was supported, in part, by a Canadian Institutes of Health Research Investigator Award to Thomas Hadjistavropoulos and by a Canadian Institutes of Health Research Senior Investigator Award to Kenneth D. Craig. Related work in our laboratories has been supported by the Canadian Institutes of Health Research, the Social Sciences and Humanities Research Council of Canada, and the Health Services Utilization and Research Commission.

We acknowledge Holly Luhning's help in preparing and formatting the manuscript for submission to the publisher. We also thank Debra Riegert of Lawrence Erlbaum Associates for her support and enthusiasm about this project.

Most importantly, we acknowledge the love and support of our families. They give us strength.

—Thomas Hadjistavropoulos
—Kenneth D. Craig

An Introduction to
Pain: Psychological Perspectives

Thomas Hadjistavropoulos
University of Regina

Kenneth D. Craig
University of British Columbia

Pain is primarily a psychological experience. It is the most pervasive and universal form of human distress and it often contributes to dramatic reductions in the quality of life. As demonstrated repeatedly in the chapters to follow, it is virtually inevitable and a relatively frequent source of distress from birth to old age. Episodes of pain can vary in magnitude from events that are mundane, but commonplace, to crises that are excruciating, sometimes intractable, and not so common, but still not rare. The costs of pain in human suffering and economic resources are extraordinary. It is the most common reason for seeking medical care, and it has been estimated that approximately 80% of physician office visits involve a pain component (Henry, 1999–2000).

The distinction between pain and nociception provides the basis for focusing on pain as a psychological phenomenon. Nociception refers to the neurophysiologic processing of events that stimulate nociceptors and are capable of being experienced as pain (Turk & Melzack, 2000). Instigation of the nociceptive system and brain processing constitute the biological substrates of the experience. But pain must be appreciated as a psychological phenomenon, rather than a purely physiological phenomenon. Specifically, it represents a perceptual process associated with conscious awareness, selective abstraction, ascribed meaning, appraisal, and learning (Melzack & Casey, 1968). Emotional and motivational states are central to understanding its nature (Price, 2000). Pain requires central integration and modulation of a number of afferent and central processes (i.e., sending messages

I

toward the central nervous system and interacting with higher components of the central nervous system) and efferent processes (i.e., sending messages away from higher centers in the central nervous system and toward muscle or gland).

This formulation acknowledges the importance of various levels of analysis of pain. The biological sciences (molecular biology, genetics, neurophysiology, pharmacological sciences, etc.) have made major advances. Indeed, they appear to be in ascendance in the study of pain. Ultimately, however, a unified theory of pain must integrate this understanding with the product of work in the behavioral and social sciences, as well as the humanities, because pain cannot be understood solely at the level of gene expression, neuronal firing, and brain circuitry. Many of the serious problems in understanding and controlling pain must be understood at the psychological and social level of analysis. The following come immediately to mind: How can we prevent pain? Why do many complaints of pain not have a medical basis? What accounts for some people reacting dispassionately and others with great distress to what appears to be the same degree of tissue damage? Why do we most often underestimate the pain of others? What accounts for general trends toward undermanagement of pain?

The discipline of psychology must play a central role in the study, assessment, and management of pain. It is not surprising that Ronald Melzack, one of the developers of the most influential theory in the field of pain, is a psychologist. Nor is it unexpected that at least 2 of the 10 most influential clinicians and researchers in the field of pain (as assessed by survey of a random sample of members of the International Association for the Study of Pain [IASP]) are psychologists (Asmundson, Hadjistavropoulos, & Antonishyn, 2001). These two individuals (Ronald Melzack and Dennis Turk) are contributors to this volume.

In this book we have tried to capture major features of the psychology of pain and the most influential contributions of psychologists to pain research and management. We are primarily interested in the ultimate impact of advances in understanding and controlling pain. Hence, although much of the volume covers applied issues, basic processes are also given careful consideration.

FROM DESCARTES TO THE NEUROMATRIX

Historical trends demonstrate the importance of psychological mechanisms. Descartes's (1644/1985) early mechanistic conceptions of pain resulted in the biomedical specificity theory that proposed that a specific pain system transmits messages from receptors to the brain. This theory is sometimes referred to as "the alarm bell" or "push button" theory (Melzack, 1973), because of its apparent simplicity. Descartes's early views were refined substantially over the years, and more complex mechanistic views gradually emerged as investigators struggled to incorporate in their models of pain the complexities and puzzles of pain that dismayed patients and clinicians struggling with pain control. Nevertheless, biomedical specificity theory continued to exert an enormous influence through the first half of the 20th century. There was little room for recognition of the importance of psychological processes such as emotion, attention, past experience, and cognitive processes in the study of pain. Patients suffering from pain without a pathophysiological basis or signs often were considered "crocks" (Melzack, 1993).

Despite dominance of sensory specificity and biomedical models of pain, clinicians were increasingly finding emotional and motivational processes to be important in understanding pain. Merskey (1998) observed that psychological explanations about motives for complaints about pain and psychodynamic theories gradually became popular during the early and middle parts of the 20th century (e.g., Ellman, Savage, Wittkower, & Rodger, 1942; Scott, 1948). Early investigation of psychiatric patients with pain had led to the erroneous conclusion that physical and psychological factors in pain were mutually exclusive and that pain is either physical or psychological (IASP Ad Hoc Subcommittee for Psychology Curriculum, 1997). Persistent pain with no identifiable causes was frequently labeled as psychogenic, a regrettable construct because it perpetuates mind/body dualistic thinking (Liebeskind & Paul, 1977) and fails to recognize that biological mechanisms are integral to all psychological phenomena, including pain.

Freud (1893–1895) viewed pain as a common conversion symptom and favored the position that pains encountered in hysteria were originally of somatic origin. In other words, he argued that the pain was not created by the neurosis, but rather the neurosis served to maintain it. Dynamic conceptions of pain emphasize the role of psychic energies derived from innate drives linked to aggression, dependency, and sexuality and postulate that the pain experience is associated with the gratification or frustration of these drives (Pilowsky, 1986). For example, pain can be construed as the product of aggression that is inflicted either on oneself or on others and can be related to the formation of a cruel superego with an associated chronic sense of guilt and low self-esteem (Pilowsky, 1986).

Although psychodynamic approaches were frequently used to characterize patients whose pain unfortunately had been labeled as "psychogenic," they have not led to any major empirically supported advances in pain management, and this perspective has been losing favor over the years (e.g., Merskey, 1998). Efforts to bolster the psychodynamic perspective come from case studies, although some work has linked suppressed anger to the experience of persistent pain. Pilowsky and Spence (1975), for example, found that a pain clinic group reported a higher incidence of anger inhibition than 40 hospital outpatients who reported pain as their most prominent symptom. It is difficult, however, to draw causal relationships from such data.

Perhaps the most significant and systematic involvement of psychologists in the field of pain began with the correspondence of Donald Hebb, a McGill University psychologist, and George A. Bishop, an American physiologist, in the early 1950s (Merskey, 1996). The starting point of their discussion was Hebb's treatment of pain in his classic text *The Organization of Behavior* (1949). Ronald Melzack, who was Hebb's student, was influenced by these ideas and began to study the effects of early experience on the pain response (Melzack & Scott, 1957). Along with Patrick Wall, Ronald Melzack later formulated the gate control theory of pain (Melzack & Wall, 1965; see also chap. 1, this volume). The theory has been the most influential and productive model of pain to date, and has led to widespread recognition of the necessity of the study of psychological factors in our understanding of pain. This work in the domain of physiological psychology was the first to account for individual variability in the pain response and to emphasize the importance of a diverse array of cognitive, emotional, environmental, and behavioral factors. These views gradually made their way into clinical practice. A large number of innovative and productive psychologists working in research and clinical capacities would acknowledge the inspiration and leadership of this work. More recently, Melzack (e.g., Melzack, 1989) proposed the concept of the "neuromatrix" to explain phenomena that could not be explained well by preexisting theories (see chap. 1, this volume).

Other psychologists and psychological theories have made major contributions. In the 1960s and 1970s, Fordyce and other behavior theorists began to construe pain behavior in terms of both operant and classical conditioning (e.g., Fordyce, Fowler, & DeLateur, 1968). Pain behaviors (e.g., complaints, inactivity, drug use) are subject to reinforcement control (i.e., through operant processes), and anxiety and other emotional reactions can become associated with certain movements and circumstances that elicit pain (i.e., through classical conditioning processes). Behavioral interventions arising from these models became fundamental to clinical practice (Fordyce, 1976). The 1980s saw an increased emphasis on cognitive processes in the conceptualization of pain with work such as the pioneering volume *Pain and Behavioral Medicine* by Turk, Meichenbaum, and Genest (1983), thereby generating interest in research and novel clinical practice. Interventions became geared toward personal beliefs about pain and its meaning, with clinicians then able to focus on modifying maladaptive thoughts. This work was complemented by further psychophysiological investigations, the study of psychophysical processes, social psychological processes, and the study of cultural and individual differences. More refined views and methodologies have since been developed and are discussed throughout this volume.

EPIDEMIOLOGY, GENDER, AND DEVELOPMENT

Although epidemiological reports vary as a function of methodology used, the population surveys of the prevalence of pain leave no question that persisting pain is of great magnitude for people of all ages (Crombie, Croft, Linton, LeResche, & von Korff, 1999). The estimated prevalence of persistent pain in the community has been found to vary from 7% to 63.5% (e.g., Crombie, 1997; Bowsher, Rigge, & Sopp, 1991; von Korff, Dworkin, & LeResche, 1990). Moreover, more than 70% of patients with cancer develop significant pain over the course of their illness, with pain being the result not only of the disease, but also of chemotherapy, surgery, and radiotherapy (Henry, 1999–2000). The Canadian National Population Health Survey (Statistics Canada, 1996–1997) showed that 15% of Canadians over the age of 15 have chronic pain, with 70% of these people rating pain as severe to the point that it would cause interference with normal activity. According to the same study, people with pain had more days off work in the week prior to the survey, and more contacts with health care services (i.e., physician visits and hospital stays in the past year). In another frequently cited study, von Korff et al. (1990) studied a probability sample of 1,016 health maintenance organization employees and found evidence of recurrent or persistent pain in 45%; severe and persistent in 8%; severe and persistent pain with 7 or more days of pain-related activity limitation in 2.7%; and persistent pain with activity limitations and three or more indicators of pain dysfunction (e.g., high family stress; health status rated as fair or poor) in 1%. Such gradations in severity were predictive of outcomes such as psychological impairment and usage of medications and health care services.

Gender and Pain Prevalence

The relationship between gender and pain is not simple. LeResche (1999) observed that patterns differ from condition to condition, and gender-specific prevalence for most conditions varies across the life span. The data with respect to back pain are inconsistent with the usual gender-related prevalence (i.e., in this special case, men often show a greater prevalence than women), and studies looking at sex differences in chest pain are lacking. LeResche (1999) reviewed the available studies and concluded that joint pain, chronic widespread pain, and fibromyalgia all increase in prevalence at least until age 65 years and all are more frequent in women than men. Abdominal pain also is more frequent in women but does not increase with age. Unruh (1996) reviewed the literature and concluded that women were more likely than men to report persistent pains in addition to the pain relating to menstruation, pregnancy, and childbirth. Unruh also concluded that these differential patterns tend to persist even under more extreme life circumstances, such as homelessness, and that gender-specific differences begin to emerge during adolescence.

The generally higher rates of pain in women relate to a variety of social factors (see chap. 7, this volume), but the pain response itself may also be mediated, in part, by biological factors (Unruh, 1996). This has been supported through headache research (Rasmussen, 1993), with pain responses and outcomes differentially affected during different stages of the menstrual cycle (Berkley, 1993; Hapidou & DeCatanzaro, 1988; Procacci et al., 1972; Rao, Ranganekar, & Safi, 1987). Animal research has supported the presence of biological factors, with male rats having significantly greater response to central morphine analgesia and systemic analgesia (Baamonde, Hidalgo, & Andres-Trelles, 1989; Kepler et al., 1991). It has been suggested that estrogen-dependent mechanisms may be responsible for some of the gender differences (Mogil, Sternberg, Kest, Marek, & Liebeskind, 1993). Ellemeyer and Westphal (1995) demonstrated that females showed greater pupil dilation at high tonic pressure levels applied to their fingers, suggesting that at least some aspects of gender differences in pain perception are beyond voluntary control. Paulson, Minoshima, Morrow, and Casey (1998) found gender differences in perceptual and neurophysiological responses to painful heat stimulation using positron emotion tomography, with females showing significantly greater activation of the contralateral prefrontal cortex, insula, and thalamus.

Pain Prevalence and Development

Pain is common in children (McAlpine & McGrath, 1999), with 15% of school-age children reporting musculoskeletal pain (Goodman & McGrath, 1991). Moreover, abdominal pain affects 75% of students and occurs weekly in 13–15% of children studied (Hyams, Burke, Davis, Rzepski, & Andrulonis, 1996). Chapter 5, by Gibson and Chambers, documents prevalence rates across the life span as well as increases in pain as a function of increasing age. Gibson and Chambers also document gender differences in pain that are evident before adulthood.

Conditions often associated with pain (musculoskeletal disease, heart disease, neoplastic disease, HIV/AIDS) increase with advancing age, as does the frequency of pain problems, although these prevalence increases stop by the seventh decade of life (Helme & Gibson, 1999). Cook and Thomas (1994) found that 50% of older adults reported experiencing daily pain and another 26% reported experiencing pain at least once in the week prior to their survey. In another survey of seniors living in the community, 86% reported experiencing significant pain in the year prior to participation in the study with close to 60% reporting multiple pain complaints (Mobily, Herr, Clark, & Wallace, 1994). In a recent investigation of 3,195 nursing home residents in three Canadian provinces, Proctor and Hirdes (2001) estimated the overall prevalence of pain in this sample as being close to 50% with approximately 24% of residents experiencing daily pain. Moreover, these investigators compared seniors with and without cognitive impairments and did not find any differences in the prevalence of potentially painful conditions. In a related study, Marzinski (1991) examined patients' charts at an Alzheimer unit and found that 43% of the patients had painful conditions, a finding consistent with the observation that cognitive impairment does not spare people from the many sources of pain that could afflict anyone (Hadjistavropoulos, von Baeyer, & Craig, 2001). Nonetheless, as is often the case in studies of the epidemiology of pain, the prevalence rates vary from study to study as a function of methodology and the questions that were investigated. This volume is intended to provide a better understanding of the complex and widespread psychological experience of pain.

THE PERSPECTIVES

In chapter 1, this volume, Melzack and Katz examine the gate control theory and transformations in our understanding of pain since it was published (Melzack & Wall, 1965). The theory integrated diverse areas we now refer to as the *neurosciences* and accommodated psychological perspectives to explain phenomena ignored by earlier sensory specific models of pain. In describing the neural bases for the complexities of pain experience, it inspired many major research and clinical advances, for example, our understanding of neuroplasticity as a basis for chronic pain (Melzack, Coderre, Katz, & Vaccarino, 2001). The theory has continued to grow, assimilating new knowledge and inspiring Melzack's recent neuromatrix model of pain. The theory and developments had major importance for the psychological and medical management of pain. Also, it opened the door for the development and popularity of the biopsychosocial model of pain, which is the focus of chapter 2, this volume, by Asmundson and Wright. This model accepts an original physical basis of pain, even when an anatomical site or pathophysiological basis cannot be established, but also recognizes the importance of affective, cognitive, behavioral, and social factors as contributors to chronic illness behavior. An overview of cognitive behavioral and psychodynamic perspectives is also provided in this chapter. The chapter provides a comprehensive overview of the model, its origins, and its empirical and theoretical support.

The chapter by Chapman focuses on motivational, perceptual, and affective mechanisms in pain and complements the chapter by Melzack and Katz. The author recognizes that pain has been defined as a distressing, complex, multidimensional experience. This requires a focus on perceptual mechanisms and the construction of conscious experience, as well as consideration of affective and motivational features. The latter are often neglected, as importance is attached to sensory mechanisms. Psychophysical and psychophysiological work provide a solid core for these investigations. Chapman's chapter develops the bridge between physiological mechanisms of pain and psychological practice by linking conscious perceptual processes with physiological functions. His concept of pain is broad (and mostly addresses "intrapersonal determinants" of the experience). Chapman's basic point is that if we want to provide good care, a more inclusive model of pain experience and its determinants needs to be employed.

Recognizing that interpersonal phenomena are often more important than intrapersonal events when pain control is the issue, we discuss in chapter 4 the communication of pain by examining both a theoretical model of pain communication (Craig, Lilley, & Gilbert, 1996; Hadjistavropoulos & Craig, 2002; Prkachin & Craig, 1995) and important findings concerning illness behavior. Social influences on the pain experience and its expression are also discussed. Communication of pain serves important adaptive functions for humans from the bioevolutionary standpoint. It can elicit rescue, protection, treatment, and longer term care to facilitate recovery. Its social purposes warn others of danger and promote delivery of culture specific care. Communication of pain is accomplished via verbal and nonverbal channels (e.g., self-report, paralinguistic vocalizations, facial expressions, and other nonverbal actions). This chapter discusses research on the expression of pain, including the importance of the entire communicative repertoire and the potential for deception, the judgmental skills and biases of potential allies and antagonists, and the advantages and disadvantages of current social systems designed to care for people communicating painful distress. Issues related to the communication of pain within families are covered, as are matters pertaining to populations with limited ability to communicate (e.g., infants, persons with cognitive or neuromuscular impairments).

Following the first part of the book that is largely focused on theoretical work, Gibson and Chambers outline important developmental considerations in the psychology of pain. Pain expression and experience transform with aging, reflecting ontogenetic maturation, socialization in specific familial and cultural settings, and the impact of experiences with pain. An understanding of the cognitive, affective, behavioral, and social challenges confronted during the various stages of life from birth to terminal illness is required. The earliest and latest stages of life presently carry substantial risk of unnecessary or undermanaged pain because of an inadequate knowledge base, underdeveloped assessment procedures, and inadequate pain management. This chapter examines and systematizes developmental processes in pain experience, expression, and communication.

A major source of individual differences (other than biological maturation) is culture. The chapter by Rollman considers the empirical and theoretical literature on the impact of culture on the experience and expression of pain, delineating observed differences and ethnocultural variations in the meaning of pain. There is a focus on mechanisms responsible for variations (acculturation and socialization), linking them to the biopsychosocial model. The chapter also addresses issues of cultural sensitivity in practice.

Individual differences in response to comparable tissue stress and injury are systematically related to known factors (gender, health anxiety, other personality traits). The chapter by Skevington and Mason provides a review of the literature and a model of social factors impacting on pain in an effort to understand the origins of individual differences. This is done with special reference to quality-of-life issues. The role of intrapersonal factors such as self-efficacy and their relationship to outcomes and recovery from pain are also considered.

The next section of the book addresses clinical issues more directly than the preceding chapters. In chapter 8, Turk et al. provide a critical overview of methods for the assessment of pain in both research and clinical settings (i.e., self-report, behavioral observation, measurement of physiological responses) and describe their relevance to a wide variety of clinical populations and phenomena. Practical suggestions for clinicians are also offered. The role of psychological assessment among pre- and postsurgical pain patients is discussed.

Bruehl and Chung move the book into an intervention focus with a state-of-the-art discussion of psychologically based interventions for acute pain (wounds, burn, other soft tissue injuries, fractures, medical procedure pain, etc.). These are examined and evaluated in terms of evidence for efficacy. Widely used behavioral and cognitive therapies and other procedures (e.g., hypnosis, placebo) are considered. Consideration is also given to life-span issues.

Heather Hadjistavropoulos and Amanda C. de C. Williams focus on interventions for chronic pain. Psychological interventions represent a necessary feature of multidisciplinary care for patients suffering from chronic pain and pain-related disability. This chapter examines the most commonly employed approaches to the treatment of chronic pain as well as the empirical evidence (or lack thereof) pertaining to their efficacy. Widely used cognitive/behavioral approaches are featured, but psychodynamic perspectives are also examined. Best practice in the context of evidence-based treatment is presented. The manner in which medication usage relates to psychological treatment (e.g., medication compliance) is addressed. More-over, a discussion of how psychological interventions can be applied with postsurgical and presurgical pain patients is included.

The last section of the volume focuses on current controversies and ethi-cal issues. The chapter by Kenneth D. Craig and Thomas Hadjistavropoulos reviews current controversies, including critical analyses of the definition of pain, frequent unavailability of psychological interventions for chronic pain, the use of self-report as a gold standard in pain assessment, fears about the implementation of certain biomedical interventions and others.

The final chapter by Thomas Hadjistavropoulos presents a discussion of ethical standards put forth by organizations of pain researchers and psy-chological associations. The presentation of these standards is supple-mented by a discussion of ethical theory traditions on which such stan-dards are based. The chapter also provides coverage of various ethical concerns that are unique to the field of pain, as well as an overview of con-cerns that are especially relevant to psychologists.

We hope that the views presented herein will provide both a better ap-preciation of state-of-the-art developments in the psychology of pain and a greater appreciation of the richness and complexity of the pain experience.

REFERENCES

Asmundson, G. J. G., Hadjistavropoulos, T., & Antonishyn, M. (2001). Profiles and perspectives of leading contributors in the field of pain. *Pain Clinic, 13*, 55–69.

Baamonde, A. I., Hidalgo, A., & Andres-Trelles, F. (1989). Sex-related differences in the effects of morphine and stress on visceral pain. *Neuropharmacology, 28*, 967–970.

Berkley, K. J. (1993, January/February). Sex and chronobiology: Opportunities for a focus on the positive. *IASP Newsletter*, 2–5.

Bowsher, D., Rigge, M., & Sopp, L. (1991). Prevalence of chronic pain in the British population: A telephone survey of 1037 households. *Pain Clinic, 4*, 223–230.

Cook, A. J., & Thomas, M. R. (1994). Pain and the use of health services among the elderly. *Journal of Aging and Health, 16*, 127–139.

Craig, K. D., Lilley, C. M., & Gilbert, C. A. (1996). Social barriers of optimal pain management in in-fants and children. *Clinical Journal of Pain, 12*, 232–242.

Crombie, I. K. (1997). Epidemiology of persistent pain. In T. S. Jensen, J. A. Turner, & Z. Wiesen-feld-Hallin (Eds.), *Proceedings of the 8th World Congress on Pain* (pp. 53–61). Seattle, WA: Inter-national Association for the Study of Pain.

Crombie, I. K., Croft, P. R., Linton, S. J., LeResche, L., & von Korff, M. (1999). *Epidemiology of pain*. Seattle, WA: International Association for the Study of Pain Press.

Descartes, R. (1985). *Treatise on man* (J. Cottingham, R. Stoothoff, & D. Murdoch, Trans.). Victo-ria, Australia: Cambridge University Press. (Original work published 1644)

Ellman, P., Savage, O. A., Wittkower, E., & Rodger, T. F. (1942). Fibrositis. A biographical study of 50 civilian and military cases. *Annals of the Rheumatic Diseases, 3*, 56–76.

Ellemeyer, W., & Westphal, W. (1995). Gender differences in pain ratings and pupil reactions to painful pressure stimuli. *Pain, 61*, 435–439.

Fordyce, W. E. (1976). *Behavioral methods for chronic pain and illness*. St. Louis, MO: Mosby.

Fordyce, W. E., Fowler, R., & DeLateur, B. (1968). An application of behavior modification technique to a problem of chronic pain. *Behavoir Research Therapy, 6*, 105–107.

Freud, S. (1893–1895). *Studies in hysteria. Complete psychological works* (Standard ed., Vol. 2). London: Hogarth Press.

Goodman, J. E., & McGrath, P. J. (1991). The epidemiology of pain in children and adolescents. A review. *Pain, 46*, 247–264.

Hadjistavropoulos, T., & Craig, K. D. (2002). A theoretical framework for understanding self-report and observational measures of pain: A communications model. *Behaviour Research and Therapy, 40*, 551–570.

Hadjistavropoulos, T., von Baeyer, C., & Craig, K. D. (2001). Pain assessment in persons with limited ability to communicate. In D. C. Turk & R. Melzack (Eds.), *Handbook of pain assessment* (2nd ed., pp. 134–149). New York: Guilford Press.

Hapidou, E. G., & DeCatanzaro, D. (1988). Sensitivity to cold pressor pain in dysmenorrheic and non-dysmenorrheic women as a function of menstrual cycle phase. *Pain, 34*, 277–283.

Hebb, D. O. (1949). *The organization of behavior.* New York: Wiley.

Helme, R. D., & Gibson, S. J. (1999). Pain in older people. In I. K. Crombie, P. R. Croft, S. J. Linton, L. LeResche, & M. von Korff (Eds.), *Epidemiology of pain* (2nd ed., pp. 103–112). Seattle, WA: International Association for the Study of Pain Press.

Henry, J. (1999–2000). *First annual report.* Montreal: Canadian Consortium on Pain Mechanisms, Diagnosis and Management.

Hyams, J. S., Burke, G., Davis, P. M., Rzepski, B., & Andrulonis, P. A. (1996). Abdominal pain and irritable bowel syndrome in adolescents: A community-based study. *Journal of Pediatrics, 129*, 220–226.

International Association for the Study of Pain Ad Hoc Subcommittee for Psychology Curriculum. (1997). *Curriculum on pain for students in psychology.* Seattle, WA: IASP Press.

Kepler, K. L., Standifer, K. M., Paul, D., Kest, B., Pasternak, G. W., & Bodnar, R. J. (1991). Gender effects and central opioid analgesia. *Pain, 45*, 87–94.

LeResche, L. (1999). Gender considerations in the epidemiology of chronic pain. In I. K. Crombie, P. R. Croft, S. J. Linton, L. LeResche, & M. von Korff (Eds.), *Epidemiology of pain* (2nd ed., pp. 43–52). Seattle, WA: International Association for the Study of Pain Press.

Liebeskind, J., & Paul, L. (1977). Psychological and physiological mechanisms of pain. *Annual Review of Psychology, 28*, 41–60.

Marzinski, L. R. (1991). The tragedy of dementia: Clinically assessing pain in the confused, nonverbal elderly. *Journal of Gerontological Nursing, 17*, 25–28.

McAlpine, L., & McGrath, P. J. (1999). Chronic and recurrent pain in children. In A. R. Block, E. F. Kremer, & E. Fernandez (Eds.), *Handbook of pain syndromes* (pp. 529–545). Mahwah, NJ: Lawrence Erlbaum Associates.

Melzack, R. (1973). *The puzzle of pain.* New York: Basic Books.

Melzack, R. (1989). Phantom limbs, the self and the brain. *Canadian Psychology, 30*, 1–16.

Melzack, R. (1993). Pain: Past, present and future. *Canadian Journal of Experimental Psychology, 47*, 615–629.

Melzack, R., & Casey, K. L. (1968). Sensory motivational and central controlled determinants of pain: A new conceptual model. In K. Shalod (Ed.), *The skin senses* (pp. 423–443). Springfield, IL: Charles C. Thomas.

Melzack, R., Coderre, T. J., Katz, J., & Vaccarino, A. L. (2001). Central neuroplasticity and pathological pain. *Annals of the New York Academy of Sciences, 933*, 157–174.

Melzack, R., & Scott, T. H. (1957). The effects of early experience on the response to pain. *Journal of Comparative Physiological Psychology, 50*, 155–161.

Melzack, R., & Wall, P. D. (1965). Pain mechanisms: A new theory. *Science, 150*, 971–979.

Merskey, H. (Ed.). (1996). *Thoughts and findings on pain: The Hebb–Bishop correspondence.* Toronto: Canadian Pain Society.

Merskey, H. (1998). History of pain research and management in Canada. *Pain Research and Management, 3,* 164–173.

Mobily, P. R., Herr, K. A., Clark, M. K., & Wallace, R. B. (1994). An epidemiologic analysis of pain in the elderly: The Iowa 65+ Rural Health Study. *Journal of Aging and Health, 6,* 139–154.

Mogil, J. S., Sternberg, W. F., Kest, B., Marek, P., & Liebeskind, J. (1983). Sex differences in the antagonism of swim stress-induced analgesia: Effects of gonadectomy and estrogen replacement. *Pain, 53,* 17–25.

Paulson, P. E., Minoshima, S., Morrow, T. J., & Casey, K. L. (1998). Gender differences in pain perception and patterns of cerebral activation during noxious heat stimulation in humans. *Pain, 76,* 223–229.

Pilowsky, I. (1986). Psychodynamic aspects of the pain experience. In R. A. Sternbach (Ed.), *The psychology of pain* (pp. 181–195). New York: Raven Press.

Pilowsky, I., & Spence, N. D. (1975). Illness behavior syndromes associated with intractable pain. *Pain, 2,* 61–71.

Price, D. D. (2000). Psychological and neural mechanisms of the affective dimension of pain. *Science, 288,* 1769–1772.

Prkachin, K. M., & Craig, K. D. (1995). Expressing pain: The communication and interpretation of facial pain signals. *Journal of Nonverbal Behavior, 19,* 191–205.

Procacci, P., Buzzelli, G., Passeri, I., Sassi, R., Voegelin, M. R., & Zoppi, M. (1972). Studies on the cutaneous pricking pain threshold in man. Cicadian and circatrigintan changes. *Headache, 3,* 260–276.

Proctor, W. R., & Hirdes, J. P. (2001). Pain and cognitive status among nursing home residents in Canada. *Pain Research and Management, 6,* 119–125.

Rao, S. S., Ranganekar, A. G., & Saifi, A. Q. (1987). Pain threshold in relation to sex hormones. *Indian Journal of Physiological Pharmacology, 31,* 250–254.

Rasmussen, B. K. (1993). Tension-type headaches. Cluster headache and miscellaneous headaches: Epidemiology. In J. Oleson, P. Tfelt-Hansen, & K. M. A. Welch (Eds.), *The headaches* (pp. 439–443). New York: Raven Press.

Scott, W. C. M. (1948). Some embryological, neurological, psychiatric and psychoanalytic implications of the body scheme. *International Journal of Psychoanalysis, 29,* 141–155.

Statistics Canada. (1996–1997). *National population health survey* (Catalogue No. 82-567-XPB). Ottawa: Statistics Canada Health Statistics Division.

Turk, D. C., Meichenbaum, D., & Genest, M. (1983). *Pain and behavioral medicine: A cognitive-behavorial perspective.* New York: Guilford Press.

Turk, D. C., & Melzack, R. (2001). *Handbook of pain assessment* (2nd ed.). New York: Guilford Press.

Unruh, A. M. (1996). Gender variations in clinical pain experience. *Pain, 65,* 123–167.

von Korff, M., Dworkin, S. F., & Le Resche, L. (1990). Graded chronic pain status: An epidemiologic evaluation. *Pain, 40,* 279–291.

1

The Gate Control Theory: Reaching for the Brain

Ronald Melzack
Department of Psychology,
McGill University

Joel Katz
Department of Psychology,
Toronto General Hospital

Theories of pain, like all scientific theories, evolve as a result of the accumulation of new facts as well as leaps of the imagination (Kuhn, 1970). The gate control theory's most revolutionary contribution to understanding pain was its emphasis on central neural mechanisms (Melzack & Wall, 1965). The theory forced the medical and biological sciences to accept the brain as an active system that filters, selects, and modulates inputs. The dorsal horns, too, were not merely passive transmission stations but sites at which dynamic activities—inhibition, excitation, and modulation—occurred. The great challenge ahead of us is to understand how the brain functions.

A BRIEF HISTORY OF PAIN IN THE 20TH CENTURY

The theory of pain we inherited in the 20th century was proposed by Descartes three centuries earlier (see Melzack & Wall, 1996). Descartes was the first philosopher to be influenced by the scientific method that flourished in the 17th century, and he achieved a major revolution by arguing that the body works like a machine that can be studied by using the experimental methods of physics pioneered by Galileo and others. Although humans, Descartes proposed, have a soul (or mind), the human body is nevertheless a machine like an animal's body.

The impact of Descartes's theory was enormous. The history of experiments on the anatomy and physiology of pain during the first half of the 20th century (reviewed in Melzack & Wall, 1996) is marked by a search for specific pain fibers and pathways and a pain center in the brain. The result was a concept of pain as a specific, straight-through sensory projection system (Fig. 1.1). This rigid anatomy of pain in the 1950s led to attempts to treat severe chronic pain by a variety of neurosurgical lesions. Descartes's specificity theory, then, determined the "facts" as they were known up to the middle of the 20th century, and even determined therapy.

Specificity theory proposed that injury activates specific pain receptors and fibers, which, in turn, project pain impulses through a spinal pain pathway to a pain center in the brain. The psychological experience of pain, therefore, was virtually equated with peripheral injury. In the 1950s, there was no room for psychological contributions to pain, such as attention, past experience, anxiety, depression, and the meaning of the situation. In-

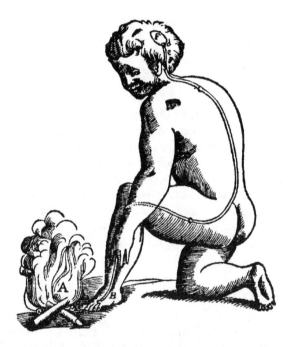

FIG. 1.1. Descartes's concept of the pain pathway. He wrote: "If for example fire (A) comes near the foot (B), the minute particles of this fire, which as you know move with great velocity, have the power to set in motion the spot of the skin of the foot which they touch, and by this means pulling upon the delicate thread CC, which is attached to the spot of the skin, they open up at the same instant the pore, d.e., against which the delicate thread ends, just as by pulling at one end of a rope one makes to strike at the same instant a bell which hangs at the other end" (Keele, 1957, p. 72).

stead, pain experience was held to be proportional to peripheral injury or pathology. Patients who suffered back pain without presenting signs of organic disease were often labeled as psychologically disturbed and sent to psychiatrists. The concept, in short, was simple and, not surprisingly, often failed to help patients who suffered severe chronic pain. To thoughtful clinical observers, specificity theory was clearly wrong.

There were several attempts to find a new theory. The major opponent to specificity was labeled as "pattern theory," but there were several different pattern theories and they were generally vague and inadequate (see Melzack & Wall, 1996). However, seen in retrospect, pattern theories gradually evolved (Fig. 1.2) and set the stage for the gate control theory. Goldscheider (1894) proposed that central summation in the dorsal horns is one of the critical determinants of pain. Livingston's (1943) theory postulated a reverberatory circuit in the dorsal horns to explain summation, referred pain, and pain that persisted long after healing was completed. Noordenbos's (1959) theory proposed that large-diameter fibers inhibited small-diameter fibers, and he even suggested that the substantia gelatinosa in the dorsal horns plays a major role in the summation and other dynamic processes described by Livingston. However, in none of these theories was there an explicit role for the brain other than as a passive receiver of messages. Nevertheless, the successive theoretical concepts moved the field in the right direction: into the spinal cord and away from the periphery as the

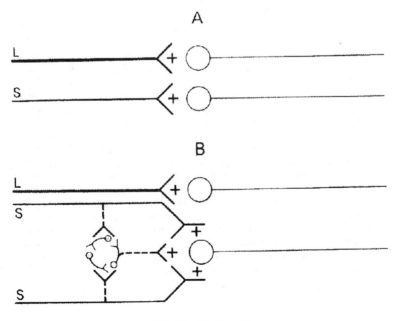

FIG. 1.2. *(Continued)*

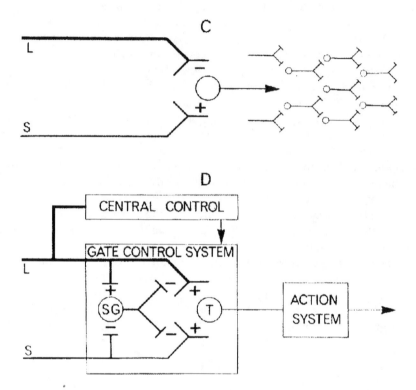

FIG. 1.2. Schematic representation of conceptual models of pain mechanisms. (A) Specificity theory. Large (L) and small (S) fibers are assumed to transmit touch and pain impulses respectively, in separate, specific, straight-through pathways to touch and pain centers in the brain. (B) Goldscheider's (1894) summation theory, showing convergence of small fibers onto a dorsal horn cell. The central network projecting to the central cell represents Livingston's (1943) conceptual model of reverberatory circuits underlying pathological pain states. Touch is assumed to be carried by large fibers. (C) Sensory interaction theory, in which large (L) fibers inhibit ( ) and small (S) fibers excite (+) central transmission neurons. The output projects to spinal cord neurons, which are conceived by Noordenbos (1959) to comprise a multisynaptic afferent system. (D) Gate control theory. The large (L) and small (S) fibers project to the substantia gelatinosa (SG) and first central transmission (T) cells. The central control trigger is represented by a line running from the large fiber system to central control mechanisms, which in turn project back to the gate control system. The T cells project to the entry cells of the action system. +, Excitation; , inhibition. From Melzack (1991), with permission.

exclusive answer to pain. At least the field of pain was making its way toward the brain.

THE GATE CONTROL THEORY OF PAIN

In 1965, Melzack and Wall proposed the gate control theory of pain. The final model, depicted in Fig. 1.2D in the context of earlier theories of pain, is the first theory of pain which incorporated the central control processes of the brain.

The gate control theory of pain (Melzack & Wall, 1965) proposes that the transmission of nerve impulses from afferent fibers to spinal cord transmission (T) cells is modulated by a gating mechanism in the spinal dorsal horn. This gating mechanism is influenced by the relative amount of activity in large- and small-diameter fibers, so that large fibers tend to inhibit transmission (close the gate) while small fibers tend to facilitate transmission (open the gate). In addition, the spinal gating mechanism is influenced by nerve impulses that descend from the brain. When the output of the spinal T cells exceeds a critical level, it activates the action system—those neural areas that underlie the complex, sequential patterns of behavior and experience characteristic of pain.

Publication of the gate control theory received an astonishing reception. The theory generated vigorous (sometimes vicious) debate as well as a great deal of research to disprove or support the theory. The search for specific pain fibers and spinal cells by our opponents now became almost frantic. It was not until the mid-1970s that the gate control theory was presented in almost every major textbook in the biological and medical sciences. At the same time, there was an explosion in research on the physiology and pharmacology of the dorsal horns and the descending control systems.

The theory's emphasis on the modulation of inputs in the spinal dorsal horns and the dynamic role of the brain in pain processes had a clinical as well as a scientific impact. Psychological factors that were previously dismissed as "reactions to pain" became seen to be an integral part of pain processing and new avenues for pain control by psychological therapies were opened. Similarly, cutting nerves and pathways was gradually replaced by a host of methods to modulate the input. Physical therapists and other health-care professionals who use a multitude of modulation techniques were brought into the picture, and TENS became an important modality for the treatment of chronic and acute pain. The current status of pain research and therapy has recently been evaluated and indicates that, despite the addition of a massive amount of detail, the conceptual components of the theory remain basically intact up to the present.

BEYOND THE GATE

We believe the great challenge ahead of us is to understand brain function. Melzack and Casey (1968) made a start by proposing that specialized systems in the brain are involved in the sensory-discriminative, motivational-affective, and cognitive-evaluative dimensions of subjective pain experience (Fig. 1.3). These names for the dimensions of subjective experience seemed strange when they were coined, but they are now used so frequently and seem so "logical" that they have become part of our language. So, too, the McGill Pain Questionnaire (Fig. 1.4), which taps into subjective experience—a function of the brain—is widely used to measure pain (Melzack, 1975a, 1987).

The gate theory also postulated that the brain exerted a tonic inhibitory effect on pain. An experiment by Melzack, Stotler, and Livingston (1958) revealed the midbrain's tonic descending inhibitory control and led directly to Reynolds's (1969) discovery that electrical stimulation of the periaqueductal gray produces analgesia. This study was followed by Liebeskind's research (Liebeskind & Paul, 1977) on pharmacological substances such as endorphins that contribute to the descending inhibition. The observation that "pain takes away pain," in which Melzack (1975b) postulated that descending inhibition tends to be activated by intense inputs, led to a series of studies on intense TENS stimulation. Later, a series of definitive studies on "diffuse noxious inhibitory controls" (DNIC) firmly established the power of descending inhibitory controls (Le Bars, Dickenson, & Besson, 1983; Fields & Basbaum, 1999).

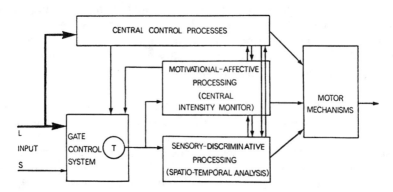

FIG. 1.3. Conceptual model of the sensory, motivational, and central control determinants of pain. The output of the T (transmission) cells of the gate control system projects to the sensory-discriminative system and the motivational-affective system. The central control trigger is represented by a line running from the large fiber system to central control processes; these, in turn, project back to the gate control system, and to the sensory-discriminative and motivational-affective systems. All three systems interact with one another, and project to the motor system. From Melzack and Casey (1968), with permission.

McGILL PAIN QUESTIONNAIRE

RONALD MELZACK

Patient's Name ————————————— Date ———————— Time————am/pm

PRI: S———— A ————— E———— M———— PRI(T)———— PPI——
   (1-10)   (11-15)   (16)   (17-20)   (1-20)

1 FLICKERING __ QUIVERING __ PULSING __ THROBBING __ BEATING __ POUNDING __ 2 JUMPING __ FLASHING __ SHOOTING __ 3 PRICKING __ BORING __ DRILLING __ STABBING __ LANCINATING __ 4 SHARP __ CUTTING __ LACERATING __ 5 PINCHING __ PRESSING __ GNAWING __ CRAMPING __ CRUSHING __ 6 TUGGING __ PULLING __ WRENCHING __ 7 HOT __ BURNING __ SCALDING __ SEARING __ 8 TINGLING __ ITCHY __ SMARTING __ STINGING __ 9 DULL __ SORE __ HURTING __ ACHING __ HEAVY __ 10 TENDER __ TAUT __ RASPING __ SPLITTING __	11 TIRING __ EXHAUSTING __ 12 SICKENING __ SUFFOCATING __ 13 FEARFUL __ FRIGHTFUL __ TERRIFYING __ 14 PUNISHING __ GRUELLING __ CRUEL __ VICIOUS __ KILLING __ 15 WRETCHED __ BLINDING __ 16 ANNOYING __ TROUBLESOME __ MISERABLE __ INTENSE __ UNBEARABLE __ 17 SPREADING __ RADIATING __ PENETRATING __ PIERCING __ 18 TIGHT __ NUMB __ DRAWING __ SQUEEZING __ TEARING __ 19 COOL __ COLD __ FREEZING __ 20 NAGGING __ NAUSEATING __ AGONIZING __ DREADFUL __ TORTURING __ PPI 0 NO PAIN __ 1 MILD __ 2 DISCOMFORTING __ 3 DISTRESSING __ 4 HORRIBLE __ 5 EXCRUCIATING __

BRIEF __	RHYTHMIC __	CONTINUOUS __
MOMENTARY __	PERIODIC __	STEADY __
TRANSIENT __	INTERMITTENT __	CONSTANT __

E = EXTERNAL
I = INTERNAL

COMMENTS:

© R. MELZACK, 1975

FIG. 1.4. McGill Pain Questionnaire. The descriptors fall into four major groups: sensory, 1–10; affective, 11–15; evaluative, 16; and miscellaneous, 17–20. The rank value for each descriptor is based on its position in the word set. The sum of the rank values is the pain rating index (PRI). The present pain intensity (PPI) is based on a scale of 0 to 5. From Melzack (1975a), with permission.

In 1978, Melzack and Loeser described severe pains in the phantom body of paraplegics with verified total sections of the spinal cord, and proposed a central "pattern-generating mechanism" above the level of the section (Melzack & Loeser, 1978). This concept, generally ignored for about 10 years, is now beginning to be accepted. It represents a revolutionary advance: It did not merely extend the gate; it said that pain could be generated by brain mechanisms in paraplegics in the absence of spinal input because the brain is completely disconnected from the cord. Psychophysical specificity, in such a concept, makes no sense; instead, we must explore how patterns of nerve impulses generated in the brain can give rise to somesthetic experience.

PHANTOM LIMBS AND THE CONCEPT
OF A NEUROMATRIX

It is evident that the gate control theory has taken us a long way. Yet, as historians of science have pointed out, good theories are instrumental in producing facts that eventually require a new theory to incorporate them. And this is what has happened. It is possible to make adjustments to the gate theory so that, for example, it includes long-lasting activity of the sort Wall has described (see Melzack & Wall, 1996). But there is a set of observations on pain in paraplegics that just does not fit the theory. This does not negate the gate theory, of course. Peripheral and spinal processes are obviously an important part of pain, and we need to know more about the mechanisms of peripheral inflammation, spinal modulation, midbrain descending control, and so forth. But the data on painful phantoms below the level of total spinal section (Melzack, 1989, 1990) indicate that we need to go above the spinal cord and into the brain.

Now let us make it clear that we mean more than the spinal projection areas in the thalamus and cortex. These areas are important, of course, but they are only part of the neural processes that underlie perception. The cortex, Gybels and Tasker (1999) made amply clear, is not the pain center and neither is the thalamus. The areas of the brain involved in pain experience and behavior must include somatosensory projections as well as the limbic system. Furthermore, cognitive processes are known to involve widespread areas of the brain. Yet the plain fact is that we do not have an adequate theory of how the brain works.

Melzack's (1989) analysis of phantom limb phenomena, particularly the astonishing reports of a phantom body and severe phantom limb pain in people after a cordectomy—that is, complete removal of several spinal cord segments (Melzack & Loeser, 1978)—led to four conclusions that point to a new conceptual nervous system. First, because the phantom limb (or other body part) feels so real, it is reasonable to conclude that the body we normally feel is subserved by the same neural processes in the brain; these brain processes are normally activated and modulated by inputs from the body but they can act in the absence of any inputs. Second, all the qualities we normally feel from the body, including pain, are also felt in the absence of inputs from the body; from this we may conclude that the origins of the patterns that underlie the qualities of experience lie in neural networks in the brain; stimuli may trigger the patterns but do not produce them. Third, the body is perceived as a unity and is identified as the "self," distinct from other people and the surrounding world. The experience of a unity of such diverse feelings, including the self as the point of orientation in the surrounding environment, is produced by central neural processes and cannot derive from the peripheral nervous system or spinal cord. Fourth, the brain processes that underlie the body-self are, to an important extent that can no longer be ignored, "built in" by genetic specification, although this built-in substrate must, of course, be modified by experience. These conclusions provide the basis of the new conceptual model (Melzack, 1989, 1990, 2001; Fig. 1.5).

Outline of the Theory

The anatomical substrate of the body-self, Melzack proposed, is a large, widespread network of neurons that consists of loops between the thalamus and cortex as well as between the cortex and limbic system. He labeled

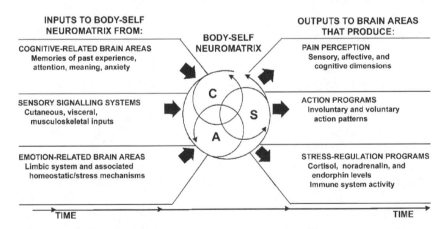

FIG. 1.5. Factors that contribute to the patterns of activity generated by the body-self neuromatrix, which is comprised of sensory, affective, and cognitive neuromodules. The output patterns from the neuromatrix produce the multiple dimensions of pain experience, as well as concurrent homeostatic and behavioral responses. From Melzack (2001), with permission.

the entire network, whose spatial distribution and synaptic links are initially determined genetically and are later sculpted by sensory inputs, as a *neuromatrix*. The loops diverge to permit parallel processing in different components of the neuromatrix and converge repeatedly to permit interactions between the output products of processing. The repeated *cyclical processing and synthesis* of nerve impulses through the neuromatrix imparts a characteristic pattern: the *neurosignature*. The neurosignature of the neuromatrix is imparted on all nerve impulse patterns that flow through it; the neurosignature is produced by the patterns of synaptic connections in the entire neuromatrix. All inputs from the body undergo cyclical processing and synthesis so that characteristic patterns are impressed on them in the neuromatrix. Portions of the neuromatrix are specialized to process information related to major sensory events (such as injury, temperature change and stimulation of erogenous tissue) and may be labeled as neuromodules that impress subsignatures on the larger neurosignature.

The neurosignature, which is a continuous output from the body-self neuromatrix, is projected to areas in the brain—the *sentient neural hub*—in which the stream of nerve impulses (the neurosignature modulated by ongoing inputs) is converted into a continually changing stream of awareness. Furthermore, the neurosignature patterns may also activate a neuromatrix to produce movement. That is, the signature patterns bifurcate so that a pattern proceeds to the *sentient neural hub* (where the pattern is transformed into the experience of movement) and a similar pattern proceeds through a neuromatrix that eventually activates spinal cord neurons to produce muscle patterns for complex actions.

The Body-Self Neuromatrix

The body is felt as a unity, with different qualities at different times. Melzack proposed that the brain mechanism that underlies the experience also comprises a unified system that acts as a whole and produces a neurosignature pattern of a whole body. The conceptualization of this unified brain mechanism lies at the heart of the new theory, and the word *neuromatrix* best characterizes it. *Matrix* has several definitions in *Webster's Dictionary* (1967), and some of them imply precisely the properties of the neuromatrix as Melzack conceived of it. First, a matrix is defined as "something within which something else originates, takes form or develops." This is exactly what Melzack implied: The neuromatrix (not the stimulus, peripheral nerves, or "brain center") is the origin of the neurosignature; the neurosignature originates and takes form in the neuromatrix. Although the neurosignature may be triggered or modulated by input, the input is only a "trigger" and does not produce the neurosignature itself. *Matrix* is also defined as a "mold" or "die," which leaves an imprint on something else. In this sense, the neuromatrix "casts" its distinctive signature on all inputs (nerve impulse patterns) that flow through it. Finally, matrix is defined as "an array of circuit elements . . . for performing a specific function as interconnected." The array of neurons in a neuromatrix, Melzack proposed, is genetically programmed to perform the specific function of producing the signature pattern. The final, integrated neurosignature pattern for the body-self ultimately produces awareness and action.

For these reasons, the term *neuromatrix* seems to be appropriate. The neuromatrix, distributed throughout many areas of the brain, comprises a widespread network of neurons that generates patterns, processes information that flows through it, and ultimately produces the pattern that is felt as a whole body. The stream of neurosignature output with constantly varying patterns riding on the main signature pattern produces the feelings of the whole body with constantly changing qualities.

Psychological Reasons for a Neuromatrix

It is difficult to comprehend how individual bits of information from skin, joints, or muscles can all come together to produce the experience of a coherent, articulated body. At any instant in time, millions of nerve impulses arrive at the brain from all the body's sensory systems, including the proprioceptive and vestibular systems. How can all this be integrated in a constantly changing unity of experience? Where does it all come together?

Melzack visualized a genetically built-in neuromatrix for the whole body, producing a characteristic neurosignature for the body that carries with it patterns for the myriad qualities we feel. The neuromatrix, as Melzack conceived of it, produces a continuous message that represents the whole body in which details are differentiated within the whole as inputs come into it. We start from the top, with the experience of a unity of the body, and look for differentiation of detail within the whole. The neuromatrix, then, is a template of the whole, which provides the characteristic neural pattern for the whole body (the body's neurosignature), as well as subsets of signature patterns (from neuromodules) that relate to events at (or in) different parts of the body.

These views are in sharp contrast to the classical specificity theory in which the qualities of experience are presumed to be inherent in peripheral nerve fibers. Pain is not injury; the *quality of pain experiences* must not be confused with the physical event of breaking skin or bone. Warmth and cold are not "out there"; temperature changes occur "out there," but the *qualities of experience* must be generated by structures in the brain. There are no external equivalents to stinging, smarting, tickling, itch; the *qualities* are produced by built-in neuromodules whose neurosignatures innately produce the qualities.

We do not learn to feel qualities of experience: Our brains are built to produce them. The inadequacy of the traditional peripheralist view becomes especially evident when we consider paraplegics with high-level complete spinal breaks. In spite of the absence of inputs from the body, virtually every quality of sensation and affect is experienced. It is known that the absence of input produces hyperactivity and abnormal firing patterns in spinal cells above the level of the break (Melzack & Loeser, 1978). But how, from this jumble of activity, do we get the meaningful experience of movement, the coordination of limbs with other limbs, cramping pain in specific (nonexistent) muscle groups, and so on? This must occur in the brain, in which neurosignatures are produced by neuromatrixes that are triggered by the output of hyperactive cells.

When all sensory systems are intact, inputs modulate the continuous neuromatrix output to produce the wide variety of experiences we feel. We may feel position, warmth, and several kinds of pain and pressure all at once. It is a single unitary feeling just as an orchestra produces a single unitary sound at any moment, even though the sound comprises violins, cellos, horns, and so forth. Similarly, at a particular moment in time we feel complex qualities from all of the body. In addition, our experience of the body includes visual images, affect, and "knowledge" of the self (versus not-self), as well as the meaning of body parts in terms of social norms and values. It is hard to conceive of all of these bits and pieces coming together to produce a unitary body-self, but we can visualize a neuromatrix that impresses a characteristic signature on all the inputs that converge on it and thereby produces the never-ending stream of feeling from the body.

The experience of the body-self involves multiple dimensions—sensory, affective, evaluative, postural, and many others. The sensory dimensions are subserved, in part at least, by portions of the neuromatrix that lie in the sensory projection areas of the brain; the affective dimensions, Melzack assumed, are subserved by areas in the brainstem and limbic system. Each major psychological dimension (or quality) of experience, he proposed, is subserved by a particular portion of the neuromatrix that contributes a distinct portion of the total neurosignature. To use a musical analogy once again, it is like the strings, tympani, woodwinds, and brasses of a symphony orchestra that each comprise a part of the whole; each makes its unique contribution yet is an integral part of a single symphony that varies continually from beginning to end.

The neuromatrix resembles Hebb's "cell assembly" by being a widespread network of cells that subserves a particular psychological function. However, Hebb (1949) conceived of the cell assembly as a network developed by gradual sensory learning, whereas Melzack, instead, proposed that the structure of the neuromatrix is predominantly determined by genetic factors, although its eventual synaptic architecture is influenced by sensory inputs. This emphasis on the genetic contribution to the brain does not diminish the importance of sensory inputs. The neuromatrix is a psychologically meaningful unit, developed by both heredity and learning, that represents an entire unified entity.

Action Patterns: The Action Neuromatrix. The output of the body-self neuromatrix, Melzack (1991, 1995, 2001) proposed, is directed at two systems: (a) the neural system that produces awareness of the output, and (b) a neuromatrix that generates overt action patterns. In this discussion, it is important to keep in mind that just as there is a steady stream of awareness, there is also a steady output of behavior.

It is important to recognize that behavior occurs only after the input has been at least partially synthesized and recognized. For example, when we respond to the experience of pain or itch, it is evident that the experience has been synthesized by the body-self neuromatrix (or relevant neuromodules) sufficiently for the neuromatrix to have imparted the neurosignature patterns that underlie the quality of experience, affect, and meaning. Apart from a few reflexes (such as withdrawal of a limb, eyeblink, and so on), behavior occurs only after inputs have been analyzed and synthesized sufficiently to produce meaningful experience. When we reach for an apple, the visual input has clearly been synthesized by a neuromatrix so that it has three-dimensional shape, color, and meaning as an edible, desirable object, all of which are produced by the brain and are not in the object "out there." When we respond to pain (by withdrawal or even by telephoning for an ambulance), we respond to an experience that has sensory qualities, affect, and meaning as a dangerous (or potentially dangerous) event to the body.

After inputs from the body undergo transformation in the body-self neuromatrix, the appropriate action patterns are activated concurrently (or nearly so) with the neural system that generates experience. Thus, in the action neuromatrix, cyclical processing and synthesis produce activation of several possible patterns and their successive elimination until one particular pattern emerges as the most appropriate for the circumstances at the moment. In this way, input and output are synthesized simultaneously, in parallel, not in series. This permits a smooth, continuous stream of action patterns.

The command, which originates in the brain, to perform a pattern such as running activates the neuromodule, which then produces firing in sequences of neurons that send precise messages through ventral horn neuron pools to appropriate sets of muscles. At the same time, the output patterns from the body-self neuromatrix that engage the neuromodules for particular actions are also projected to the neural "awareness system" and produce experience. In this way, the brain commands may produce the experience of movement of phantom limbs even though there are no limbs to move and no proprioceptive feedback. Indeed, reports by paraplegics of terrible fatigue due to persistent bicycling movements, like the painful fatigue in a tightly clenched phantom fist in arm amputees (Katz, 1993), indicate that feelings of effort and fatigue are produced by the neurosignature of a neuromodule rather than particular input patterns from muscles and joints.

The phenomenon of phantom limbs has allowed us to examine some fundamental assumptions in psychology. One assumption is that sensations are produced only by stimuli and that perceptions in the absence of stimuli are psychologically abnormal. Yet phantom limbs, as well as phantom seeing (Schultz & Melzack, 1991), indicate that this notion is wrong. The brain does more than detect and analyze inputs; it generates perceptual experience even when no external inputs occur.

Another entrenched assumption is that perception of one's body results from sensory inputs that leave a memory in the brain, and that the total of these signals becomes the body image. But the existence of phantoms in people born without a limb or who have lost a limb at an early age suggests that the neural networks for perceiving the body and its parts are built into the brain (Melzack, 1989, 1990, 1995; Melzack et al., 1997). The absence of inputs does not stop the networks from generating messages about missing body parts; they continue to produce such messages throughout life. In short, phantom limbs are a mystery only if we assume the body sends sensory messages to a passively receiving brain. Phantoms become comprehensible once we recognize that the brain generates the experience of the body. Sensory inputs merely modulate that experience; they do not directly cause it.

PAIN AND STRESS

We are so accustomed to considering pain as a purely sensory phenomenon that we have ignored the obvious fact that injury does not merely produce pain; it also disrupt the brain's homeostatic regulation systems, thereby producing "stress" and initiating complex programs to reinstate homeostasis. By recognizing the role of the stress system in pain processes, we discover that the scope of the puzzle of pain is vastly expanded and new pieces of the puzzle provide valuable clues in our quest to understand chronic pain (Melzack, 1998, 1999).

Hans Selye, who founded the field of stress research, dealt with stress in the biological sense of physical injury, infection, and pathology, and also recognized the importance of psychological stresses (Selye, 1956). In recent years, the latter sense of the word has come to dominate the field. However, it is important for the purpose of understanding pain to keep in mind that stress is a biological system that is activated by physical injury, infection, or any threat to biological homeostasis, as well as by psychological threat and insult of the body-self. Both are correct and important.

The disruption of homeostasis by injury activates programs of neural, hormonal, and behavioral activity aimed at a return to homeostasis. The particular programs that are activated are selected from a genetically determined repertoire of programs and are influenced by the extent and severity of the injury. When injury occurs, sensory information rapidly alerts the brain and begins the complex sequence of events to reinstate homeostasis. Cytokines are released within seconds after injury. These substances, such as gamma-interferon, interleukins 1 and 6, and tumor necrosis factor, enter the bloodstream in 1 to 4 minutes and travel to the brain. The cytokines, therefore, are able to activate fibers that send messages to the brain and, concurrently, to breach the blood–brain barrier at specific sites and have an immediate effect on hypothalamic cells. The cytokines together with evaluative information from the brain rapidly begin a sequence of activities aimed at the release and utilization of glucose for necessary actions, such as removal of debris, the repair of tissues, and (sometimes) fever to destroy bacteria and other foreign substances. At sufficient severity of injury, the noradrenergic system is activated: Adrenalin is released into the blood stream and the powerful locus ceruleus/norepinephrine (LC/NE) system in the brainstem projects information upward throughout the brain and downward through the descending efferent sympathetic nervous system. Thus the whole sympathetic system is activated to produce readiness of the heart, blood vessels, and other viscera for complex programs to reinstate homeostasis (Chrousos & Gold, 1992; Sapolsky, 1994).

At the same time, the perception of pain activates the hypothalamic-pituitary-adrenal (HPA) system, in which corticotropin-releasing hormone (CRH) produced in the hypothalamus enters the local bloodstream, which carries the hormone to the pituitary, causing the release of adrenocorticotropic hormone (ACTH) and other substances. The ACTH then activates the adrenal cortex to release cortisol, which may play a powerful role in determining chronic pain. Cortisol also acts on the immune system and the endogenous opioid system. Although these opioids are released within minutes, their initial function may be simply to inhibit or modulate the release of cortisol. Experiments with animals suggest that their analgesic effects may not appear until as long as 30 minutes after injury.

Cortisol, together with noradrenergic activation, sets the stage for response to life-threatening emergency. If the output of cortisol is prolonged, or excessive, or of abnormal patterning, it may produce destruction of muscle, bone, and neural tissue and produce the conditions for many kinds of chronic pain.

Cortisol is an essential hormone for survival after injury because it is responsible for producing and maintaining high levels of glucose for rapid response after injury, threat, or other emergency. However, cortisol is potentially a highly destructive substance because, to ensure a high level of glucose, it breaks down the protein in muscle and inhibits the ongoing replacement of calcium in bone. Sustained cortisol release, therefore, can produce myopathy, weakness, fatigue, and decalcification of bone. It can also accelerate neural degeneration of the hippocampus during aging and suppress the immune system (Sapolsky, 1994). It may also affect the central nervous system (Lariviere & Melzack, 2000).

A major clue to the relationships among injury, stress, and pain is that many autoimmune diseases, such as rheumatoid arthritis and scleroderma, are also pain syndromes (Melzack, 1998, 1999). Furthermore, more women than men suffer from autoimmune diseases as well as chronic pain syndromes. Among the 5% of adults who suffer from an autoimmune disease, two out of three are women. Pain diseases also show a sex difference, as Berkley and Holdcroft (1999) argued, with the majority prevalent in women, and a smaller number prevalent in men. Of particular importance is the change in sex ratios concurrently with changes in sex hormone output as a function of age. Estrogen increases the release of peripheral cytokines, such as gamma-interferon, which in turn produce increased cortisol. This may explain, in part, why more females than males suffer from most kinds of chronic pain as well as painful autoimmune diseases such as multiple sclerosis and lupus.

Some forms of chronic pain may occur as a result of the cumulative destructive effect of cortisol on muscle, bone, and neural tissue. Furthermore, loss of fibers in the hippocampus due to aging reduces a natural brake on cortisol release that is normally exerted by the hippocampus. As a result, cortisol is released in larger amounts, producing a greater loss of hippocampal fibers and a cascading deleterious effect. This is found in aging primates and presumably also occurs in humans. It could explain the increase of chronic pain problems among older people.

The cortisol output by itself may not be sufficient to cause any of these problems, but rather provides the conditions so that other contributing factors may, all together, produce them. Sex-related hormones, genetic predispositions, psychological stresses derived from social competition, and the hassles of everyday life may act together to influence cortisol release, its amount and pattern, and the effects of the target organs.

These speculations are supported by strong evidence. Chrousos and Gold (1992) documented the effects of dysregulation of the cortisol system: effects on muscle and bone, to which they attribute fibromyalgia, rheumatoid arthritis, and chronic fatigue syndrome. They proposed that they are caused by hypocortisolism, which could be due do depletion of cortisol as a result of prolonged stress. Indeed, Sapolsky (1994) attributed myopathy, bone decalcification, fatigue, and accelerated neural degeneration during aging to prolonged exposure to stress.

Clearly, consideration of the relationship between stress-system effects and chronic pain leads directly to examination of the effects of suppression of the immune system and the development of autoimmune effects. The fact that several autoimmune diseases are also classified as chronic pain syndromes—such as Crohn's disease, multiple sclerosis, rheumatoid arthritis, scleroderma, and lupus—suggests that the study of these syndromes in relation to stress effects and chronic pain could be fruitful. Immune suppression, which involves prolonging the presence of dead tissue, invading bacteria and viruses, could produce a greater output of cytokines, with a consequent increase in cortisol and its destructive effects. Furthermore, prolonged immune suppression may diminish gradually and give way to a rebound, excessive immune response. The immune system's attack on its own body's tissues may produce autoimmune diseases that are also chronic pain syndromes. Thorough investigation may provide valuable clues for understanding at least some of the terrible chronic pain syndromes that now perplex us and are beyond our control.

PAIN AND NEUROPLASTICITY

There was no place in the specificity concept of the nervous system for "plasticity," in which neuronal and synaptic functions are capable of being molded or shaped so that they influence subsequent perceptual experiences. Plasticity related to pain represents persistent functional changes, or "somatic memories," (Katz & Melzack, 1990), produced in the nervous system by injuries or other pathological events. The recognition that such changes can occur is essential to understanding the chronic pain syndromes, such as low back pain and phantom limb pain, that persist and often destroy the lives of the people who suffer them.

Denervation Hypersensitivity
and Neuronal Hyperactivity

Sensory disturbances associated with nerve injury have been closely linked to alterations in CNS function. Markus, Pomeranz, and Krushelnycky (1984) demonstrated that the development of hypersensitivity in a rat's hindpaw following sciatic nerve section occurs concurrently with the expansion of the saphenous nerve's somatotopic projection in the spinal cord. Nerve injury may also lead to the development of increased neuronal activity at every level of the somatosensory system (see review by Coderre, Katz,

Vaccarino, & Melzack, 1993). In addition to spontaneous activity generated from the neuroma, peripheral neurectomy also leads to increased spontaneous activity in the dorsal root ganglion and spinal cord. Furthermore, after dorsal rhizotomy, there are increases in spontaneous neural activity in the dorsal horn, the spinal trigeminal nucleus, and the thalamus.

Clinical neurosurgery studies reveal a similar relationship between denervation and CNS hyperactivity. Neurons in the somatosensory thalamus of patients with neuropathic pain display high spontaneous firing rates, abnormal bursting activity, and evoked responses to stimulation of body areas that normally do not activate these neurons (Lenz et al., 1987; Lenz, Kwan, Dostrovsky, & Tasker, 1989). The site of abnormality in thalamic function appears to be somatotopically related to the painful region. In patients with complete spinal cord transection and dysesthesias referred below the level of the break, neuronal hyperactivity was observed in thalamic regions that had lost their normal sensory input, but not in regions with apparently normal afferent input (Lenz et al., 1987). Furthermore, in patients with neuropathic pain, electrical stimulation of subthalamic, thalamic, and capsular regions may evoke pain and in some instances even reproduce the patient's pain (Nathan, 1985; Tasker, 1989). Direct electrical stimulation of spontaneously hyperactive cells evokes pain in some but not all pain patients, raising the possibility that in certain patients the observed changes in neuronal activity may contribute to the perception of pain (Lenz, Kwan, Dostrovsky, & Tasker, 1987). Studies of patients undergoing electrical brain stimulation during brain surgery reveal that pain is rarely elicited by test stimuli unless the patient suffers from a chronic pain problem. However, brain stimulation can elicit pain responses in patients with chronic pain that does not involve extensive nerve injury or deafferentation. Nathan (1985) described a patient who underwent thalamic stimulation for a movement disorder. The patient had been suffering from a toothache for 10 days prior to the operation. Electrical stimulation of the thalamus reproduced the toothache.

It is possible that receptive field expansions and spontaneous activity generated in the CNS following peripheral nerve injury are, in part, mediated by alterations in normal inhibitory processes in the dorsal horn. Within 4 days of a peripheral nerve section there is a reduction in the dorsal root potential and, therefore, in the presynaptic inhibition it represents (Wall & Devor, 1981). Nerve section also induces a reduction in the inhibitory effect of A-fiber stimulation on activity in dorsal horn neurons (Woolf & Wall, 1982). Furthermore, nerve injury affects descending inhibitory controls from brainstem nuclei. In the intact nervous system, stimulation of the locus ceruleus (Segal & Sandberg, 1977) or the nucleus raphe magnus (Oliveras, Guilbaud, & Besson, 1979) produces an inhibition of dorsal horn neurons. Following dorsal rhizotomy, however, stimulation of these areas produces excitation, rather than inhibition, in half the cells studied (Hodge, Apkarian, Owen, & Hanson, 1983).

Recent advances in our understanding of the mechanisms that underlie pathological pain have important implications for the treatment of both acute and chronic pain. Because it has been established that intense noxious stimulation produces a sensitization of CNS neurons, it is possible to direct treatments not only at the site of peripheral tissue damage, but also at the site of central changes. Furthermore, it may be possible in some instances to prevent the development of central changes which contribute to pathological pain states. The fact that amputees are more likely to develop phantom limb pain if there is pain in the limb prior to amputation (Katz & Melzack, 1990), combined with the finding that the incidence of phantom limb pain is reduced if patients are rendered pain free by epidural blockade with bupivacaine and morphine prior to amputation (Bach, Noreng, & Tjellden, 1988) suggests that the development of neuropathic pain can be prevented by reducing the potential for central sensitization at the time of amputation. Although the latter finding is contentious (McQuay, 1992; McQuay, Carroll, & Moore, 1988), the conclusions by Bach et al. remain valid (Katz et al., 1992, 1994).

The evidence that postoperative pain is also reduced by premedication with regional and/or spinal anesthetic blocks and/or opiates (McQuay et al., 1988; Tversky, Cozacov, Ayache, Bradley, & Kissin, 1990; Katz et al., 1992) suggests that acute postoperative pain can also benefit from the blocking of the afferent barrage arriving within the CNS and the central sensitization it may induce (Katz, Jackson, Kavanagh, & Sandler, 1996). Whether chronic postoperative problems such as painful scars, postthoracotomy chest-wall pain, and phantom limb and stump pain can be reduced by blocking nociceptive inputs during surgery remains to be determined. Furthermore, additional research is required to determine whether multiple-treatment approaches (involving local and epidural anesthesia, as well as pretreatment with opiates and anti-inflammatory drugs) that produce an effective blockade of afferent input may also prevent or relieve other forms of severe chronic pain such as postherpetic neuralgia and reflex sympathetic dystrophy. It is hoped that a combination of new pharmacological developments, careful clinical trials, and an increased understanding of the contribution and mechanisms of noxious stimulus-induced neuroplasticity, will lead to improved clinical treatment and prevention of pathological pain.

THE MULTIPLE DETERMINANTS OF PAIN

The neuromatrix theory of pain proposes that the neurosignature for pain experience is determined by the synaptic architecture of the neuromatrix, which is produced by genetic and sensory influences. The neurosignature pattern is also modulated by sensory inputs and by cognitive events, such as psychological stress. Furthermore, stressors, physical as well as psychological, act on stress-regulation systems, which may produce lesions of muscle, bone, and nerve tissue, thereby contributing to the neurosignature patterns that give rise to chronic pain. In short, the neuromatrix, as a result of homeostasis-regulation patterns that have failed, may produce the destructive conditions that give rise to many of the chronic pains that so far have been resistant to treatments developed primarily to manage pains that are triggered by sensory inputs. The stress regulation system, with its complex, delicately balanced interactions, is an integral part of the multiple contributions that give rise to chronic pain.

The neuromatrix theory guides us away from the Cartesian concept of pain as a sensation produced by injury or other tissue pathology and toward the concept of pain as a multidimensional experience produced by multiple influences. These influences range from the existing synaptic architecture of the neuromatrix to influences from within the body and from other areas in the brain. Genetic influences on synaptic architecture may determine—or predispose toward—the development of chronic pain syndromes. Figure 1.5 summarizes the factors that contribute to the output pattern from the neuromatrix that produce the sensory, affective, and cognitive dimensions of pain experience and the resultant behavior.

Multiple inputs act on the neuromatrix programs and contribute to the *output* neurosignature. They include (a) sensory inputs (cutaneous, visceral, and other somatic receptors); (b) visual and other sensory inputs that influence the cognitive interpretation of the situation; (c) phasic and tonic cognitive and emotional inputs from other areas of the brain; (d) intrinsic neural inhibitory modulation inherent in all brain function; and (e) the activity of the body's stress regulation systems, including cytokines as well as the endocrine, autonomic, immune, and opioid systems. We have traveled a long way from the psychophysical concept that seeks a simple one-to-one relationship between injury and pain. We now have a theoretical framework in which a genetically determined template for the body-self is modulated by the powerful stress system and the cognitive functions of the brain, in addition to the traditional sensory inputs.

REFERENCES

Bach, S., Noreng, M. F., & Tjellden, N. U. (1988). Phantom limb pain in amputees during the first 12 months following limb amputation, after preoperative lumbar epidural blockade. *Pain, 33,* 297–301.

Berkley, K. J., & Holdcroft, A. (1999). Sex and gender differences in pain. In P. D. Wall & R. Melzack (Eds.), *Textbook of pain* (4th ed., pp. 951–965). Edinburgh: Churchill Livingstone.

Chrousos, G. P., & Gold, P. W. (1992). The concepts of stress and stress system disorders. *J. Am. Med. Assoc., 267*, 1244–1252.

Coderre, T. J., Katz, J., Vaccarino, A. L., & Melzack, R. (1993). Contribution of central neuroplasticity to pathological pain: Review of clinical and experimental evidence. *Pain, 52*, 259–285.

Fields, H. L., & Basbaum, A. I. (1999). Central nervous system mechanisms of pain modulation. In P. D. Wall & R. Melzack (Eds.), *Textbook of pain* (4th ed., pp. 309–329). Edinburgh: Churchill Livingstone.

Goldscheider, A. (1894). *Uber den schmerzs in physiologischer und klinischer hinsicht.* Berlin: Hirschwald.

Gybels, J. M., & Tasker, R. R. (1999). Central neurosurgery. In P. D. Wall & R. Melzack (Eds.), *Textbook of pain* (4th ed., pp. 1307–1339). Edinburgh: Churchill Livingstone.

Hebb, D. O. (1949). *The organization of behavior.* New York: Wiley.

Hodge, C. J., Apkarian, A. V., Owen, M. P., & Hanson, B. S. (1983). Changes in the effects of stimulation of locus coeruleus and nucleus raphe magnus following dorsal rhizotomy. *Brain Research, 288*, 325–329.

Katz, J. (1993). The reality of phantom limbs. *Emotion and Motivation, 17*, 147–178.

Katz, J., Claireux, M., Kavanagh, B. P., Roger, S., Nierenberg, H., Redahan, C., & Sandler, A. N. (1994). Pre-emptive lumbar epidural anaesthesia reduces postoperative pain and patient-controlled morphine consumption after lower abdominal surgery. *Pain, 59*, 395–403.

Katz, J., Jackson, M., Kavanagh, B. P., & Sandler, A. N. (1996). Acute pain after thoracic surgery predicts long-term post-thoracotomy pain. *Clinical Journal of Pain, 12*, 50–55.

Katz, J., Kavanagh, B. P., Sandler, A. N., Nierenberg, H., Boylan, J. F., & Shaw, B. F. (1992). Pre-emptive analgesia: Clinical evidence of neuroplasticity contributing to postoperative pain. *Anesthesiology, 77*, 439–446.

Katz, J., & Melzack, R. (1990). Pain "memories" in phantom limbs: Review and clinical observations. *Pain, 43*, 319–336.

Keele, K. D. (1957). *Anatomies of pain.* Oxford: Blackwell Scientific Publications.

Kuhn, T. S. (1970). *The structure of scientific revolutions* (2nd ed.). Chicago: University of Chicago Press.

Lariviere, W. R., & Melzack, R. (2000). The role of corticotropin-releasing factor in pain and analgesia. *Pain, 84*, 1–12.

Le Bars, D., Dickenson, A. H., & Besson, J. M. (1983). Opiate analgesia and descending control systems. In J. J. Bonica, U. Lindblom, & A. Iggo (Eds.), *Advances in pain research and therapy: Proceedings of the IIIrd World Congress on Pain* (Vol. 5, pp. 341–372). New York: Raven Press.

Lenz, F. A., Kwan, H. C., Dostrovsky, J. O., & Tasker, R. R. (1989). Characteristics of the bursting pattern of action potential that occurs in the thalamus of patients with central pain. *Brain Research, 496*, 357–360.

Lenz, F. A., Tasker, R. R., Dostrovsky, J. O., Kwan, H. C., Gorecki, J., Hirayama, T., & Murphy, J. T. (1987). Abnormal single-unit activity recorded in the somatosensory thalamus of a quadriplegic patient with central pain. *Pain, 31*, 225–236.

Liebeskind, J. C., & Paul, L. A. (1977). Psychological and physiological mechanisms of pain. *Annual Review of Psychology, 28*, 41–60.

Livingston, W. K. (1943). *Pain mechanisms.* New York: Macmillan.

Markus, H., Pomeranz, B., & Krushelnycky, D. (1984). Spread of saphaneous somatotopic projection map in spinal cord and hypersensitivity of the foot after chronic sciatic denervation in adult rat. *Brain Research, 296*, 27–39.

McQuay, H. J. (1992). Pre-emptive analgesia. *British Journal of Anaesthesiology, 69*, 1–3.

McQuay, H. J., Carroll, D., & Moore, R. A. (1988). Post-operative orthopaedic pain—The effect of opiate premedication and local anaesthetic blocks. *Pain, 33*, 291–295.

Melzack, R. (1975a). The McGill pain questionnaire: Major properties and scoring methods. *Pain, 1*, 277–299.

Melzack, R. (1975b). Prolonged relief of pain by brief, intense transcutaneous somatic stimulation. *Pain, 1,* 357–373.

Melzack, R. (1987). The short-form McGill pain questionnaire. *Pain, 30,* 191–197.

Melzack, R. (1989). Phantom limbs, the self and the brain (The D. O. Hebb Memorial Lecture). *Canadian Psychology, 30,* 1–14.

Melzack, R. (1990). Phantom limbs and the concept of a neuromatrix. *Trends in Neuroscience, 13,* 88–92.

Melzack, R. (1991). The gate control theory 25 years later: New perspectives on phantom limb pain. In M. R. Bond, J. E. Charlton, & C. J. Woolf (Eds.), *Pain research and therapy: Proceedings of the VIth world congress on pain* (pp. 9–21). Amsterdam: Elsevier.

Melzack, R. (1995). Phantom limb pain and the brain. In B. Bromm & J. E. Desmedt (Eds.), *Pain and the brain* (pp. 73–82). New York: Raven Press.

Melzack, R. (1998). Pain and stress: Clues toward understanding chronic pain. In M. Sabourin, F. Craik, & M. Robert (Eds.), *Advances in psychological science, Vol. 2, Biological and cognitive aspects* (pp. 63–85). Hove: Psychology Press.

Melzack, R. (1999). Pain and stress: A new perspective. In R. J. Gatchel & D. C. Turk (Eds.), *Psychological factors in pain* (pp. 89–106). New York: Guilford Press.

Melzack, R. (2001). Pain and the neuromatrix in the brain. *Journal of Dental Education, 65,* 1378–1382.

Melzack, R., & Casey, K. L. (1968). Sensory, motivational and central control determinants of pain: A new conceptual model. In D. Kenshalo (Ed.), *The skin senses* (pp. 423–443). Springfield, IL: Charles C. Thomas.

Melzack, R., Israel, R., Lacroix, R., & Schultz, G. (1997). Phantom limbs in people with congenital limb deficiency or amputation in early childhood. *Brain, 120,* 1603–1620.

Melzack, R., & Loeser, J. D. (1978). Phantom body pain in paraplegics: Evidence for a central "pattern generating mechanism" for pain. *Pain, 4,* 195–210.

Melzack, R., Stotler, W. A., & Livingston, W. K. (1958). Effects of discrete brainstem lesions in cats on perception of noxious stimulation. *Journal of Neurophysiology, 21,* 353–367.

Melzack, R., & Wall, P. D. (1965). Pain mechanisms: A new theory. *Science, 150,* 971–979.

Melzack, R., & Wall, P. D. (1996). *The challenge of pain* (2nd ed.). London: Penguin.

Nathan, P. W. (1985). Pain and nociception in the clinical context. *Philosophical Transactions of the Royal Society of London, 308,* 219–226.

Noordenbos, W. (1959). *Pain.* Amsterdam: Elsevier.

Oliveras, J. L., Guilbaud, G., & Besson, J. M. (1979). A map of serotonergic structures involved in stimulation produced analgesia in unrestrained freely moving cats. *Brain Research, 164,* 317–322.

Reynolds, D. V. (1969). Surgery in the rat during electrical analgesia induced by focal brain stimulation. *Science, 164,* 444–445.

Sapolsky, R. M. (1994). *Why zebras don't get ulcers.* New York: W. H. Freeman.

Schultz, G., & Melzack, R. (1991). The Charles Bonnet syndrome: "Phantom visual images." *Perception, 20,* 809–825.

Segal, M., & Sandberg, D. (1977). Analgesia produced by electrical stimulation of catecholamine nuclei in the rat brain. *Brain Research, 123,* 369–372.

Selye, H. (1956). *The stress of life.* New York: McGraw-Hill.

Tasker, R. R. (1989). Stereotactic surgery. In P. D. Wall & R. Melzack (Eds.), *Textbook of pain* (pp. 840–855). Edinburgh: Churchill Livingstone.

Tverskoy, M., Cozacov, C., Ayache, M., Bradley, E. L., & Kissin, I. (1990). Postoperative pain after inguinal hemiorraphy with different types of anesthesia. *Anesthesia and Analgesia, 70,* 29–35.

Wall, P. D., & Devor, M. (1981). The effect of peripheral nerve injury on dorsal root potentials and on transmission of afferent signals into the spinal cord. *Brain Research, 209,* 95–111.

Webster's Seventh New Collegiate Dictionary. (1967). p. 522. Springfield, MA: G and C Merriam.

Woolf, C. J., & Wall, P. D. (1982). Chronic peripheral nerve section diminishes the primary afferent A fibre mediated inhibition of rat dorsal horn neurons. *Brain Research, 242,* 77–85.

2

Biopsychosocial Approaches to Pain

Gordon J. G. Asmundson
Faculty of Kinesiology and Health Studies
and Department of Psychology, University of Regina

Kristi D. Wright
Department of Psychology, University of Regina

If we liken models of pain to facial displays of emotion, it becomes readily apparent that many expressions have evolved. Indeed, over the years there have been a large number of models proffered by individuals from varying intellectual traditions. Most of these models can be grouped within one of several general categories—traditional biomedical, psychodynamic, and biopsychosocial. The intent of all models, without exception, has been to address the enduring questions of "What is pain?" and "How do we best alleviate pain and the suffering associated with it?" The primary purpose of this chapter is to gain insight into answers to these questions by exploring various iterations of the biopsychosocial approach and related empirical literature.

To date, there have been a number of reviews written on biopsychosocial approaches to pain (e.g., Robinson & Riley, 1999; Turk, 1996a; Turk & Flor, 1999; Waddell, 1991, 1992). Nonetheless, the face of pain, or at least the way we as clinical and research psychologists view it, is constantly changing. Indeed, many of the earlier models have proven inadequate for patient care, and more recent research has superseded initial formulations. Take, for example, the advancement of the original conceptualizations of the gate control theory (Melzack & Casey, 1968; Melzack & Wall, 1965, 1982)—the first to integrate physiological and psychological mechanisms of pain—to the current neuromatrix model as described by Melzack and Katz in chapter 1 of this volume. Similar progress has occurred in the context of biopsychosocial approaches that have emerged from postulates of the gate control theory, such that our answers to the "what" and "how" questions just posed are, in our opinion, becoming more clear. To this end, the concepts presented herein provide an important piece of the foundation on which the assessment and treatment approaches described in other chapters of this volume are built.

Our intent in this chapter is to provide an overview and critical analysis of the traditional biomedical and psychodynamic models, summarize elements of the gate control theory that strongly influenced current conceptualizations of pain, and review important details of models that fall under the biopsychosocial rubric. Within the context of the latter, we include discussion of some of the most influential behavioral, cognitive, and cognitive-behavioral models and associated empirical findings. We conclude by positing a synthesis of the various iterations of the biopsychosocial approach, place this in the context of a comprehensive diathesis–stress model (i.e., a model in which dispositional tendencies to respond to stressors in a certain way interacts with stressors to produce illness behavior), and briefly discuss its implications for future research.

TRADITIONAL BIOMEDICAL MODEL

The traditional biomedical model of pain dates back hundreds of years. Descartes (1596–1650) modernized it in the 17th century (Bonica, 1990; Turk, 1996a), and in that form it held considerable influence through to the mid 20th century. The model holds, in essence, that pain is a sensory experience that results from stimulation of specific noxious receptors, usually from physical damage due to injury or disease (see Fig. 2.1). Consistent with Cartesian dualism (i.e., the idea that mind and body are nonoverlapping entities), the model has been described by some (e.g., Engel, 1977; Turk & Flor, 1999) as being both reductionistic (i.e., assumes that all disease is directly linked to specific physical pathology) and exclusionary (i.e., assumes that social, psychological, behavioral mechanisms of illness are not of primary importance).

Consider the case of Jamie, a middle-aged person with strained muscles in the low back. Applying the traditional biomedical model, the method of

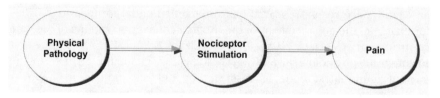

FIG. 2.1. Schematic of traditional medical model.

diagnosing and subsequently treating Jamie should be, for all practical purposes (and notwithstanding availability of adequate diagnostic, surgical, and pharmacologic technology), straightforward. Jamie's physical pathology would be confirmed by data obtained from objective tests of physical damage and, if thorough, tests of impairment. Medical interventions would then be directed toward rectifying the muscle strain. The impact of the strain on Jamie's social, psychological, and behavioral functioning would not be given much weight in any intervention. Indeed, other symptoms reported by Jamie, such as depressed mood, hypervigilance to somatic sensations, *and pain*, would not be viewed as significant but, rather, as secondary reactions to (or symptoms of) the muscle strain. These would be expected to subside after the muscle strain had healed.

In Jamie's case, intervention was targeted at healing the muscle strain and all symptoms subsided within 5 weeks. But, for every Jamie there is another person for whom application of an identical intervention does not resolve pain and other symptoms, including disability, despite eventual healing of physical pathology. Why? As becomes evident in this chapter, the reductionistic and exclusionary assumptions of the biomedical models have not been upheld. We now know that pain involves more than sensation arising from physical pathology. Indeed, many people with persistent pain, including perhaps the majority with low back pain, will never have had an identifiable medical diagnosis of tissue damage.

Most 20th-century models of pain, including amendments to the traditional biomedical model (e.g., Bonica, 1954; Hardy, Wolff, & Goodell, 1952), recognize to some degree that factors such as cognition and emotional state are important in the experience of pain. These models were not without criticism. For example, they posited a primary role for sensation and did not recognize the possibility that sensation and affect might be processed in parallel (Craig, 1984). Still, they demarcated a beginning to the recognition of the interplay between biological, psychological, and sociocultural factors in the pain experience. Before turning attention to integrated multidimensional models of pain, we lay more of the groundwork by taking a look at models of the psychodynamic tradition.

PSYCHODYNAMIC MODELS

The psychodynamic model can be considered to be among the first to posit a *central role* for psychological factors in pain (see Merskey & Spear, 1967), albeit with an emphasis on persistent (or chronic) rather than acute presentations. A number of psychodynamic models have been proposed over the years (e.g., Blumer & Heilbronn, 1981; Breuer & Freud, 1893–1895/1957; Engel, 1959). These models are similar in that, unlike the traditional biomedical model, they shift focus from physical pathology by conceptualizing persistent pain as an expression of emotional conflict. Rather than review all of the psychodynamic models, we provide an overview of the influential models of Freud (Breuer & Freud, 1893–1895/1957) and Engel (1959).

Freud (Breuer & Freud, 1893–1895/1957) held that persistent pain was maintained by an emotional loss or conflict, most often at the unconscious level. Central to Freud's model was the process of conversion, or expressing *emotional pain* (i.e., the unresolved conflict) by converting it into physical symptoms that were a symbolic and more tolerable expression of the underlying emotional issues. To illustrate, a women reporting dyspareunia (i.e., persistent genital pain associated with sexual intercourse) may be thought to be expressing some unresolved unconscious conflict regarding taboo sexual urges, such as having sex with her sister's husband. Freud believed that the somatic expression of pain would subside with resolution of the emotional issues. These ideas have been subsequently modified and adapted by other theorists working within the framework of the psychodynamic tradition.

In 1959 Engel introduced the concepts of *psychogenic pain* and the *pain-prone personality* to further explain the nature of persistent pain. The key elements of Engel's position were that (a) persistent pain can, but need not, have a basis in physical pathology, and (b) in some people, it is a psychological phenomenon that serves a self-protective function. It is pain in the absence of identifiable physical pathology that has, since Engel's (1959) contribution, been referred to by many as psychogenic, or of psychological origin. Most often the decision is made on the basis of exclusion; that is, in the absence of identifiable pathology, it is presumed emotional conflict must explain the symptoms.

Engel framed his model from a developmental perspective in which a person amasses a large set of experiences wherein pain is associated with, and derives meaning from, the context in which it has occurred. For example, early in life a person may learn to associate pain with others' responses to his or her behavior (e.g., affection in response to crying, punishment in response to inappropriate behavior, aggression). Later in life, the person may use pain as an unconscious defense against various bouts of emotional distress he or she experiences (much as posited by Freud). Although the former of these propositions was supported in part by findings from empirical tests of social learning influences on pain (e.g., Craig, 1978), the latter remains controversial.

What type of person is most likely to do this or, in other words, to have a pain-prone personality? Engel (1959) suggested that those with psychiatric conditions, as described by diagnostic nomenclature of the day (e.g., *DSM–I* provided for the possibilities of hysteria, major depression, hypochondriasis, or paranoid schizophrenia), were particularly prone to experience persistent pain. Amendments to Engel's model, such as Blumer and Heilbroon's (1982) position on chronic pain as a variant of major depressive disorder, or *masked depression*, added depressed affect, alexithymia, family history of depression and chronic pain, and discrete biological markers (e.g., response to antidepressants) to the list of contributors to the pain-prone personality. The results of a large number of studies suggest that the prevalence of current psychiatric conditions is, indeed, elevated in patients with chronic pain relative to base rates in the general population (e.g., Asmundson, Jacobson, Allerdings, & Norton, 1996; Dersh, Gatchel, Polatin, & Mayer, 2002; Katon, Egan, & Miller, 1985; Large, 1986). It is questionable, however, whether the presence of psychiatric morbidity makes one more likely to use pain as an unconscious defense mechanism and, thereby, more prone to persistent pain (see, e.g., the July 1982 issue of *The Journal of Nervous and Mental Disease*, and Large, 1986).

With few exceptions (Adler, Zlot, Hürny, Minder, 1989), the psychodynamic formulations have not fared well against empirical scrutiny (see reviews by Gamsa, 1994; Large, 1986; Roth, 2000; Roy, 1985), and now have diminished popularity in mainstream psychology. Notwithstanding, they did play a key role in drawing attention to the importance of psychological (and contextual) factors in the experience of pain at a time when treatment for pain was primarily directed by the biomedical model. This attention led to increased and continuing research into a wide array of psychosocial variables (e.g., birth order, childhood abuse, interpersonal and marital difficulties, depression, anxiety, personality disorders, illness behavior), their role in the development and maintenance of chronic pain, and their importance in contemporary psychological treatment formulations. Indeed, the interest in psychological factors spawned by psychodynamic theorists served as an essential precursor to the development of contemporary biopsychosocial approaches. However, using Roth's (2000) analogy of the double-edged sword, it is noteworthy that there are lingering and unwanted scars of this psychodynamic thrust. These include the general tendency to assume (a) that all cases of pain in the absence of identifiable physical pathology are the result of psychological factors, and (b) that these are equally relevant to *all* people with persistent pain. Although incorrect, these assumptions can (and still often do) have a negative impact on opinions and general treatment of people who suffer from persistent pain conditions.

GATE CONTROL THEORY

As noted earlier, Melzack and colleagues' seminal papers on the gate control theory of pain (Melzack & Casey, 1968; Melzack & Wall, 1965) are frequently cited as the first to integrate physiological and psychological mechanisms of pain within the context of a single model. It is beyond the scope of this chapter to provide a detailed synopsis of the theory; however, given its contribution to current conceptualizations of pain, a brief overview is warranted.

Melzack and Wall (1965) proposed that a hypothetical gating mechanism within the dorsal horn of the spinal cord is responsible for allowing or disallowing the passage of ascending nociceptive information from the periphery to the brain. These essential elements are as follows:

- The gating mechanism is influenced by the relative degree of excitatory activity in the spinal cord transmission cells, with excitation along the large-diameter, myelinated fibers closing the gate and along the small-diameter, unmyelinated fibers opening the gate.

- Descending transmissions (i.e., from the brain to the gating mechanism) regarding current cognition and affective state also influence the gating mechanism (suggesting the importance of higher level brain activities and processes).

- The summation of information traveling along the different types of ascending fibers from the periphery with that traveling on descending fibers from the brain determines whether the gate is open or closed and, as such, influences the perception of pain.

Since this original proposal we have, of course, moved beyond believing that the key to understanding pain is knowing what happens in the dorsal horn. Melzack and Casey (1968) further proposed that three different neural networks (i.e., sensory-discriminative, motivational-affective, and cognitive-evaluative) influence the modulation of sensory input. They also recognized that processing of input could occur in parallel, at least at the sensory and affective level. This revised model allowed for "perceptual information regarding the location, magnitude, and spatiotemporal properties of the noxious stimulus, motivational tendency toward escape or attack, and cognitive information based on analysis of multimodal information, past experience, and probability of outcome of different response strategies" (pp. 427–428).

Think back to the case of Jamie, who had pain associated with muscle strain in the low back. Applying the postulates of the gate control theory, Jamie's pain experience might be understood as follows: Stimulation of nociceptors in the region of muscle strain facilitated transmission of information along ascending fibers, through an open gate, and on to Jamie's brain. At the same time, Jamie's brain was sending information about her current cognitions and emotional state (i.e., depressed and hypervigilant) back to the gate along descending fibers. The summation of the ascending nociceptive input and descending information regarding cognition and emotion, in this case, kept the gate open. This process was ongoing (i.e., it lasted for many days) and involved an interaction between physiological, cognitive, and affective inputs that continuously modified Jamie's perception of the pain. Medical and behavioral interventions ultimately served to close the gate, reducing pain, and improving Jamie's mood state and overall functional ability.

Based on this brief overview it should be apparent that the gate control theory challenged the primary assumptions of the traditional biomedical and psychodynamic models. Rather than being exclusively conceptualized as sensation arising from physical pathology or somatic manifestation of unresolved emotional conflicts, the experience of pain came to be viewed as a combination of both pathophysiology and psychological factors. On this basis, then, Jamie's depressed mood would not be viewed as a secondary reaction to pain, nor would the pain be viewed as a result of depressed mood. Rather, each would be seen as having a reciprocal influence on the other.

The assumptions of the gate control theory have not gone unchallenged, and advances in our understanding of the anatomy and structure of the gating mechanism have led to various revisions. The details of the changing views of the physiology of the gating mechanism are beyond the intent and scope of this chapter. We recommend that interested readers refer to articles in Supplement 6 of the 1999 volume of *Pain* entitled "A Tribute to Patrick D. Wall" and to recent reviews written by Turk and Flor (1999) and Wall (1996). Notwithstanding, the essential elements of the model, as described earlier, have proven a heuristic of considerable value to both basic scientists and clinical scientist-practitioners.

Melzack's (1999) own words most accurately describe the most important contribution of the theory:

> Never again, after 1965, could anyone try to explain pain exclusively in terms of peripheral factors. The theory forced the medical and biological sciences to accept the brain as an active system that filters, selects and modulates inputs . . . we highlighted the central nervous system as an essential component in the process. (p. S123)

Since 1965, but particularly over the past 25 years, there have been many advances to our understanding of the specific nature of the psychological and sociocultural factors of pain. For example, Price (2000) proposed a parallel-serial model of pain affect that is consistent with existing literature. This model details a central network of brain structures (e.g., anterior cingulate cortex, hypothalamus, insular cortex) and pathways (e.g., spino-hypothalamic pathway, cortico-limbic somatosensory pathway), comprising both serial and parallel connections, as the mechanism through which the emotional valance of pain is determined and subsequently expressed. Other important advances are succinctly captured in the context of Melzack's neuromatrix theory (see chap. 1, this volume), as well as in other general models that focus on the cognitive, affective, and behavioral aspects of the pain experience.

THE BIOPSYCHOSOCIAL APPROACH

Turk and Flor (1999) have accurately and succinctly captured the basic premises of the biopsychosocial approach to pain. They stated:

> Predispositional factors and current biological factors may initiate, maintain, and modulate physical perturbations; predispositional and current psychological factors influence the appraisal and perception of internal physiological signs; and social factors shape the behavioral responses of patients to the perceptions of their physical perturbations. (p. 20)

In short, the biopsychosocial approach holds that the experience of pain is determined by the interaction among biological, psychological (which include cognition, affect, behavior), and social factors (which include the social and cultural contexts that influence a person's perception of and response to physical signs and symptoms). Compared to either of the traditional biomedical or psychodynamic positions, the biopsychosocial approach posits a much broader, multidimensional, and complex perspective on pain. This is true for both acute and chronic pain, although it is in the case of the latter that the model has proven most heuristic.

A number of specific iterations of the general biopsychosocial approach to pain have been put forth over the years. Like similar models proposed to account for other chronic health conditions (e.g., asthma, functional dyspepsia; tinnitus, Meniere's disease; Asmundson, Wright, & Hadjistavropoulos, 2000), these iterations are based on several assumptions, as follows:

- Unlike the traditional biomedical model, the focus is not on *disease* per se but rather on *illness*, where illness is viewed as a type of behavior (Parsons, 1951). *Illness behavior* is a term used to describe the "ways in which given symptoms may be differently perceived, evaluated, or acted (or not acted) upon by different kinds of persons" (Mechanic, 1962, p. 189). This definition implies that there are individual differences in responses to somatic sensations, and that these can be understood in the context of psychological and social processes (Mechanic, 1962).
- Illness behavior is considered a dynamic processes, with the role of biological, psychological, and social factors changing in relative impor-

tance as the condition evolves (also see Engel, 1977; Lipowski, 1983). Although a condition may be initiated by biological factors, the psychological and social factors may come to play a primary role in maintenance and exacerbation. Also, as suggested earlier, there are individual differences in the relative importance of any given factor at any given time during the course of a condition.

With these assumptions in mind, we now turn to several of the most influential biopsychosocial approaches to chronic pain. These include the operant model, Glasgow model, biobehavioral model, and fear avoidance models. We organize our presentation of these models in an ascending chronological order. Empirical evidence is grouped according to degree of relevance to the model under consideration; however, it should be noted that the findings of some investigations have implications for more than one model.

THE OPERANT MODEL

Model Summary

Fordyce and colleagues (Fordyce, 1976; Fordyce, Shelton, & Dundore, 1982) detailed an operant conditioning model that describes how positive and negative reinforcement (i.e., presentation or removal of a stimulus, respectively) serve as mechanisms through which acute pain behaviors are maintained over time and thus become chronic. The premises of this model are as follows:

- In response to an acute injury, people employ certain behaviors (e.g., escape or withdrawal, avoidance of activity, limping) that serve an adaptive function in reducing likelihood of further tissue damage.
- Behaviors that reduce pain are negatively reinforced, in the short term, by the reduction of suffering associated with stimulation of nociceptors.
- These behaviors can become persistent and *maladaptive* when reinforcement shifts from the reduction of nociceptive input to various external positive (e.g., increases social attention from family and friends) and negative (e.g., reduced degree of responsibility for completing tasks) reinforcers.

Accordingly, chronic pain is viewed as a set of observable behaviors that persist beyond the time required for healing of physical pathology and lead to declines in physical activity and associated deconditioning, increases in use of analgesic medications, and the development of additional illness behaviors.

Empirical Overview

Evidence in support of the operant model has come primarily from studies supporting operant-based treatment approaches (Block, Kremer, & Gaylor, 1980; Cairns & Pasino, 1977; also see recent meta-analysis by Morley, Eccleston, & Williams, 1999), although this evidence is viewed by some as equivocal (Sharp, 2001; Turk, 1996b). Despite this treatment-based evidence, there have been few empirical tests of the validity of the operant model. Linton and Götestam (1985), for example, conducted an experiment with adult hospital employees exposed to a constant-level noxious stimulus while either increases or decreases in verbal reports of pain from ischemic stimuli were reinforced. Significant differences between reinforced increases and decreases in pain reports within subjects were observed. More recently, Flor and colleagues (Flor, Knost, & Birbaumer, 2002) reinforced increases and decreases in verbal pain reports in chronic back pain patients and matched healthy controls exposed to electrical stimulation. Numerous physiological indices were also evaluated. Results indicated that, despite similar learning rates, the patients were influenced more by operant conditioning factors than were the control subjects. Specifically, they were more likely to maintain elevated pain ratings and cortical responsivity (N150) during extinction. Others, however, have failed to show clear-cut operant conditioning effects (Lousberg, Groenman, Schmidt, & Gielen, 1996).

THE GLASGOW MODEL

Model Summary

In an attempt to give equal emphasis to all components of the biopsychosocial approach, Waddell and colleagues (Waddell, 1987, 1991, 1992; Waddell, Main, Morris, Di Paoloa, & Gray, 1984; Waddell, Newton, Henderson, Somerville, & Main, 1993) applied the construct of illness behavior to chronic low back pain. They view chronic low back pain as a form of illness behavior stemming from physiological impairment (defined as "pathologic, anatomic, or physiologic abnormality of structure or function leading to loss of normal body ability"; Waddell, Somerville, Henderson, & Netwon, 1992) and influenced by cognition, affect, and social factors. In Fig. 2.2 we depict the essential features of the model as they relate to the case of Kelly, who, like Jamie described earlier, had chronic back pain as well as depressed mood and hypervigilance to somatic sensations subsequent to a muscle strain. Unlike Jamie, Kelly's pain persisted over several years.

The illustration shows how biological and psychological factors interact (within the context of a larger social environment) in a manner that pro-

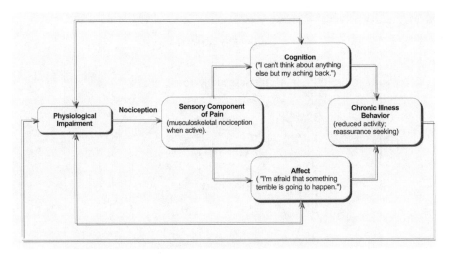

FIG. 2.2. Application of the Glasgow model of chronic low back pain to illustrate Kelly's clinical presentation.

motes chronic illness (or pain) behavior and, ultimately, disability. Social factors, although not explicit, impact on the interpretation of nociception as well as illness behaviors. The elements of the model can also be illustrated as a biopsychosocial cross section of a person's clinical presentation at a single point in time (see Fig. 2.3). Although not evident in either Fig. 2.2 or 2.3, it is noteworthy that the Glasgow model recognizes that physical pathology (whether or not currently identifiable) plays an important precipitating role, and that the ongoing physiological impairment (e.g., muscular deconditioning) can give rise to nociception that is distinct from the original physical pathology.

Empirical Overview

Waddell (1991, 1992) reviewed the literature related to the Glasgow model. Empirical investigations examining the importance of active exercise in rehabilitation of low back pain have, for the most part, yielded results that provide confirmation of its validity. Waddell (1992) identified 13 out of 17 controlled studies that showed statistically and clinically significant benefits in pain, disability, physical impairment, cardiovascular fitness, psychological distress, or work loss as a result of the implementation of the active exercise approach (i.e., progressive increase in activity through exercise). Additionally, controlled trials comparing a combined behavioral/rehabilitation approach to physical exercise alone in the treatment of low back pain have also provided support for this model.

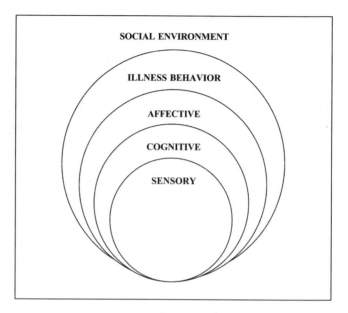

FIG. 2.3. Cross-sectional representation of the Glasgow model. Reprinted from Waddell et al. (1993), "A Fear-Avoidance Beliefs Questionnaire (FABQ) and the role of fear-avoidance beliefs in chronic low back pain and disability," p. 164. Copyright 1993. Reproduced with kind permission from Elsevier Science.

Through theoretical analysis and literature review, coupled with results from pilot studies, Waddell and colleagues (1993) concluded that the concept of fear avoidance is a significant and driving factor within the context of the biopsychosocial model of low back pain and disability. As such, the core features of the Glasgow model were recently subsumed as a part of the fear-avoidance models. The fear-avoidance literature is reviewed in more detail later.

THE BIOBEHAVIORAL MODEL

Model Summary

The first model of pain to comprehensively incorporate both cognitive and behavioral elements was proposed by Turk, Meichenbaum, and Genest (1983). The initial model was an attempt to extend the behavioral conceptualization posed by Fordyce (1976), based on the influential writings on cognitive therapy published in the latter part of the 1970s (e.g., Beck, 1976; Meichenbaum, 1977). More recently, Turk and colleagues (Turk, 2002; Turk & Flor, 1999) described the model using the term *biobehavioral*, where *bio* refers to biological factors and *behavioral* to a broad spectrum of psychological and sociocultural factors. The key elements of the model are summarized as follows:

- Some people have a diathesis, or predisposition, for a reduced threshold for nociceptive activation and a tendency to respond with fear to bodily sensations. This diathesis may result from genetic makeup, social learning, prior trauma, or some combination of each.
- Aversive stimulation, whether related to nociception or some other stressor (e.g., marital conflict, too many time demands), interacts with the diathesis.
- The diathesis–stress interaction leads to conditioned and unconditioned autonomic nervous system (comprising sympathetic and parasympathetic divisions), sensitization of central nervous system structures, and muscular responsivity, as well as avoidance behavior, when appraisals are negative and coping resources are insufficient.
- The type (i.e., the specific symptom manifestation) and persistence of the illness problem that develops are determined, in part, by the way in which one attends and responds to nociception.
- A variety of learning processes, the meaning ascribed to symptoms (through processes such as expectancies, hypervigilance, preoccupation, misinterpretations of catastrophic nature, fear), avoidance behavior, social interaction (e.g., the way in which one's significant others respond to their pain), and subsequent alterations in physiological responsivity (e.g., persistent sympathetic nervous system activation; persistent muscular reactivity) play an important role in maintenance and exacerbation of symptoms.

To summarize, the biobehavioral model suggests that chronic pain problems are the product of an *interaction* between a necessary predisposition and specific (learned) cognitive, behavioral, social, and physiological response patterns to pain sensations and other stressors as well as subsequent maladaptive responses to resulting distress. In this context, then, it is the person's anticipation of and response to distress, not nociceptive input itself, that leads some to experience chronic pain and associated disability.

Empirical Overview

Empirical studies of postulates of the biobehavioral model were recently reviewed by Turk and Flor (1999) and Turk (2002). Research in a number of areas substantiates the applicability of the biobehavioral model to the genesis, maintenance, and exacerbation of pain. With respect to the notion of diathesis, or predisposition, the presence of anxiety sensitivity (i.e., a disposition to respond with fear to somatic sensations) was suggested as a predisposing factor in chronic pain (Asmundson, 1999; Asmundson, Norton, & Norton, 1999; Muris, Vlaeyen, & Meesters, 2001). A positive association was identified between anxiety sensitivity and pain-specific anxiety, avoidance behaviors, fear of negative consequences of pain, and negative affect (Turk, 2000; also see Asmundson, 1999; Asmundson et al., 1999). In terms of the impact of learning on behavior and pain perception, memories of somatosensory pain specific to a particular pain site have been found to form as a result of chronic pain (Flor, Braun, Elbert, & Birbaumer, 1997). This formation was shown to manifest itself in an exaggerated portrayal of the affected pain site in the primary somatosensory cortex. Further, learned memory for pain was demonstrated in patients with phantom limb pain, such that the amount of reorganization in cortical structures was shown to be proportional to the magnitude of phantom leg pain (Flor et al., 1995).

Turk and Flor (1999) suggested that pain management programs that aim to facilitate a patient's ability to attribute success to his or her own volition will result in long-term behavioral changes, and these, in turn, will impact affective, cognitive, and sensory aspects of pain experience. Investigations showed that these types of treatment programs do promote changes in pain-specific beliefs, coping style, and behavior, as well as pain severity (e.g., Arnstein, Caudill, Mandle, Norris, & Beasly, 1999; Buckelew et al., 1996; Dolce, Crocker, Moletteire, & Doleys, 1986). Indeed, it was specifically demonstrated that increased perceived control over pain and decreased catastrophizing are associated with decreases in pain severity ratings, functional disability, and physiological activity (e.g., Jensen & Bodin, 1998; Jensen, Turner, & Romano, 1991; Jensen, Turner, Romano, & Karoly, 1991; Sullivan et al., 2001).

FEAR-AVOIDANCE MODELS

Model Summary

The role of fear and avoidance behavior as they relate to chronic pain have received considerable attention over the past decade (for recent reviews, see Asmundson et al., 1999; Vlaeyen & Linton, 2000). Indeed, the literature in this area has grown to the point where state-of-the-art theory and research are being published in the form of an edited book (Asmundson, Vlaeyen, & Crombez, 2003). The postulates of fear-avoidance models have their roots in early observations of significant anxiety in the pathology of pain (e.g., Paulett, 1947; Rowbotham, 1946), as well as in operant conditioning theory (Linton, Melin, & Götestam, 1984; Fordyce, 1976) and its illness behavior reformulations (Turk & Flor, 1999; Waddell et al., 1993).

Several fear-avoidance models have been proposed to account for chronic pain behavior. The fear-avoidance model of exaggerated pain perception (Lethem, Slade, Troup, & Bentley, 1983), for example, attempted to explain the process by which the emotional and sensory components of pain become desynchronous (i.e., why fear and avoidance remain while tissue damage remits) in some patients with chronic pain. Extending postulates of the operant model of chronic pain, Philips (1987) incorporated elements of the cognitive theory of avoidance (Seligman & Johnson, 1973) to explain cases where behavioral withdrawal was observed to continue in the absence of adequate reinforcement. Avoidance was viewed as a product of pain severity, a preference for minimizing discomfort, and cognitions (comprising expectancies, feelings of self-efficacy, and memories of past exposures) that reexposure to certain experiences or activities will result in pain and suffering.

Influenced by the work of Waddell et al. (1993), Letham et al. (1983), and Philips (1987), and building on their earlier work (Linton et al., 1984; Vlaeyen, Kole-Snijders, Boeren, & van Eek, 1995), Vlaeyen and Linton (2000) proposed a comprehensive fear-avoidance model of chronic musculoskeletal pain. This model, illustrated in Fig. 2.4, can be summarized as follows:

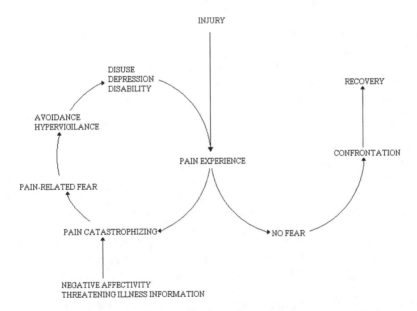

FIG. 2.4. Fear-avoidance model. Reprinted from Vlaeyen and Linton, "Fear-avoidance and its consequences in chronic musculoskeletal pain: A state of the art," p. 329. Copyright 2000. Reproduced with kind permission from the International Association for the Study of Pain, 909 NE 43rd Ave, Suite 306, Seattle, WA, USA.

- Injury initiates the experience of pain.
- If the experience is appraised as nonthreatening (e.g., viewed as a temporary hindrance that can be overcome), it is confronted and dealt with in an adaptive manner that allows the person to proceed toward recovery.
- If the experience is appraised as threatening (e.g., a catastrophic event that will never resolve), it may be dealt with in a maladaptive manner that perpetuates a vicious fear–avoidance cycle that, in turn, promotes disability.

In this context, then, confrontation is conceptualized as an adaptive response that is associated with behaviors that promote recovery. Avoidance, on the other hand, is viewed as a maladaptive response that leads to a number of undesirable consequences. These include limitations in activity, physical and psychological consequences that contribute to disability, continued nociceptive input (which, like the Glasgow model, may not necessarily be related to original injury; also see Norton & Asmundson, 2003), and further catastrophizing and fear.

Empirical Overview

Vlaeyen and Linton (2000) published a state-of-the-art review showing an ever-increasing number of findings that corroborate postulates of fear-avoidance models. Precursors of pain-related fear, including anxiety sensitivity and health anxiety (i.e., the belief that bodily signs and symptoms are indicative of serious illness), have been clearly identified. For example, in a sample of chronic musculoskeletal pain patients, Asmundson and Taylor (1996) found that anxiety sensitivity directly influences fear of pain, which, in turn, directly influences self-reported escape/avoidance behavior. These findings were replicated in adolescents (Muris et al., 2001) and adults with heterogeneous pain complaints (Zvolensky, Goodie, McNeil, Sperry, & Sorrell, 2001). There is converging evidence demonstrating that fear of pain affects the way people attend and respond to information about pain (Asmundson, Kuperos, & Norton, 1997; Eccleston & Crombez, 1999; Hadjistavropoulos, Craig, & Hadjistavropoulos, 1998; McCracken, 1997; Peters, Vlaeyen, & Kunnen, 2002; Snider, Asmundson, & Weise, 2000). Likewise, there is mounting evidence that fear of pain influences physical performance and is more strongly related to functional disability than are indices of pain severity (Crombez, Vervaet, Lysens, Baeyens, & Eelen, 1998; Crombez, Vlaeyen, Heuts, & Lysens, 1999; McCracken, Zayfert, & Gross, 1992; Vlaeyen et al., 1995; Waddell et al., 1993). Finally, at the practical level, specifically treating the "fear" component using techniques known to be effective in reducing fears (i.e., graded exposure) has been shown to be most effective in reducing avoidance behavior and associated disability in patients with chronic musculoskeletal pain (Linton, Overmeer, Janson, Vlaeyen, & de Jong, 2002; Vlaeyen, de Jong, Geilen, Heuts, & van Breukelen, 2001; Vlaeyen, de Jong, Onghena, Kerckhoffs-Hanssen, & Kole-Snidjers, 2002).

TOWARD AN INTEGRATED DIATHESIS–STRESS MODEL

Our presentation of the various faces of pain shows, to a large degree, a developmental progression from the simplistic notions of somatogenic and psychogenic causation through to the increasingly elaborate yet parsimonious postulates of the contemporary multidimensional, biopsychosocial approaches. In scanning the essential elements of the various models considered under the rubric of "biopsychosocial," certain consistencies and themes are apparent. These include recognition of the importance of (a) some physiological pathology (which may not remain the same as that associated with initial nociception), (b) some form of vulnerability (diathesis), (c) a tendency to catastrophically misinterpret somatic sensations and respond to them in maladaptive ways, and (d) the development of a self-reinforcing vicious cycle that serves to exacerbate and maintain symptoms and functional disability. Taking an approach similar to that employed by Sharp (2001) in his recent reformulation of Turk and colleagues biobehavioral model of pain (Turk, 2002; Turk & Flor, 1999; Turk et al., 1983), we propose a model that integrates empirically supported elements of the operant, Glasgow, biobehavioral, and contemporary fear-avoidance models. This integrated stress–diathesis model is illustrated in Fig. 2.5.

It is important to keep in mind that pain and pain behaviors do not occur in isolation. Rather, they are communicated in (see Hadjistavropoulos & Craig, 2002) and influenced, for better or worse, by one's social, interpersonal, and cultural milieu (e.g., Bates, Edwards, & Anderson, 1993; Craig, 1978). For example, a supportive environment can facilitate efforts to cope with pain; however, if there is not enough or, indeed, too much support (i.e., where the "supporter" is overly solicitous), the overall pain experience is likely to be aggravated. This appears to hold true for interactions with significant others as well as those responsible for medical care, litigation, and other such responses (see Sharp, 2001). Similarly, social modeling and social learning experiences influence strongly the way in which one interprets and responds to signs and symptoms of illness (e.g., Chambers, Craig, & Bennet, 2002; Craig & Prkachin, 1978; Martin, Lemos, & Leventhal, 2001). So, interpretation and behavioral responses to pain depend, to some degree, on what is learned from seeing others in pain and from cultural norms. This is recognized, to varying degrees, in all of the biopsychosocial models discussed earlier and provides the umbrella under which our model is placed.

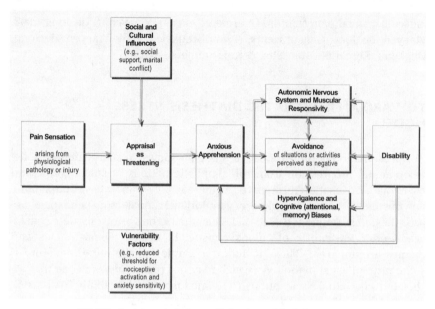

FIG. 2.5. An integrated stress–diathesis model of chronic pain.

As illustrated, our integrated diathesis–stress model recognizes the importance of physiological, psychological, and sociocultural factors in the etiology, exacerbation, and maintenance of chronic pain. Interactions between various factors are clearly indicated and, importantly, can lead to a vicious, self-reinforcing cycle that influences and is influenced by distress and functional disability. An initial physical pathology or injury is recognized as necessary to nociception and the appraisal that set the cycle in motion. Also necessary is a predispositional vulnerability factor (diathesis). The difference between those who become distressed and disabled (like Kelly) and those who don't (like Jamie) is presumed to lie in the manner in which nociception is appraised and responded to. Those with a predisposition that reduces threshold for nociceptive activation and increases the tendency to respond with fear to bodily sensations (i.e., anxiety sensitivity, illness sensitivity) are more likely to respond to pain sensations with anxious apprehension (i.e., a future-oriented *preparedness* to cope with upcoming negative events or experiences). In turn, they develop cognitive and behavioral repertoires that serve to maintain this preparedness. Also, physiological stimulation shifts from nociceptive input of the precipitating pathology or injury to that stemming from autonomic nervous system and muscular activation. Learning processes contribute not only to the maintenance of the vicious cycle, but to anxious anticipation regarding events only remotely associated with pain-specific distress and disability. Thus, a general sense of perceived readiness for and inability to influence personally relevant events and outcomes develops. Those without the necessary predisposition appraise their pain sensation as nonthreatening, do not respond with maladaptive cognitive or behavioral repertoires, and in most cases recover.

CONCLUSIONS

The primary intent of this chapter was to provide an overview of the various expressions of pain that have been prominent over the years in addressing the enduring questions of "What is pain?" and "How can we alleviate it?" Early models, whether physiological or psychological in focus, were based on a unidimensional conceptualization. Subsequent to the seminal contributions of Melzack and colleagues (Melzack & Casey, 1968; Melzack & Wall, 1965), models moved toward a multidimensional conceptualization, recognizing a complex interplay between physiological, psychological, and sociocultural mechanisms in the pain experience. Today there are a number of heuristic biopsychosocial models, each holding (sometimes overlapping) implications for understanding, assessing, and treating pain that persists in the absence of identifiable physical pathology.

We have presented an integrated diathesis–stress model of chronic pain founded, in part, on empirical support garnered from tests of other models, in an attempt to emphasize the importance of interplay between biology, cognition, affect, and social factors, as well as the key role of learning and associated self-reinforcing feedback loops. In this context it should be clear that simplistic notions of somatogenesis and psychogenesis are obsolete. Our model, like its predecessors, yields a number of questions that, should they be answered systematically, will serve to guide further advances in both pain assessment and intervention strategies. What is the precise nature of the diathesis? Is it genetic or learned? Can it be modified? To what extend does anxious apprehension for pain-specific events and experiences generalize to other sectors of a person's life? Can we apply the models in a way that allows identification of vulnerable or at-risk people prior to development of chronic pain and associated disability? In other words, is prevention feasible? In what ways do physiological reactivity serve to perpetuate the cycle? What is the best method of intervention for those who become mired in the vicious cycle? Graded in vivo exposure appears to have great potential, but is there more to learn from the effective interventions of fundamental fears? How do we best address the influence of social influences in the context of intervention? These are but a few of the questions that await further investigation.

REFERENCES

Adler, R. H., Zlot, S., Hürny, C., & Minder, C. (1989). Engel's "Psychogenic pain and the pain-prone patient": A retrospective, controlled clinical study. *Psychosomatic Medicine, 51*, 87–101.

Arnstein, P., Caudill, M., Mandle, C., Norris, A., & Beasly, R. (1999). Self efficacy as a mediator of the relationship between pain intensity, disability and depression in chronic pain patients. *Pain, 80*, 483–491.

Asmundson, G. J. G. (1999). Anxiety sensitivity and chronic pain: Empirical findings, clinical implications, and future directions. In S. Taylor (Ed.), *Anxiety sensitivity: Theory, research and treatment of the Fear of Anxiety* (pp. 269–285). Mahwah, NJ: Lawrence Erlbaum Associates.

Asmundson, G. J. G., Jacobson, S. J., Allerdings, M. D., & Norton, G. R. (1996). Social phobia in disabled workers with chronic musculoskeletal pain. *Behaviour Research and Therapy, 34*, 939–943.

Asmundson, G. J. G., Kuperos, J. L., & Norton, G. R. (1997). Do patients with chronic pain selectively attend to pain-related information?: Preliminary evidence for mediating role of fear. *Pain, 72*, 27–32.

Asmundson, G. J. G., Norton, P. J., & Norton, G. R. (1999). Beyond pain: The role of fear and avoidance in chronicity. *Clincial Psychology Review, 19*, 97–119.

Asmundson, G. J. G., & Taylor, S. (1996). Role of anxiety sensitivity in pain-related fear and avoidance. *Journal of Behavioral Medicine, 19*, 577–586.

Asmundson, G. J. G., Vlaeyen, J. W. S., & Crombez, G. (2003). *Understanding and treating fear of pain*. New York: Oxford University Press.

Asmundson, G. J. G., Wright, K. D., & Hadjistavropoulos, H. D. (2000). Anxiety sensitivity and disabling chronic health conditions: State of the art and future directions. *Scandinavian Journal of Behaviour Therapy, 29*, 100–117.

Bates, M., Edwards, W., & Anderson, K. (1993). Ethnocultural influences on variation in chronic pain perception. *Pain, 52*, 101–112.

Beck, A. (1976). *Cognitive therapy and emotional disorders*. New York: International University Press.

Block, A., Kremer, E., & Gaylor, M. (1980). Behavioral treatment of chronic pain: The spouse as a discriminitive cue for pain behavior. *Pain, 9*, 243–252.

Blumer, D., & Heilbronn, M. (1982). Chronic pain as a variant of depressive disease: The pain-prone disorder. *Journal of Nervous and Mental Disease, 170*, 381–406.

Bonica, J. J. (1954). *The management of pain*. Philadelphia: Lea & Febiger.

Bonica, J. J. (1990). *The management of pain* (2nd ed.). Philadelphia: Lea & Febiger.

Breuer, J., & Freud, S. (1957). *Studies on hysteria* (J. Strachey, Ed. and Trans.). New York: Basic Books. (Original work published 1893–1895)

Buckelew, S. P., Huyser, B., Hewett, J. E., Parker, J. C., Johnson, J. C., Conway, R., & Kay, D. (1996). Self-efficacy predicting outcome among fibromyalgia subjects. *Arthritis Care and Research, 9*, 97–104.

Cairns, D., & Pasino, J. (1977). Comparison of verbal reinforcement and feedback in the operant treatment of disability due to chronic low back pain. *Behavior Therapy, 8*, 621–630.

Chambers, C. T., Craig, K. D., & Bennett, S. M. (2002). The impact of maternal behavior on children's pain experiences: An experimental analysis. *Journal of Pediatric Psychology, 27*, 293–301.

Craig, K. (1978). Social modeling influences on pain. In R. Sternback (Ed.), *The psychology of pain* (pp. 67–95). New York: Raven Press.

Craig, K. D. (1984). Emotional aspects of pain. In P. D. Wall & R. Melzack (Eds.), *Textbook of pain* (pp. 261–274). Edinburgh: Churchill-Livingston.

Craig, K. D., & Prkachin, K. M. (1978). Social modeling influences on sensory decision theory and psychophysiological indexes of pain. *Journal of Personality and Social Psychology, 36*, 805–815.

Crombez, G., Vervaet, L., Lysens, R., Baeyens, F., & Eelen, P. (1998). Avoidance and confrontation of painful, back straining movements in chronic back pain patients. *Behavior Modification, 22,* 62–77.

Crombez, G., Vlaeyen, J. W. S., Heuts, P. H. T. G., & Lysens, R. (1999). Fear of pain is more disabling than pain itself. Evidence on the role of pain-related fear in chronic back pain disability. *Pain, 80,* 329–339.

Dersh, J., Gatchel, R. J., Polatin, P., & Mayer, T. (2002). Prevalence of psychiatric disorders in patients with chronic work-related musculoskeletal pain disability. *Journal of Occupational and Environmental Medicine, 44,* 459–468.

Dolce, J. J., Crocker, M. F., Moletteire, C., & Doleys, D. M. (1986). Exercise, quotas, anticipatory concern and self efficacy expectancies in chronic pain: A preliminary report. *Pain, 24,* 365–372.

Eccleston, C., & Crombez, G. (1999). Pain demands attention: A cognitive-affective model of the interruptive function of pain. *Psychological Bulletin, 125,* 209–215.

Engel, G. L. (1959). "Psychogenic" pain and pain-prone patient. *American Journal of Medicine, 26,* 899–918.

Engel, G. L. (1977). The need for a new medical model: A challenge for biomedicine. *Science, 196,* 129–135.

Flor, H., Braun, C., Elbert, T., & Birbaumer, N. (1997). Extensive reorganization of primary somatosensory cortex in chronic back pain patients. *Neuroscience Letters, 224,* 5–8.

Flor, H., Elbert, T., Wienbruch, C., Pantev, C., Knecht, S., Birbaumer, N., Larbig, W., & Taub, E. (1995). Phantom limb pain as a perceptual correlate of cortical reorganization. *Nature, 357,* 482–484.

Flor, H., Knost, B., & Birbaumer, N. (2002). The role of operant conditioning in chronic pain: An experimental investigation. *Pain, 95,* 111–118.

Fordyce, W. E. (1976). *Behavioural methods for chronic pain and illness.* St. Louis, MO: C. V. Mosby.

Fordyce, W. E., Shelton, J. L., & Dundore, D. E. (1982). The modification of avoidance learning pain behaviours. *Journal of Behavioural Medicine, 5,* 405–414.

Gamsa, A. (1994). The role of psychological factors in chronic pain. I. A half century of study. *Pain, 57,* 5–15.

Hadjistavropoulos, H. D., Craig, K. D., & Hadjistavropoulos, T. (1998). Cognitive and behavioral responses to illness information: The role of health anxiety. *Behavioural Research and Therapy, 36,* 149–164.

Hadjistavropoulos, T., & Craig, K. D. (2002). A theoretical framework for understanding self-report and observational measures of pain: A communications model. *Behaviour Research and Therapy, 40,* 551–570.

Hardy, J. D., Wollf, H. G., & Goodell, H. (1952). *Pain sensations and reactions.* Baltimore, MD: Williams & Wilkins.

Jensen, I. B., & Bodin, L. (1998). Multimodal cognitive-behavioural treatment for workers with chronic spinal pain: A matched cohort study with an 18-month follow-up. *Pain, 76,* 35–44.

Jensen, M. P., Turner, J. A., & Romano, J. M. (1991). Self-efficacy and outcome expectancies: Relationship to chronic pain coping strategies and adjustment. *Pain, 44,* 263–269.

Jensen, M. P., Turner, J. A., Romano, J. M., & Karoly, P. (1991). Coping with chronic pain: A critical review of the literature. *Pain, 47,* 249–283.

Katon, W., Egan, K., & Miller, D. (1985). Chronic pain: Lifetime psychiatric diagnoses and family history. *American Journal of Psychiatry, 142,* 1156–1160.

Large, R. (1986). DSM–III diagnosis in chronic pain. Confusion or clarity? *Journal of Nervous and Mental Disease, 174,* 295–303.

Lethem, J., Slade, P. D., Troup, J. D. G., & Bentley, G. (1983). Outline of a fear-avoidance model of exaggerated pain perception—I. *Behaviour Research and Therapy, 21,* 401–408.

Linton, S. J., & Götestam, K. G. (1985). Controlling pain reports through operant conditioning: A laboratory demonstration. *Perceptual and Motor Skills, 60,* 427–437.

Linton, S. J., Melin, L., & Götestam, K. G. (1984). *Behavioral analysis of chronic pain and its management* (Progress in behavior modification, Vol. 18). New York: Academic Press.

Linton, S. J., Overmeer, T., Janson, M., Vlaeyen, J. W. S., & de Jong, J. R. (2002). Graded in-vivo exposure treatment for fear-avoidant pain patients with functional disability: A case study. *Cognitive Behavior Therapy, 31,* 49–58.

Lipowski, Z. J. (1983). Psychosocial reactions to physical illness. *Canadian Medical Association Journal, 128,* 1069–1072.

Lousberg, R., Groenman, N. H., Schmidt, A. J., & Gielen, A. A. (1996). Operant conditioning of the pain experiences. *Perceptual and Motor Skills, 83,* 883–900.

Martin, R., Lemos, K., & Leventhal, H. (2001). The psychology of physical symptoms and illness behavior. In G. J. G. Asmundson, S. Taylor, & B. J. Cox (Eds.), *Health Anxiety: Clinical and research perspectives on hypochondriasis and related disorders* (pp. 23–45). London: Wiley.

McCracken, L. M. (1997). "Attention" to pain in persons with chronic pain. A behavioral approach. *Behavior Therapy, 28,* 271–284.

McCracken, L. M., Zayfert, C., & Gross, R. T. (1992). The pain anxiety symptoms scale: Development and validation of a scale to measure fear of pain. *Pain, 50,* 67–73.

Mechanic, D. (1962). The concept of illness behavior. *Journal of Chronic Disease, 15,* 189–194.

Meichenbaum, D. (1977). *Cognitive behavior modification: An integrative approach.* New York: Plenum.

Melzack, R. (1999). From the gate to the neuromatrix. *Pain, Suppl 6,* S121–S126.

Melzack, R., & Casey, K. L. (1968). Sensory, motivational, and central control determinants of pain. A new conceptual model. In D. R. Kenshalo (Ed.), *The skin senses* (pp. 423–443). Springfield, IL: Charles C. Thomas.

Melzack, R., & Wall, P. D. (1965). Pain mechanisms. *Science, 150,* 971–979.

Melzack, R., & Wall, P. D. (1982). *The challenge of pain.* New York: Basic Books.

Merskey, H., & Spear, F. D. (1967). The concept of pain. *Journal of Psychosomatic Research, 11,* 59–67.

Morley, S., Eccleston, C., & Williams, A. (1999). A systematic review and meta-analysis of randomized controlled trials of cognitive-behaviour therapy and behaviour therapy for chronic pain in adults, excluding headaches. *Pain, 80,* 1–13.

Muris, P., Vlaeyen, J., & Meesters, C. (2001). The relationship between anxiety sensitivity and fear of pain in healthy adolescents. *Behavior Research and Therapy, 39,* 1357–1368.

Norton, G. R., & Asmundson, G. J. G. (2003). Physiological arousal in fear-avoidance models of chronic pain. *Behavior Therapy, 34,* 17–30.

Parsons, T. (1951). Illness and the role of the physician: A sociological perspective. *American Journal of Orthopsychiatry, 21,* 452–460.

Paulett, J. D. (1947). Low back pain. *Lancet, 253,* 272–276.

Peters, M. L., Vlaeyen, J. W. S., & Kunnen, A. M. W. (2002). Is pain-related fear a predictor of somatosensory hypervigilance in chronic low back pain patients? *Behaviour Research and Therapy, 40,* 85–103.

Philips, H. C. (1987). Avoidance behaviour and its role in sustaining chronic pain. *Behaviour Research and Therapy, 25,* 273–279.

Price, D. D. (2000). Psychological and neural mechanisms of the affective dimension of pain. *Science, 288,* 1769–1772.

Robinson, M. E., & Riley, J. L. III. (1999). Models of pain. In A. R. Block, E. F. Kremer, & E. Fernandez (Eds.), *Handbook of pain syndromes: Biopsychosocial perspectives* (pp. 23–40). Mahwah, NJ: Lawrence Erlbaum Associates.

Roth, R. (2000). Psychogenic models of chronic pain. A selective review and critique. In M. Massie (Ed.), *Psychogenic models of chronic pain* (pp. 89–131). Washington, DC: American Psychiatric Press.

Rowbotham, G. F. (1946). Pain and its underlying pathology. *Journal of Mental Science, 92,* 595–604.

Roy, R. (1985). Engel's pain-prone disorder patient: 25 Years after. *Psychotherapy and Psychosomatics, 43*, 126–135.

Seligman, M., & Johnson, J. C. (1973). A cognitive theory of avoidance learning. In F. J. McGuigan & D. B. Lumsden (Eds.), *Contemporary approaches to conditioning and learning* (pp. 69–110). New York: Wiley.

Sharp, T. J. (2001). Chronic pain: A reformulation of the cognitive-behavioural model. *Behaviour Research and Therapy, 39*, 787–800.

Snider, B., Asmundson, G. J. G., & Weise, K. (2000). Automatic and strategic processing of threat cues in patients with chronic pain: A modified Stroop evaluation. *Clinical Journal of Pain, 16*, 144–154.

Sullivan, M. J. L., Thorn, B., Haythornthwaite, J. A., Keefe, F., Martin, M., Bradley, L. A., & Lefebre, J. C. (2001). Theoretical perspectives on the relation between catastrophizing and pain. *Clinical Journal of Pain, 17*, 52–64.

Turk, D. C. (1996a). Biopsychosocial perspective on chronic pain. In R. J. Gatchel & D. C. Turk (Eds.), *Psychological approaches to pain management* (pp. 3–32). New York: Guilford Press.

Turk, D. C. (1996b). Cognitive factors in chronic pain and disability. In K. Dobson & K. Craig (Eds.), *Advances in cognitive-behavioral therapy* (pp. 83–115). Newbury Park, CA: Sage.

Turk, D. C. (2002). A diathesis-stress model of chronic pain and disability following traumatic injury. *Pain Research and Management, 7*, 9–19.

Turk, D. C., & Flor, H. (1999). The Biobehavioral perspective of pain. In R. J. Gatchel & D. C. Turk (Eds.), *Psychosocial factors in pain. Clinical perspectives* (pp. 18–34). New York: Guilford Press.

Turk, D. C., Meichenbaum, D., & Genest, M. (1983). *Pain and behavioral medicine: A cognitive-behavioral perspective.* New York: Guilford Press.

Vlaeyen, J. W. S., de Jong, J., Geilen, M., Heuts, P. H. T. G., & van Breukelen, G. (2001). Graded exposure in vivo in the treatment of pain-related fear: A replicated single-case experimental design in four patients with chronic low back pain. *Behaviour Research and Therapy, 39*, 151–156.

Vlaeyen, J. W. S., de Jong, J., Onghena, P., Kerckhoffs-Hanssen, M., & Kole-Snijders, A. M. J. (2002). Can pain-related fear be reduced? The application of cognitive-behavioural exposure in vivo. *Pain Research and Management, 7*, 144–153.

Vlaeyen, J. W. S., Kole-Snijders, A. M. J., Boerem, R. G. B., & van Eek, H. (1995). Fear of movement/(re)injury in chronic low back pain and its relation to behavioral performance. *Pain, 62*, 363–372.

Vlaeyen, J. W. S., & Linton, S. J. (2000). Fear-avoidance and its consequences in chronic musculoskeletal pain: A state of the art. *Pain, 85*, 317–332.

Waddell, G. (1987). A new clinical model for the treatment of low back pain. *Spine, 12*, 632–644.

Waddell, G. (1991). Low back disability. A syndrome of Western civilization. *Neurosurgery Clinics of North America, 2*, 719–738.

Waddell, G. (1992). Biopsychosocial analysis of low back pain. *Clinical Rheumatology, 6*, 523–557.

Waddell, G., Main, C. J., Morris, E. W., Di Paola, M. P., & Gray, I. C. M. (1984). Chronic low back pain, psychological distress, and illness behavior. *Spine, 9*, 209–213.

Waddell, G., Newton, M., Henderson, I., Somerville, D., & Main, C. J. (1993). A Fear-Avoidance Beliefs Questionnaire (FABQ) and the role of fear-avoidance in chronic low back pain and disability. *Pain, 52*, 157–168.

Waddell, G., Somerville, D., Henderson, I., & Newton, M. (1992). Objective clinical evaluation of physical impairment in chronic low back pain. *Spine, 17*, 617–628.

Wall, P. D. (1996). Comments after 30 years of the gate control theory of pain. *Pain Forum, 5*, 12–22.

Zvolensky, M. J., Goodie, J. L., McNeil, D. W., Sperry, J. A., & Sorrell, J. T. (2001). Anxiety sensitivity in the prediction of pain-related fear and anxiety in a heterogeneous chronic pain population. *Behaviour Research and Therapy, 39*, 683–696.

3

Pain Perception, Affective Mechanisms, and Conscious Experience

C. Richard Chapman
Pain Research Center,
Department of Anesthesiology,
University of Utah

Pain has afflicted humankind since the dawn of human self-awareness, yet we are still struggling to understand its nature. Young physicians in training, whose job it will be to prevent or relieve pain in myriad medical settings, listen to instructors who teach about pain receptors, pain pathways, and mechanisms that gate pain at the dorsal horn of the spinal cord. Continuing medical education efforts sustain and enhance the same message, implying that pain is a primitive sensory signal. Specific sensory end organs transduce injury and transmit "pain," and along the pathway from the periphery to the brain, descending modulatory pathways gate this transmission. Curiously, these same lecturers and teachers are quick to agree that pain is subjective and that it exists only in the brain and when the perceiver is conscious. They point out that they merely equate nociception, the transduction and signal transmission of tissue injury, with pain itself. Surely, they reason, when injury occurs, some message of tissue trauma moves from the periphery to the somatosensory cortex, and when that message reaches the somatosensory cortex, something "realizes" it and pain happens. They further reason that, because pain is intrinsically unpleasant, it causes negative emotional responses that we recognize as emotional reactions to pain.

I emphasize this to point out that a large gap exists between what science now knows about pain and what we understand in day-to-day life, apply in medical practice, and teach future health care providers. Current evidence makes it clear that nociception and pain are far from synonyms. Pain is conscious; nociception is not. Pain can exist in the absence of nociception, and nociception can take place without pain. Importantly, pain has emotional features and nociception does not.

Although nociception can occur in an unconscious individual, pain cannot. Like other phenomena of consciousness, pain is an emergent product of complex, distributed activity within the brain. It is not a signal that "enters" consciousness, but rather an aspect of the moment-to-moment construction of consciousness, which comprises awareness of both the external and internal, or somatic, environment. Put succinctly, pain is a complex, consciousness-dependent, unpleasant somatic experience with cognitive and emotional as well as sensory features.

Pain does not occur alone but rather against a background of complex bodily awareness. We experience a range of somatic perceptions that signal ill-being (e.g., nausea, fatigue, vertigo) as opposed to well-being, and pain is one of these. Pain is the somatic perception of tissue damage; it entails sensory awareness, negative emotional arousal (threat), and cognition (attention, appraisal, attribution, and more). Persons in pain become emotional, not because reactions occur when the sensory message reaches the somatosensory cortex, but because nociception triggers multiple limbic processes in parallel with central sensory processes.

These considerations indicate that pain is inherently psychological in nature; it is not a primitive sensory message of tissue trauma. One can pursue its mechanisms reductionistically, focusing on neuron, neurotransmitter, or even calcium channel, but at the end of the day, human pain is always a complex psychological experience. It follows that the prevention and control of pain are inherently psychological maneuvers.

This chapter begins by reviewing some historical lines of thought that have shaped today's beliefs about pain. I then define and consider the nature of emotion and cognition, as they apply to pain as a psychological experience. Turning to the limbic brain, I introduce the concept of nociception-driven emotion, describe the central neuroanatomy of such emotion, and review literature that reveals the mechanisms by which nociception triggers central mechanisms for negative feeling. This includes functional brain imaging studies of patients and volunteers in pain. Finally, I briefly describe the potential relationship of nociception and pain to stress and sickness. A concluding section considers the clinical implications of a psychological view of pain.

THE MIND–BODY PROBLEM

Our current understanding of the relationship between mental processes and the body stems directly from Descartes' notions of mind–body dualism. Descartes, a 17th-century philosopher and mathematician, viewed human beings as dualistic creatures: The mind and body are separate entities (Descartes, 1649/1967). The immaterial soul, he reasoned, must reside in the pineal body because this is the only unpaired organ in the brain. He described the life processes of the body itself as something akin to clockwork mechanisms. The actions of the mind were, in Cartesian thinking, the workings of the soul.

Descartes held that the awareness of pain, like awareness of other bodily sensations, must take place in a special location where the mind observes the body. Dennett (1991) termed this hypothetical seat of the mind the *Cartesian theater*. In this theater, the mind observes and interprets the constantly changing array of multimodality signals that the body produces. The body is a passive environment; the mind is the nonphysical activity of the soul.

Today, most scholars avow that a theater of the mind cannot exist. Scientifically, the activity of the brain and the mind are inseparable. Nonetheless, Cartesian dualism is endemic in Western thought and culture. Classical approaches to emotion and pain stemmed from Cartesian thinking, as did psychophysics. Early work on psychosomatic disorders focused on mind–body relationships. Today, much of the popular movement favoring alternative medicine emphasizes "the mind–body connection," keeping oneself healthy through right thinking, and the power of the mind to control the immune system. It is hard to avoid Cartesian thinking when the very fabric of our language threads it through our thinking as we reason and speak.

Cartesian assumptions erect a subtle but powerful barrier for someone seeking to understand the affective dimension of pain. Relegating emotions to the realm of the mind and their physiological consequences to the body is classical Descartes. It prevents us from appreciating the intricate interdependence of subjective feelings and physiology, and it detracts from our ability to comprehend how the efferent properties of autonomic nervous function can contribute causally to the realization of an emotional state. Mental processes and physiology are interdependent. What we call the mind is consciousness, and consciousness is an emergent property of the activity of the brain. In a feedback-dependent manner, the brain regulates the physiological arousal of the body, and emotion is a part of this process.

PAIN AS EMOTION

What Is Emotion?

Descartes (1649) introduced the term *emotion* in his essay on "Passion of the Soul." It allowed him to distinguish specific bodily sensations from more complex feeling states such as fear, hate, and joy. Understanding pain as an emotion must begin with an appreciation for the origins and purposes of emotion.

Many physicians who treat pain problems regard emotions as epiphenomenal feeling states associated with mental activity, subjective in character, and largely irrelevant to the state of a patient's physical health and functional capability. In fact, emotions are primarily physiological and only secondarily subjective. To the extent that they are subjective, we experience them in terms of bodily awareness and judge the events that provoke them as good or bad according to how our bodies feel. Because they can strongly affect cardiovascular function, visceral motility, and genitourinary function, emotions can have an important role in health overall and especially in pain management. Simple negative emotional arousal can exacerbate certain pain states such as sympathetically maintained pain, angina, and tension headache. It contributes significantly to musculoskeletal pain, pelvic pain, and other pain problems in some patients.

Emotions are complex states of physiological arousal and awareness that impute positive or negative hedonic qualities to a stimulus (event) in the internal or external environment. Behaviorally, they serve as action dispositions. A rich and complex literature exists on the nature of emotion, with many competing perspectives. I cannot cover it here and instead offer what is necessarily an overly simplistic summary of the field, as I think it should apply to pain research and theory.

One objective aspect of emotion is autonomically and hormonally mediated physiological arousal. Another objective aspect is behavioral, as defined by observation. The subjective aspects of emotion, "feelings," are phenomena of consciousness. Emotion represents in consciousness the biological importance or meaning of an event to the perceiver.

Emotion as a whole has two defining features: valence and arousal. *Valence* refers to the hedonic quality associated with an emotion: the positive or negative feeling attached to perception. *Arousal* refers to the degree of heightened activity in the central nervous system and autonomic nervous system associated with perception.

Although emotions as a whole can be either positive or negative in valence, pain research addresses only negative emotion. Viewed as an emotion, pain represents threat to the biological, psychological, or social integrity of the person. In this respect, the emotional aspect of pain is a protective response that normally contributes to adaptation and survival. If uncontrolled or poorly managed in patients with severe or prolonged pain, it produces suffering.

Emotion and Evolution

There are many frameworks for studying the psychology of emotion. I favor a sociobiological (evolutionary) framework because this way of thinking construes feeling states, related physiology, and behavior as mechanisms of adaptation and survival. Nature has equipped us with the capability for negative emotion for a purpose; bad feelings are not simply accidents of human consciousness. They are protective mechanisms that normally serve us well, but, like uncontrolled pain, sustained and uncontrolled negative emotions can become pathological states that can produce both maladaptive behavior and physiological pathology.

By exploring the emotional dimension of pain from the sociobiological perspective, the reader may gain some insight about how to prevent or control the negative affective aspect of pain, which fosters suffering. Unfortunately, implementing this perspective requires that we change conventional language habits that involve describing pain as a transient sensory event. I suggest the following: *Pain is a compelling and emotionally negative state of the individual that has as its primary defining feature awareness of, and homeostatic adjustment to, tissue trauma.*

Emotions including the emotional dimension of pain characterize mammals exclusively, and they foster mammalian adaptation by making possible complex behaviors and adaptations. Importantly, they play a strong role in consciousness and serve the function of producing and summarizing information that is important for selection among alternative behaviors. According to MacLean (1990), emotions "impart subjective information that is instrumental in guiding behavior required for self-preservation and preservation of the species." The subjective awareness that is an affect consists of a sense of bodily pervasiveness or of *feelings localized to certain parts of the body.* Because negative emotion such as fear evolved to facilitate adaptation and survival, emotion plays an important defensive role. The ability to experience threat when encountering injurious events protects against life-threatening injury.

Cognition and Emotion

The strength of emotional arousal associated with an injury indicates, and expresses, the magnitude of perceived threat to the biological integrity of the person. Within the contents of consciousness, threat is a strong negative feeling state and not a pure informational appraisal. In humans, threatening events such as injury that are not immediately present can exist as emotionally colored somatosensory images.

Phenomenal awareness consists largely of the production of images. Visual images are familiar to everyone: We can readily imagine seeing things. We can also produce auditory images by imaging a familiar tune or taste images by imaging sucking a lemon or tasting a familiar drink or food. Similarly, we can generate somatosensory images. Everyone can, for example, imagine the feeling of a full bladder, the sensation of a particular shoe on a foot, or a familiar muscle tension or a familiar ache. Interpretation of images often takes the form of self-talk, which employs language. The use of language allows the individual to quickly communicate private experience to others. Apart from language and self-talk, cognition operates largely on images.

Patients can react emotionally to the mental image of a painful event before it happens (e.g., venipuncture), or for that matter they can respond emotionally to the sight of another person's tissue trauma. The emotional intensity of such a feeling marks the adaptive significance of the event that produced the experience for the perceiver. In general, the threat of a minor injury normally provokes less feeling than one that incurs a risk of death. The emotional magnitude of a pain is the internal representation of the threat associated with the event that produced the pain.

At more abstract levels, patients make meaning of tissue injury or painful events of any sort by interpreting them in a broader context. This process is unique to the individual, although culture can shape the process. In some cases, the meaning that the patient creates for an event can itself become a stimulus for negative emotion, and this can interact with, and amplify, the affective component of the pain. For example, consider two hypothetical young women who suffer identical injuries. The first woman, who works as a fashion model, expresses great anguish immediately after an injury that may leave a scar. Another young woman, whose passion is riding a trail bike on rocky mountainsides, expresses much less anguish. She commonly suffers falls that lead to injuries and scars, which she regards without concern. The scar that will follow the tissue trauma is a threat to one, but not to the other, and the threat that the first woman experiences combines additively with the emotional arousal inherent in the pain itself. She will experience more pain and express more anguish than the first because a secondary factor amplifies the affective dimension of her pain. This illustrates a basic psychological principle: Emotion and cognition are interdependent determinants of behavior and subjective well-being.

THE LIMBIC BRAIN AND MECHANISMS OF EMOTION

The limbic brain represents an anatomical common denominator across mammalian species (MacLean, 1990), and emotion is a common feature of mammals. Consequently, investigators can learn much about human emotion by studying mammalian laboratory animals. The limbic brain is very complex, and it is the central mechanism of emotion.

Early investigators focused on the role of olfaction in limbic function, and this led them to link the limbic brain to emotion. Emotion may have evolutionary roots in olfactory perception. MacLean introduced the somewhat controversial term "limbic system" and characterized its functions (MacLean, 1952). He identified three main subdivisions of the limbic brain: amygdala, septum and thalamocingulate (MacLean, 1990) that represent sources of afferents to parts of limbic cortex (see Fig. 3.1). MacLean postulated that the limbic brain responds to two basic types of input: interoceptive and exteroceptive. These refer to sensory information from internal and external environments, respectively. Because nociception by definition involves signals of tissue trauma, it excites the limbic brain via interoceptive signaling.

Pain research has yet to address the links between nociception and limbic processing definitively. However, anecdotal medical evidence implicates limbic structures in the distress that characterizes the experience of pain. Radical frontal lobotomies, once performed on patients for psychosurgical purposes, typically interrupted pathways projecting from hypothalamus to cingulate cortex and putatively relieved the suffering of intractable pain without destroying sensory awareness (Fulton, 1951). Such neurosurgical records help clarify recent positron emission tomographic observations of human subjects undergoing painful cutaneous heat stimulation: Noxious stimulation activates contralateral cingulate cortex and sev-

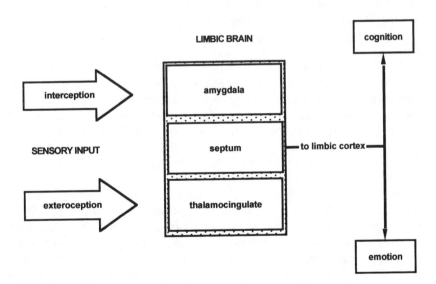

FIG. 3.1.   Three divisions of the limbic brain, according to MacLean (1990). The amygdalal and septal divisions are phylogenetically older than the thalamocingulate division. The amygdalar division contributes to self-preservation (feeding, attack, defense). The septal division is concerned with sexual behavior and procreation. The thalamocingulate division contributes to sexual and family-related behaviors, including nurturance, autonomic arousal, and probably some cognitive processes such as attention.

eral other limbic areas. Later, I describe progress in functional brain imaging research on pain that further elucidates the relationship of limbic activity to pain.

The Autonomic Nervous System and Emotion

The autonomic nervous system (ANS) plays an important role in regulating the constancy of the internal environment, and it does so in a feedback-regulated manner under the direction of the hypothalamus, the solitary nucleus, the amygdala, and other central nervous system structures (LeDoux, 1986, 1996). In general, it regulates activities that are not normally under voluntary control. The hypothalamus is the principal integrator of autonomic activity. Stimulation of the hypothalamus elicits highly integrated patterns of response that involve the limbic system and other structures (Morgane, 1981).

Many researchers hold that the ANS comprises three divisions, the sympathetic, the parasympathetic, and the enteric (Burnstock & Hoyle, 1992; Dodd & Role, 1991). Others subsume the enteric under the other two divisions. Broadly, the sympathetic nervous system makes possible the arousal needed for fight and flight reactions, whereas the parasympathetic system governs basal heart rate, metabolism, and respiration. The enteric nervous system innervates the viscera via a complex network of interconnected plexuses.

The sympathetic and parasympathetic systems are largely mutual physiological antagonists—if one system inhibits a function, the other typically augments it. There are, however, important exceptions to this rule that demonstrate complementary or integratory relationships. The mechanism most heavily involved in the affective response to tissue trauma is the sympathetic nervous system.

During emergency or injury to the body, the hypothalamus uses the sympathetic nervous system to increase cardiac output, respiration rate, and blood glucose. It also regulates body temperature, causes piloerection, alters muscle tone, provides compensatory responses to hemorrhage, and dilates pupils. These responses are part of a coordinated, well-orchestrated response pattern called the defense response (Cannon, 1929; Sokolov, 1963, 1990). It resembles the better known orienting response in some respects, but it can only occur following a strong stimulus that is noxious or frankly painful. It sets the stage for escape or confrontation, thus serving to protect the organism from danger. In a conscious cat, both electrical stimulation of the hypothalamus and infusion of norepinephrine into the hypothalamus elicit a rage reaction with hissing, snarling, and attack posture with claw exposure, and a pattern of sympathetic nervous system arousal accompanies this (Barrett, Shaikh, Edinger, & Siegel, 1987; Hess, 1936; Hilton, 1966). Circulating epinephrine produced by the adrenal medulla during activation of the hypothalamo-pituitary-adrenocortical axis accentuates the defense response, fear responses, and aversive emotional arousal in general.

Because the defense response and related changes are involuntary in nature, we generally perceive them as something that the environment does to us. We generally describe such physiological changes, not as the bodily responses that they are, but rather as feelings. We might describe a threatening and physiologically arousing event by saying that "It scared me" or that "It made me really mad."

Phenomenologically, feelings seem to happen to us; we do not "do" them in the sense that we think thoughts or choose actions. They are not volitional. Emotions are who we are in a given circumstance rather than choices we make, and we commonly interpret events and circumstances in terms of the emotions that they elicit. ANS arousal, therefore, plays a major role in the complex psychological experience of injury and is a part of that experience.

Early views of the ANS followed the lead of Cannon (1929) and held that emergency responses and all forms of intense aversive arousal are undifferentiated, diffuse patterns of sympathetic activation. Although this is broadly true, research has shown that definable patterns characterize emotional arousal, and that these are related to the emotion involved, the motor activity required, and perhaps the context (LeDoux, 1986, 1996). An investigator attempting to understand how humans experience emotions must remember that the brain not only recognizes patterns of arousal; it also creates them.

One of the primary mechanisms in the creation of emotion is feedback-dependent sympathetic efferent activation. The ANS has both afferent and efferent functions. The afferent mechanisms signal changes in the viscera and other organs, whereas efferent activity conveys commands to those organs. Consequently, the ANS can maintain feedback loops related to viscera, muscle, blood flow, and other responses. The visceral feedback system exemplifies this process. In addition, feedback can occur via the endocrine system, which under the control of the ANS releases neurohormones into the systemic circulation. Because feedback involves both autonomic afferents and endocrine responses, and because some feedback occurs at the level of unconscious homeostatic balance and other feedback involves awareness, the issue of how visceral change contributes to the creation of an emotional state is complex. The mechanisms are almost certainly pattern dependent, dynamical, and at least partly specific to the emotion involved. Moreover, they occur in parallel with sensory information processing.

The feedback concept is central to emotion research: Awareness of physiological changes elicited by a stimulus is a primary mechanism of emotion. The psychiatric patient presenting with panic attack, phobia, or anxiety is reporting a subjective state based on patterns of physiological signals and not an existential crisis that exists somewhere in the domain of the mind, somehow apart from the body. Similarly, the medical patient expressing emotional distress during a painful procedure, or during uncontrolled postoperative pain, is experiencing the sensory features of that pain against the background of a cacophony of sympathetic arousal signals.

The concept of feedback underscores an essential point: A sensory stimulus does not have purely sensory effects. It undergoes parallel processing at the affective level. When a neural signal involves threat to biological integrity, it elicits strong patterns of sympathetic and neuroendocrine response. These, in turn, contribute to the awareness of the perceiver. Sensory processing provides information about the environment, but this information exists in awareness against a background of emotional arousal, either positive or negative, and that arousal may vary from mild to extreme.

Nociception and the Limbic Brain

Central sensory and affective pain processes share common sensory mechanisms in the periphery. A-delta and C fibers serve as tissue trauma transducers (nociceptors) for both, the chemical products of inflammation sensitize these nociceptors, and peripheral neuropathic mechanisms such as ectopic firing excite both processes. In some cases neuropathic mechanisms may substitute for transduction as we classically define it, producing afferent signal volleys that appear, to the central nervous system, like signals originating in nociceptors. Differentiation of sensory and affective processing begins at the dorsal horn of the spinal cord. Sensory transmission follows spinothalamic pathways, and transmission destined for affective processing takes place in spinoreticular pathways. For more detail on the sensory processing of nociception, see Willis and Westlund (1997).

Nociceptive centripetal transmission engages multiple pathways: spinoreticular, spinomesencephalic, spinolimbic, spinocervical, and spinothalamic tracts (Villanueva, Bing, Bouhassira, & Le Bars, 1989; Willis & Westlund, 1997). The spinoreticular tract contains somatosensory and viscerosensory afferent pathways that arrive at different levels of the brain stem. Spinoreticular axons possess receptive fields that resemble those of spinothalamic tract neurons projecting to medial thalamus, and, like their spinothalamic counterparts, they transmit tissue injury information (Craig, 1992; Villanueva, Cliffer, Sorkin, Le Bars, & Willis, 1990). Most spinoreticular neurons carry nociceptive signals, and many of them respond preferentially to noxious activity (Bing, Villanueva, & Le Bars, 1990; Bowsher, 1976). The spinomesencephalic tract comprises several projections that terminate in multiple midbrain nuclei, including the periaqueductal gray, the red nucleus, nucleus cuniformis, and the Edinger–Westphal nucleus (Willis & Westlund, 1997). Spinolimbic tracts include the spinohypothalamic tract, which reaches both lateral and medial hypothalamus (Burstein, Cliffer, & Giesler, 1988; Burstein, Dado, Cliffer, & Giesler, 1991) and the spinoamygdalar tract that extends to the central nucleus of the amygdala (Bernard & Besson, 1990). The spinocervical tract, like the spinothalamic tract, conveys signals to the thalamus. All of these tracts transmit tissue trauma signals rostrally.

Central processing of nociceptive signals to produce affect undoubtedly involves multiple neurotransmitter systems. Four extrathalamic afferent pathways project to neocortex: the noradrenergic medial forebrain bundle originating in the locus ceruleus (LC); the serotonergic fibers that arise in the dorsal and median raphé nuclei; the dopaminergic pathways of the ventral tegmental tract that arise from substantia nigra; and the acetylcholinergic neurons that arise principally from the nucleus basalis of the substantia innominata (Foote & Morrison, 1987). Of these, the noradrenergic and serotonergic pathways link most closely to negative emotional states (Bremner, Krystal, Southwick, & Charney, 1996; Gray, 1982, 1987). The set of structures receiving projections from this complex and extensive network corresponds to classic definition of the limbic brain (Isaacson, 1982; MacLean, 1990; Papez, 1937).

Although other processes governed predominantly by other neurotransmitters almost certainly play important roles in the complex experience of emotion during pain, I emphasize the role of central noradrenergic processing and the medial forebrain bundle here. This limited perspective offers the advantage of simplicity, and the literature on the role of central noradrenergic pathways in anxiety, panic, stress, and posttraumatic stress disorder provides a strong basis (Bremner et al., 1996; Charney & Deutch, 1996). This processing involves the medial forebrain bundle that subdivides into two central noradrenergic pathways: the dorsal and ventral noradrenergic bundles.

Locus Ceruleus and the Dorsal Noradrenergic Bundle

Substantial evidence supports the hypothesis that noradrenergic brain pathways are major mechanisms of anxiety and stress (Bremner et al., 1996). The majority of noradrenergic neurons originate in the locus ceruleus (LC). This pontine nucleus resides bilaterally near the wall of the fourth ventricle. The locus has three major projections: ascending, descending, and cerebellar. The ascending projection, the dorsal noradrenergic bundle (DNB), is the most extensive and important pathway for our purposes (Fillenz, 1990). Projecting from the LC throughout limbic brain and to all of neocortex, the DNB accounts for about 70% of all brain norepinephrine (Svensson, 1987). The LC gives rise to most central noradrenergic fibers in spinal cord, hypothalamus, thalamus, hippocampus (Aston-Jones, Foote, & Segal, 1985), and, in addition, it projects to limbic cortex and

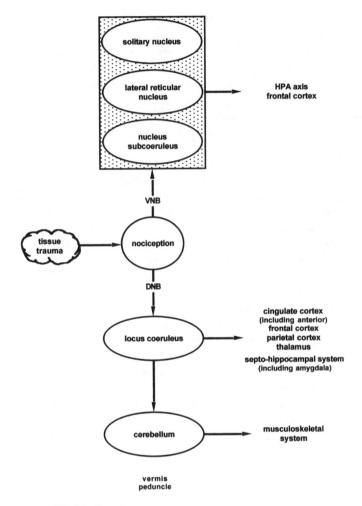

FIG. 3.2. Noradrenergic pathways activated by nociception.

neocortex. Consequently, the LC exerts a powerful influence on higher level brain activity. Figure 3.2 illustrates the relationships among central noradrenergic pathways and structures.

The *noradrenergic stress response hypothesis* holds that any stimulus that threatens the biological, psychological, or psychosocial integrity of the individual increases the firing rate of the LC, and this in turn results in increased release and turnover of norepinephrine in the brain areas involved in noradrenergic innervation. Studies show that the LC reacts to signaling from sensory stimuli that potentially threaten the biological integrity of the individual or signal damage to that integrity (Elam, Svensson, & Thoren, 1986b;

Svensson, 1987). Spinal-cord lamina one cells terminate in the LC (Craig, 1992). The major sources of LC afferent input are the paragigantocellularis and prepositus hypoglossi nuclei in the medulla, but destruction of these nuclei does not block LC response to somatosensory stimuli (Rasmussen & Aghajanian, 1989). Other sources of afferent input to the locus include the lateral hypothalamus, the amygdala, and the solitary nucleus. Whether nociception stimulates the LC directly or indirectly is still uncertain.

Nociception inevitably and reliably increases activity in neurons of the LC, and LC excitation appears to be a consistent response to nociception (Korf, Bunney, & Aghajanian, 1974; Morilak, Fornal, & Jacobs, 1987; Stone, 1975; Svensson, 1987). Notably, this does not require cognitively mediated attentional control because it occurs in anesthetized animals. Foote, Bloom, and Aston-Jones (1983) reported that slow, tonic spontaneous activity at the locus in rats changed under anesthesia in response to noxious stimulation. Experimentally induced phasic LC activation produces alarm and apparent fear in primates (Redmond & Huang, 1979), and lesions of the LC eliminate normal heart-rate increases to threatening stimuli (Redmond, 1977). In a resting animal, LC neurons discharge in a slow, phasic manner (Rasmussen, Morilak, & Jacobs, 1986).

The LC reacts consistently, but it does not respond exclusively, to nociception. LC firing rates increase following nonpainful but threatening events such as strong cardiovascular stimulation (Elam, Svensson, & Thoren, 1985; Morilak et al., 1987) and certain visceral events such as distention of the bladder, stomach, colon, or rectum (Svensson, 1987; Aston-Jones et al., 1985). Highly novel and sudden stimuli that could represent potential threat, such as loud clicks or light flashes, can also excite the LC in experimental animals (Rasmussen et al., 1986). Thus, the LC responds to biologically threatening or potentially threatening events, of which tissue injury is a significant subset. Amaral and Sinnamon (1977) described the LC as a central analog of the sympathetic ganglia. Viewed in this way, it is an extension of the autonomic protective mechanism described earlier.

Invasive studies confirm the linkage between LC activity and threat. Direct activation of the DNB and associated limbic structures in laboratory animals produces sympathetic nervous system response and elicits emotional behaviors such as defensive threat, fright, enhanced startle, freezing, and vocalization (McNaughton & Mason, 1980). This indicates that enhanced activity in these pathways corresponds to negative emotional arousal and behaviors appropriate to perceived threat. LC firing rates increase two- to threefold during the defense response elicited in a cat that has perceived a dog (Barrett et al., 1987). Moreover, infusion of norepinephrine into the hypothalamus of an awake cat elicits a defensive rage reaction that includes activation of the LC noradrenergic system. In general, the mammalian defense response involves increased regional turnover and release of norepinephrine in the brain regions that the LC innervates. The LC response to threat, therefore, may be a component of the partly "prewired" patterns associated with the defense response.

Increased alertness is a key element in early stages of the defense response. Normally, activity in the LC increases alertness. Tonically enhanced LC and DNB discharge corresponds to hypervigilance and emotionality (Bremner et al., 1996; Butler, Weiss, Stout, & Nemeroff, 1990; Foote et al., 1983). The DNB is the mechanism for vigilance and defensive orientation to affectively relevant and novel stimuli. It also regulates attentional processes and facilitates motor responses (Foote & Morrison, 1987; Gray, 1987; Svensson, 1987; Elam, Svensson, & Thoren, 1986a). In this sense, the LC influences the stream of consciousness on an ongoing basis and readies the individual to respond quickly and effectively to threat when it occurs.

LC and DNB support biological survival by making possible global vigilance for threatening and harmful stimuli. Siegel and Rogawski (1988) hypothesized a link between the LC noradrenergic system and vigilance, focusing on rapid eye movement (REM) sleep. They noted that LC noradrenergic neurons maintain continuous activity in both normal waking state and non-REM sleep, but during REM sleep, these neurons virtually cease discharge activity. Moreover, an increase in REM sleep ensues either after lesion of the DNB or following administration of clonidine, an alpha-2 adrenoceptor agonist. Because LC inactivation during REM sleep permits rebuilding of noradrenergic stores, REM sleep may be necessary preparation for sustained periods of high alertness during subsequent waking. Conversely, reduced LC activity periods (REM sleep) allow time for a suppression of sympathetic tone.

Both adaptation and sensitization can alter the LC response to threat. Abercrombie and Jacobs (1987a, 1987b) demonstrated a noradrenergically mediated increase in heart rate in cats exposed to white noise. Elevated heart rate decreased with repeated exposure, as did LC activation and circulating levels of norepinephrine. Libet and Gleason (1994) found that stimulation via permanently implanted LC electrodes did not elicit indefinite anxiety. This indicates that the brain either adapts to locus excitation or engages a compensatory response to excessive LC activation under some circumstances. In addition, central noradrenergic responsiveness changes as a function of learning. In the cat, pairing a stimulus with a noxious air puff results in increased LC firing with subsequent presentations of the stimulus, but previous pairing of that stimulus with a food reward produces no alteration in LC firing rates with repeated presentation (Rasmussen et al., 1986). These studies show that, despite its apparently "prewired" behavioral subroutines, the noradrenergic brain shows substantial neuroplasticity. The emotional response of animals and people to a painful stimulus can adapt, and it can change as a function of experience.

From a different perspective, Bremner et al. (1996) postulated that chronic stress can affect regional norepinephrine turnover and thus contribute to the *response sensitization* evident in panic disorder and post-traumatic stress disorder. Chronic exposure to a stressor (including perseverating nociception) could create a situation in which noradrenergic synthesis cannot keep up with demand, thus depleting brain norepinephrine levels. Animals exposed to inescapable shock demonstrate greater LC responsiveness to an excitatory stimulus than animals that have experienced escapable shock (Weiss & Simson, 1986). In addition, such animals display "learned helplessness" behaviors—they cease trying to adapt to, or cope with, the source of shock (Seligman, Weiss, Weinraub, & Schulman, 1980). From an evolutionary perspective, this is a failure of the defense response as adaptation; it represents surrender to suffering. Extrapolating this and related observations to patients, Bremner and colleagues (1996) suggested that persons who have once encountered overwhelming stress and suffered exhaustion of central noradrenergic resources may respond excessively to similar stressors that they encounter later.

The Ventral Noradrenergic Bundle and the Hypothalamo-Pituitary-Adrenocortical (HPA) Axis

The ventral noradrenergic bundle (VNB) originates in the LC and enters the medial forebrain bundle. Neurons in the medullary reticular formation project to the hypothalamus via the VNB (Sumal, Blessing, Joh, Reis, & Pickel, 1983). Sawchenko and Swanson (1982) identified two VNB-linked noradrenergic and adrenergic pathways to paraventricular hypothalamus in the rat: the A1 region of the ventral medulla (lateral reticular nucleus, LRN), and the A2 region of the dorsal vagal complex (the nucleus tractus solitarius, or solitary nucleus), which receives visceral afferents. These medullary neuronal complexes supply 90% of catecholaminergic innervation to the paraventricular hypothalamus via the VNB (Assenmacher, Szafarczyk, Alonso, Ixart, & Barbanel, 1987).

The noradrenergic axons in the VNB respond to noxious stimulation (Svensson, 1987), as does the hypothalamus itself (Kanosue, Nakayama, Ishikawa, & Imai-Matsumura, 1984). Moreover, nociception-transmitting neurons at all segmental levels of the spinal cord project to medial and lateral hypothalamus and several telencephalic regions (Burstein et al., 1988, 1991; Willis & Westlund, 1987). These projections link tissue injury and the hypothalamic response, as do hormonal messengers in some circumstances.

The hypothalamic paraventricular nucleus (PVN) coordinates the HPA axis. Neurons of the PVN receive afferent information from several reticular areas including ventrolateral medulla, dorsal raphé nucleus, nucleus raphé magnus, LC, dorsomedial nucleus, and the nucleus tractus solitarius (Lopez,

Young, Herman, Akil, & Watson, 1991; Peschanski & Weil-Fugacza, 1987; Sawchenko & Swanson, 1982). Still other afferents project to the PVN from the hippocampus, septum, and amygdala (Feldman, Conforti, & Weidenfeld, 1995). Nearly all hypothalamic and preoptic nuclei send projections to the PVN. This suggests that limbic connections mediate endocrine responses during stress. Feldman et al. noted that limbic stimulation always increases adrenocortical activity in rats.

In responding to potentially or frankly injurious stimuli, the PVN initiates a complex series of events regulated by feed back mechanisms. These processes ready the organism for extraordinary behaviors that will maximize its chances to cope with the threat at hand (Selye, 1978). Although laboratory studies often involve highly controlled and specific noxious stimulation, real-life tissue trauma usually involves a spectrum of afferent activity, and the pattern of activity may be a greater determinant of the stress response than the specific receptor system involved (Lilly & Gann, 1992). Traumatic injury, for example, might involve complex signaling from the site of injury including inflammatory mediators, baroreceptor signals from blood volume changes, and hypercapnea. Tissue trauma normally initiates much more than nociception.

Diminished nociceptive transmission during stress or injury helps people and animals to cope with threat without the distraction of pain. Laboratory studies with rodents indicate that animals placed in restraint or subjected to cold water develop analgesia (Amir & Amit, 1979; Bodnar, Glusman, Brutus, Spiaggia, & Kelly, 1979; Kelly, Silverman, Glusman, & Bodner, 1993). Lesioning the PVN attenuates such stress-induced analgesia (Truesdell & Bodnar, 1987).

The medullary mechanisms involved in this are complex and include the response of the solitary nucleus to baroreceptor stimulation (Ghione, 1996). Stressor-induced, increased blood pressure stimulates carotid baroreceptors, and these in turn activate the solitary nucleus, which then initiates activity in descending pathways that gate incoming nociceptive traffic at the dorsal horn of the spinal cord. This mechanism links psychophysiological response to a stressor with endogenous pain modulation.

Some investigators emphasize that neuroendocrine arousal mechanisms are not limited to emergency situations, even though most research emphasizes that such situations elicit them (Grant, Aston-Jones, & Redmond, 1988; Henry, 1986). In complex social contexts, submission, dominance, and other transactions can elicit neuroendocrine and autonomic responses, modified perhaps by learning and memory. This suggests that neuroendocrine processes accompany all sorts of emotion-eliciting situations.

The hypothalamic PVN supports stress-related autonomic arousal through neural as well as hormonal pathways. It sends direct projections to the sympathetic intermediolateral cell column in the thoracolumbar spinal cord and the parasympathetic vagal complex, both sources of preganglionic autonomic outflow (Krukoff, 1990). In addition, it signals release of epinephrine and norepinephrine from the adrenal medulla. ACTH (adrenocorticotrophic hormone) release, although not instantaneous, is quite rapid: It occurs within about 15 seconds (Sapolsky, 1992). These considerations implicate the HPA axis in the neuroendocrinologic and autonomic manifestations of emotion associated with tissue trauma.

In addition to controlling neuroendocrine and autonomic nervous system reactivity, the HPA axis coordinates emotional arousal with behavior (Panksepp, 1986). As noted earlier, stimulation of the hypothalamus can elicit well-organized action patterns, including defensive threat behaviors and autonomic arousal (Jänig, 1985). The existence of demonstrable behavioral subroutines in animals suggests that the hypothalamus plays a key role in matching behavioral reactions and bodily adjustments to challenging circumstances or biologically relevant stimuli. Moreover, stress hormones at high levels, especially glucocorticoids, may affect central emotional arousal, lowering startle thresholds and influencing cognition (Sapolsky, 1992). Saphier (1987) observed that cortisol altered the firing rate of neurons in limbic forebrain. Clearly, stress regulation is a complex, feedback-dependent, and coordinated process. The hypothalamus appears to take executive responsibility for coordinating behavioral readiness with physiological capability, awareness, and cognitive function.

Chapman and Gavrin (1999) suggested that prolonged nociception may cause a sustained, maladaptive stress response in patients. Signs of this include fatigue, dysphoria, myalgia, nonrestorative sleep, somatic hypervigilance, reduced appetite and libido, impaired physical functioning, and impaired concentration. In this way, the emotional dimension of persisting pain may, through its physiological manifestation, contribute heavily to the disability associated with chronic or unrelieved cancer pain.

Central Serotonergic Pathways

The serotonergic system is the most extensive monoaminergic system in the brain. It originates in the raphé nuclei of the medulla, the pons, and the mesencephalon (Grove, Coplan, & Hollander, 1997; Watson, Khachaturian, Lewis, & Akil, 1986). Descending projections from the raphé nuclei modulate nociceptive traffic at laminae I and II in the spinal cord and also motor neurons. The raphé nuclei of the midbrain and upper pons project via the medial forebrain bundle to multiple limbic sites such as hypothalamus, septum and hippocampus, cingulate cortex, and cerebral cortex, including frontal cortex.

The potential role of serotonergic mechanisms in affective disorders, particularly depression and panic disorder, continues to receive a great deal of attention (Grove et al., 1997; van Praag, 1996). These are important for pain perception because descending endogenous modulatory pathways from the nucleus raphé magnus, the solitary nucleus, and other mesencephalic structures can attenuate or gate nociceptive signaling at the level of the dorsal horn, and these pathways are largely serotonergic. Longstanding, but thinly supported, speculation holds that depletion of serotonin may result in diminished endogenous modulation of nociception and hypersensitivity to noxious events.

Currently, the major antidepressant medications are selective serotonin (5-hydroxytryptamine; 5-HT) reuptake inhibitors, often called SSRIs (Asberg & Martensson, 1993). Increased receptor selectivity in the newer drugs helps to maximize benefit and minimize side effects of these medications.

It is now clear that the older assumptions of simple bioamine deficiency are insufficient to account for the role of serotonin in affective disorders. Although a definitive understanding is still at issue, it has become clear that the serotonergic system influences the actions of the HPA axis, particularly by augmenting cortisol-induced feedback inhibition (Bagdy, Calogero, Murphy, & Szemeredi, 1989; Dinan, 1996; Korte, Van, Bouws, Koolhaas, & Bohus, 1991). Moreover, it interacts with noradrenergic pathways in complex ways, including attenuation of firing in LC neurons (Aston-Jones et al., 1991). The interdependence of the monoamine systems and the HPA axis indicates that we cannot hope to account for complex patterns of brain or behavioral responses by considering these elements individually. They appear to be components of a larger system that we have yet to conceptualize.

TWO STAGES IN THE EMOTIONAL ASPECT OF PAIN

The physiology of emotion suggests that the affective dimension of pain involves a two-stage mechanism. The primary mechanism generates an immediate experience akin to hypervigilance or fear; put simply, it is threat. In nature, this rapid response to injury serves to disrupt ongoing attentional and behavioral patterns. At the same time, efferent messages from the hypothalamus, amygdala, and other limbic structures excite the autonomic nervous system, which in turn alters bodily states. Cardiac function, muscle tension, altered visceral function, respiration rate, and trembling all occur, and awareness of these reactions creates a strong negative subjective experience. This body state awareness is the second mechanism of the affective dimension of pain.

Damasio (1994) submitted that visceral and other event-related, autonomically mediated body state changes constitute "somatic markers." That is, they serve as messengers, delivering affective evaluations of perceptual experiences that either confirm or deny the potential threat inherent in an event. A somatic marker is essentially a somatic image. Perceptually, the brain operates on images that are symbolic representations of external and internal objects or events. Just as it is more efficient for a listener to work with words in language as opposed to phonemes, cognition is more efficient when it uses images rather than simple sensations. The somatic marker images associated with tissue trauma are often complex patterns of physiological arousal. They serve as symbolic representations of threat to the biological (and sometimes the psychological or social) integrity of the person. Like other images, they can enter into complex patterns of association. Because the secondary stage of the affective response involves images and symbols, it represents cognition as well as emotion.

PAIN, STRESS, AND SICKNESS

The defensive response of the central nervous system to injury or disease is complex. We have already seen that it is not limited to simple sensory signaling of tissue trauma, awareness of such signaling, and conscious response. Much of the information processing is unconscious, and physiological responses are initially unconscious, producing affective changes and subsequent awareness of emotional arousal. The HPA axis plays a strong role in emotional arousal and the defense response, and it helps govern the immune system (Sternberg, 1995). The immune system does much more than identifying and destroying foreign substances: It may function as a sense organ that is diffusely distributed throughout the body (Blalock, Smith, & Meyer, 1985; Willis & Westlund, 1997).

Some investigators contend that the brain and immune system form a bidirectional communication network (Lilly & Gann, 1992; Maier & Watkins, 1998). First, products of the immune system communicate injury-related events and tissue pathology to the brain. The key products are cytokines such as interleukin-1 (IL-1) and interleukin-6 (IL-6) released by macrophages and other immune cells. They appear to do this not by functioning as blood-borne messengers, but by activating the vagus nerve. Paraganglia surrounding vagal terminals have dense binding sites for IL-1, and they synapse on vagal fibers that terminate in the solitary nucleus. Thus, cytokines appear to excite (albeit indirectly) vagal afferents that terminate in one of the major control centers for the autonomic nervous system.

Second, the brain controls the immune system via the actions of the sympathetic nervous system and the hypothalamic secretion into the bloodstream of releasing factors that activate the anterior pituitary via the HPA axis (Sternberg, 1995). The pituitary body releases peptides related to pro-opiomelanocortin, such as ACTH and beta-endorphin, and these in turn trigger the release of glucocorticoids. Because the cells and organs of the immune system express receptors for these hormones, they can respond to humoral messenger molecules of central origin. This system is important for pain research because, according to Maier and Watkins (1998), activation of these pathways by a stressor such as tissue trauma produces a constellation of adaptive behaviors and physiological changes that correspond to the "sickness" response.

The *sickness response* is a negative experience, but it evolved to promote recuperation and survival. It includes fever, increased slow-wave sleep, increased leucocytosis, reduced exploration, diminished sexual interest, reduced activity, depressed mood, and somewhat diminished cognitive abilities. Collectively, these responses conserve energy and foster its redirection to increased body temperature, which suppresses the reproduction of microbial organisms. Sickness tends to occur with both microbial infection and tissue injury because an open wound normally invites infection. Viewed broadly, sickness is an unpleasant motivational state that promotes recuperation.

These considerations suggest that feeling sick is a part of the brain's defense against microbial invasion. Tissue trauma can provoke it, and thus it tends to accompany the experience of pain. Obviously, chronic sickness in the absence of definable injury of pathology serves no biological purpose. The role of the sickness response in chronic pain states merits study.

CLINICAL IMPLICATIONS

The preceding review reveals that the brain deals in complex ways with signals of tissue trauma. Figure 3.3 provides a simple overview of this complexity and indicates how different types of intervention for pain act at different levels of the neuraxis. It is rarely reasonable to assume that psychological processes are incidental to pain; indeed, pain is itself a psychological experience, and the expression of pain is a behavior.

Highly organized patterns of protective response occur during pain, and they involve the autonomic nervous system, the HPA axis, and the immune system, as well as subjective awareness. Negative emotion is a major feature of pain and a direct consequence of complex central nociceptive processing involving sympathetic activation and activity in the HPA axis. Emotion is not purely subjective, and its psychophysiology can be medically significant. Cognitive processes invariably accompany human emotion, so they are a part of the pain experience.

If the emotional component of pain is an integral part of the experience of pain, with its own physiological mechanisms, then it stands to reason that medicine should incorporate the affective dimension into diagnosis of

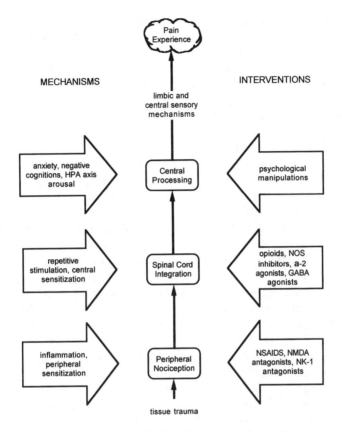

FIG. 3.3. Mechanisms of pain and related interventional strategies, organized according to levels of the neuraxis.

pain states and direct therapeutic intervention toward pain affect. Most physicians try to look around or beyond the negative emotion that the patient in pain presents in an attempt to discern whether the pain sensation signals an undiagnosed injury or disease process. This is a necessary first step, but when the results are negative, it is important to assess the patient's affective status. This should entail more than asking about the patient's spirits or mood. The goal is to discern whether the patient produces excessive sympathetic activity in everyday life, and whether there is endocrinological evidence for HPA axis arousal.

Reports of poor or nonrestorative sleep, diminished appetite, general ongoing fatigue, and sore muscles or "ache all over" feelings are often indicators of excessive or prolonged negative affect. Nociception-driven affective arousal maybe the cause of the patient's suffering, a complicating factor in the pain syndrome (e.g., contributing secondarily to sympathetic mechanisms), or the cause of many of the debilitating complications of persisting pain. There is a pressing need for further research on the role of pain affect in generating and perpetuating the constellation of symptoms that accompany chronic pain or cancer pain such as fatigue, sleep disorder, impaired concentration, general myalgia, and negative mood.

The progress of acute pain to disabling chronic pain may depend, in some cases, heavily on the affective dimension of pain. Such dependence can be psychological (e.g., involving classical and operant conditioning), but it can also be physiological because negative emotion involves sympathetic arousal, and this may interact with the mechanisms of some complex regional pain syndromes, angina, or other disorders.

The best way to control the affective dimension of pain medically, when possible, is to prevent or stop the nociceptive or neuropathic neural traffic. When this is not possible, then the affective dimension of pain should be a target for intervention in its own right. The physiological consequences of prolonged sympathetic arousal and HPA axis arousal are negative, and the patient is suffering.

Many clinicians think first of benzodiazepines for controlling negative emotions, but these work primarily at cortical areas. They may quiet the patient and change behavior, but this does not mean that they reduce the physiological consequences of the nociception at lower levels of the neuraxis. There is a need for further research on the potential prophylactic benefits of alpha-2 agonists, which may help prevent or blunt the sympathetic response to acute pain states such as postoperative pain or procedural pain. Patients with chronic pain could potentially benefit from these drugs as well if they have complex regional pain syndrome, angina, headache, or a variety of other conditions in which sympathetic activation helps sustain the pain.

Psychological training in deep relaxation may assist the rehabilitation of chronic pain patients by helping them to limit the affective dimension of their pain. In addition, clinicians can sometimes attenuate negative emotional overlay by providing information to patients and by listening patiently to the patient's concerns. Patients who feel that they can trust their providers are less anxious. Many respond positively to clinician awareness of suffering and bad feelings.

Because pain is a complex psychological experience, psychology should have a strong role in pain research and pain management. Although psychologists have contributed to the field in such areas as pain assessment and cognitive-behavioral therapy, they have not yet built a bridge between the physiological mechanisms of pain and psychological practice. Such a bridge is important not only for scientific reasons, but also for communication. Psychology needs to be at the center of the pain field where it can integrate progress in basic science with clinical pain assessment and treatment.

This will require a combination of strong theory and a psychophysiological basis for psychological constructs. Strong effort in this direction is crucial for the pain field because no other discipline can properly characterize and comprehensively study pain.

REFERENCES

Abercrombie, E. D., & Jacobs, B. L. (1987a). Single-unit response of noradrenergic neurons in the locus coeruleus of freely moving cats. I. Acutely presented stressful and nonstressful stimuli. *Journal of Neuroscience, 7*(9), 2837–2843.

Abercrombie, E. D., & Jacobs, B. L. (1987b). Single-unit response of noradrenergic neurons in the locus coeruleus of freely moving cats. II. Adaptation to chronically presented stressful stimuli. *Journal of Neuroscience, 7*(9), 2844–2848.

Amaral, D. B., & Sinnamon, H. M. (1977). The locus coeruleus: Neurobiology of a central noradrenergic nucleus. *Progress in Neurobiology, 9*, 147–196.

Amir, S., & Amit, Z. (1979). The pituitary gland mediates acute and chronic pain responsiveness in stressed and non-stressed rats. *Life Sciences, 24*, 439–448.

Asberg, M., & Martensson, B. (1993). Serotonin selective antidepressant drugs: Past, present, future. *Clinical Neuropharmacology, 16*(Suppl. 3), S32–S44.

Assenmacher, I., Szafarczyk, A., Alonso, G., Ixart, G., & Barbanel, G. (1987). Physiology of neuropathways affecting CRH secretion. In W. F. Ganong, M. F. Dallman, & J. L. Roberts (Eds.), *The hypothalamic-pituitary-adrenal axis revisited* (Vol. 512, pp. 149–161). New York: New York Academy of Sciences.

Aston-Jones, G., Foote, S. L., & Segal, M. (1985). Impulse conduction properties of noradrenergic locus coeruleus axons projecting to monkey cerebrocortex. *Neuroscience, 15*, 765–777.

Aston-Jones, G., Shipley, M. T., Chouvet, G., Ennis, M., Van, B. E., Pieribone, V., Shiekhattar, R., Akaoka, H., Drolet, G., Astier, B., et al. (1991). Afferent regulation of locus coeruleus neurons: Anatomy, physiology and pharmacology. *Progress in Brain Research, 88*, 47–75.

Bagdy, G., Calogero, A. E., Murphy, D. L., & Szemeredi, K. (1989). Serotonin agonists cause parallel activation of the sympathoadrenomedullary system and the hypothalamo-pituitary-adrenocortical axis in conscious rats. *Endocrinology, 125*(5), 2664–2669.

Barrett, J. A., Shaikh, M. B., Edinger, H., & Siegel, A. (1987). The effects of intrahypothalamic injections of norepinephrine upon affective defense behavior in the cat. *Brain Research, 426*(2), 381–384.

Bernard, J. F., & Besson, J. M. (1990). The spino(trigemino)pontoamygdaloid pathway: Electrophysiological evidence for an involvement in pain processes. *Journal of Neurophysiology, 63*(3), 473–490.

Bing, Z., Villanueva, L., & Le Bars, D. (1990). Ascending pathways in the spinal cord involved in the activation of subnucleus reticularis dorsalis neurons in the medulla of the rat. *Journal of Neurophysiology, 63*, 424–438.

Blalock, J. E., Smith, E. M., & Meyer, W. J., 3rd. (1985). The pituitary-adrenocortical axis and the immune system. *Clinics in Endocrinology and Metabolism, 14*(4), 1021–1038.

Bodnar, R. J., Glusman, M., Brutus, M., Spiaggia, A., & Kelly, D. (1979). Analgesia induced by cold-water stress: Attenuation following hypophysectomy. *Physiology & Behaviour, 23*, 53–62.

Bowsher, D. (1976). Role of the reticular formation in responses to noxious stimulation. *Pain, 2*, 361–378.

Bremner, J. D., Krystal, J. H., Southwick, S. M., & Charney, D. S. (1996). Noradrenergic mechanisms in stress and anxiety: I. Preclinical studies. *Synapse, 23*(1), 28–38.

82 CHAPMAN

Burnstock, G., & Hoyle, C. H. V. (Eds.). (1992). *Autonomic neuroeffector mechanisms*. Philadelphia: Harwood Academic.

Burstein, R., Cliffer, K. D., & Giesler, G. J. (Eds.). (1988). *The spinohypothalamic and spinotelecephalic tracts: Direct nociceptive projections from the spinal cord to the hypothalamus and telencephalon*. New York: Elsevier.

Burstein, R., Dado, R. J., Cliffer, K. D., & Giesler, G. J. J. (1991). Physiological characterization of spinohypothalamic tract neurons in the lumbar enlargement of rats. *Journal of Neurophysiology, 66*(1), 261–284.

Butler, P. D., Weiss, J. M., Stout, J. C., & Nemeroff, C. B. (1990). Corticotropin-releasing factor produces fear-enhancing and behavioral activating effects following infusion into the locus coeruleus. *Journal of Neuroscience, 10*, 176–183.

Cannon, W. B. (1929). *Bodily changes in pain, hunger, fear and rage*. New York: Appleton.

Chapman, C. R., & Gavrin, J. (1999). Suffering the contributions of persisting pain. *Lancet, 353*, 2233–2237.

Charney, D. S., & Deutch, A. (1996). A functional neuroanatomy of anxiety and fear: Implications for the pathophysiology and treatment of anxiety disorders. *Critical Reviews of Neurobiology, 10*(3–4), 419–446.

Craig, A. D. (1992). Spinal and trigeminal lamina I input to the locus coeruleus anterogradely labeled with *Phaseolus vulgaris* leucoagglutinin (PHA-L) in the cat and the monkey. *Brain Research, 584*(1–2), 325–328.

Damasio, A. R. (1994). *Descartes' error: Emotion and reason in the human brain*. New York: Grosset/Putnam.

Dennett, D. (1991). *Consciousness explained*. Boston: Little, Brown.

Descartes, R. (1967). The passions of the soul. In *The philosophical works of Descartes* (Vol. 1, pp. 219–327, Trans. E. S. Haldane & G. T. R. Ross). New York: Dover. (Original work published 1649)

Dinan, T. G. (1996). Serotonin and the regulation of hypothalamic-pituitary-adrenal axis function. *Life Sciences, 58*(20), 1683–1694.

Dodd, J., & Role, L. W. (1991). The anatomic nervous system. In E. R. Kandel, J. H. Schwartz, & T. M. Jessell (Eds.), *Principles of neural science* (3rd ed., pp. 761–775). New York: Elsevier.

Elam, M., Svensson, T. H., & Thoren, P. (1985). Differentiated cardiovascular afferent regulation of locus coeruleus neurons and sympathetic nerves. *Brain Research, 358*, 77–84.

Elam, M., Svensson, T. H., & Thoren, P. (1986a). Locus coeruleus neurons and sympathetic nerves: Activation by cutaneous sensory afferents. *Brain Research, 366*, 254–261.

Elam, M., Svensson, T. H., & Thoren, P. (1986b). Locus coeruleus neurons and sympathetic nerves: Activation by visceral afferents. *Brain Research, 375*, 117–125.

Feldman, S., Conforti, N., & Weidenfeld, J. (1995). Limbic pathways and hypothalamic neurotransmitters mediating adrenocortical responses to neural stimuli. *Neuroscience and Biobehavioural Reviews, 19*(2), 235–240.

Fillenz, M. (1990). *Noradrenergic neurons*. Cambridge: Cambridge University Press.

Foote, S. L., & Morrison, J. H. (1987). Extrathalamic modulation of corticofunction. *Annual Review of Neuroscience, 10*, 67–95.

Foote, S. L., Bloom, F. E., & Aston-Jones, G. (1983). Nucleus locus ceruleus: New evidence of anatomical and physiological specificity. *Physiology Review, 63*, 844–914.

Fulton, J. E. (1951). *Frontal lobotomy and affective behavior*. New York: W. W. Norton.

Ghione, S. (1996). Hypertension-associated hypalgesia. Evidence in experimental animals and humans, pathophysiological mechanisms, and potential clinical consequences. *Hypertension, 28*(3), 494–504.

Grant, S. J., Aston-Jones, G., & Redmond, D. E., Jr. (1988). Responses of primate locus coeruleus neurons to simple and complex sensory stimuli. *Brain Research Bulletin, 21*(3), 401–410.

Gray, J. A. (1982). *The neuropsychology of anxiety: An enquiry into the functions of the septohippocampal system*. New York: Oxford University Press.

Gray, J. A. (1987). *The psychology of fear and stress* (2nd ed.). Cambridge: Cambridge University Press.

Grove, G., Coplan, J. D., & Hollander, E. (1997). The neuroanatomy of 5-HT dysregulation and panic disorder. *Journal of Neuropsychiatry and Clinical Neurosciences, 9*(2), 198–207.

Henry, J. P. (1986). Neuroendocrine patterns of emotional response. In R. Plutchik & H. Kellerman (Eds.), *Emotion: Theory, research and practice* (Vol. 3, pp. 37–60). Orlando, FL: Academic Press.

Hess, W. R. (1936). Hypothalamus und die Zantren des autonomen Nervensystems: Physiologie. *Archiv fuer Psychiatrie und Nervenkrankheiten, 104*(548–557).

Hilton, S. M. (1966). Hypothalamic regulation of the cardiovascular system. *British Medical Bulletin, 22*, 243–248.

Isaacson, R. L. (1982). *The limbic system* (2nd ed.). New York: Plenum Press.

Jänig, W. (1985). Systemic and specific autonomic reactions in pain: Efferent, afferent and endocrine components. *European Journal of Anaesthesiology, 2*, 319–346.

Kanosue, K., Nakayama, T., Ishikawa, Y., & Imai-Matsumura, K. (1984). Responses of hypothalamic and thalamic neurons to noxious and scrotal thermal stimulation in rats. *Journal of Thermal Biology, 9*, 11–13.

Kelly, D. D., Silverman, A. J., Glusman, M., & Bodner, R. J. (1993). Characterization of pituitary mediation of stress-induced antinociception in rats. *Physiology & Behaviour, 53*, 769–775.

Korf, J., Bunney, B. S., & Aghajanian, G. K. (1974). Noradrenergic neurons: Morphine inhibition of spontaneous activity. *European Journal of Pharmacology, 25*, 165–169.

Korte, S. M., Van, D. S., Bouws, G. A., Koolhaas, J. M., & Bohus, B. (1991). Involvement of hypothalamic serotonin in activation of the sympathoadrenomedullary system and hypothalamo-pituitary-adrenocortical axis in male Wistar rats. *European Journal of Pharmacology, 197*(2–3), 225–228.

Krukoff, T. L. (1990). Neuropeptide regulation of autonomic outflow at the sympathetic preganglionic neuron: Anatomical and neurochemical specificity. *Annals of the New York Academy of Science, 579*, 162–167.

LeDoux, J. E. (1986). The neurobiology of emotion. In J. E. Ledoux & W. Hirst (Eds.), *Mind and brain: Dialogs in cognitive neuroscience* (pp. 301–354). Cambridge, MA: Cambridge University Press.

LeDoux, J. E. (1996). *The emotional brain: The mysterious underpinnings of emotional life.* New York: Simon & Schuster.

Libet, B., & Gleason, C. A. (1994). The human locus coeruleus and anxiogenesis. *Brain Research, 634*(1), 178–180.

Lilly, M. P., & Gann, D. S. (1992). The hypothalamic-pituitary-adrenal-immune axis. A critical assessment. *Archives of Surgery, 127*(12), 1463–1474.

Lopez, J. F., Young, E. A., Herman, J. P., Akil, H., & Watson, S. J. (1991). Regulatory biology of the HPA axis: An integrative approach. In S. C. Risch (Ed.), *Central nervous system peptide mechanisms in stress and depression* (pp. 1–52). Washington, DC: American Psychiatric Press.

MacLean, P. D. (1952). Some psychiatric implications of physiological studies on frontotemporal portion of limbic system (visceral brain). *Electroencephalography and Clinical Neurophysiology, 4*, 407–418.

MacLean, P. D. (1990). *The triune brain in evolution: Role in paleocerebral functions.* New York: Plenum Press.

Maier, S. F., & Watkins, L. R. (1998). Cytokines for psychologists: Implications of bidirectional immune-to-brain communication for understanding behavior, mood, and cognition. *Psychological Review, 105*(1), 83–107.

McNaughton, N., & Mason, S. T. (1980). The neuropsychology and neuropharmacology of the dorsal ascending noradrenergic bundle—A review. *Progress in Neurobiology, 14*, 157–219.

Morgane, P. J. (1981). Historical and modern concepts of hypothalamic organization and function. In P. J. Morgan & J. Panksepp (Eds.), *Handbook of the hypothalamus* (Vol. 1, pp. 1–64). New York: Marcel Dekker.

Morilak, D. A., Fornal, C. A., & Jacobs, B. L. (1987). Effects of physiological manipulations on locus coeruleus neuronal activity in freely moving cats. II. Cardiovascular challenge. *Brain Research, 422,* 24–31.

Panksepp, J. (1986). The anatomy of emotions. In R. Plutchik & H. Kellerman (Eds.), *Emotion: Theory, research and experience* (Vol. 3, pp. 91–124). Orlando, FL: Academic Press.

Papez, J. W. (1937). A proposed mechanism of emotion. *Archives of Neurology and Psychiatry, 38,* 725–743.

Peschanski, M., & Weil-Fugacza, J. (1987). Aminergic and cholinergic afferents to the thalamus: Experimental data with reference to pain pathways. In J. M. Besson, G. Guilbaud, & M. Paschanski (Eds.), *Thalamus and pain* (pp. 127–154). Amsterdam: Excerpta Medica.

Rasmussen, K., & Aghajanian, G. K. (1989). Withdrawal-induced activation of locus coeruleus neurons in opiate-dependent rats: Attenuation by lesions of the nucleus paragigantocellularis. *Brain Research, 505*(2), 346–350.

Rasmussen, K., Morilak, D. A., & Jacobs, B. L. (1986). Single unit activity of locus coeruleus neurons in the freely moving cat. I. During naturalistic behaviors and in response to simple and complex stimuli. *Brain Research, 371*(2), 324–334.

Redmond, D. E. J. (1977). Alteration in the functions of the nucleus locus coeruleus: A possible model for studies of anxiety. In I. Hannin & E. Usdin (Eds.), *Animal models in psychiatry and neurology* (pp. 293–306). New York: Pergamon Press.

Redmond, D. E. J., & Huang, Y. G. (1979). Current concepts. II. New evidence for a locus coeruleus-norepinephrine connection with anxiety. *Life Sciences, 25,* 2149–2162.

Saphier, D. (1987). Cortisol alters firing rate and synaptic responses of limbic forebrain units. *Brain Research Bulletin, 19,* 519–524.

Sapolsky, R. M. (1992). *Stress, the aging brain, and the mechanisms of neuron death.* Cambridge: MIT Press.

Sawchenko, P. E., & Swanson, L. W. (1982). The organization of noradrenergic pathways from the brain stem to the paraventricular and supraoptic nuclei in the rat. *Brain Research, 273*(3), 275–325.

Seligman, M. E., Weiss, J., Weinraub, M., & Schulman, A. (1980). Coping behavior: Learned helplessness, physiological change and learned inactivity. *Behaviour Research and Therapy, 18,* 459–512.

Selye, H. (1978). *The stress of life.* New York: McGraw-Hill.

Siegel, J. M., & Rogawski, M. A. (1988). A function for REM sleep: Regulation of noradrenergic receptor sensitivity. *Brain Research Reviews, 13,* 213–233.

Sokolov, E. N. (1963). *Perception and the conditioned reflex.* Oxford: Pergamon Press.

Sokolov, E. N. (1990). The orienting response, and future directions of its development. *Pavlovian Journal of Biological Science, 25*(3), 142–150.

Sternberg, E. M. (1995). Neuroendocrine factors in susceptibility to inflammatory disease: Focus on the hypothalamic-pituitary-adrenal axis. *Hormone Research, 43*(4), 159–161.

Stone, E. A. (1975). Stress and catecholamines. In A. J. Friedhoff (Ed.), *Catecholamines and behavior* (Vol. 2, pp. 31–72). New York: Plenum Press.

Sumal, K. K., Blessing, W. W., Joh, T. H., Reis, D. J., & Pickel, V. M. (1983). Synaptic interaction of vagal afference and catecholaminergic neurons in the rat nucleus tractus solitarius. *Journal of Brain Research, 277,* 31–40.

Svensson, T. H. (1987). Peripheral, autonomic regulation of locus coeruleus noradrenergic neurons in brain: Putative implications for psychiatry and psychopharmacology. *Psychopharmacology, 92,* 1–7.

Truesdell, L. S., & Bodner, R. J. (1987). Reduction in cold-water swim analgesia following hypothalamic paraventricular nucleus lesions. *Physiology & Behaviour, 39,* 727–731.

van Praag, H. M. (1996). Faulty cortisol/serotonin interplay. Psychopathological and biological characterisation of a new, hypothetical depression subtype (SeCA depression). *Psychiatry Research, 65*(3), 143–157.

Villanueva, L., Bing, Z., Bouhassira, D., & Le Bars, D. (1989). Encoding of electrical, thermal, and mechanical noxious stimuli by subnucleus reticularis dorsalis neurons in the rat medulla. *Journal of Neurophysiology, 61,* 391–402.

Villanueva, L., Cliffer, K. D., Sorkin, L. S., Le Bars, D., & Willis, W. D. J. (1990). Convergence of heterotopic nociceptive information onto neurons of caudal medullary reticular formation in monkey (Macaca fascicularis). *Journal of Neurophysiology, 63,* 1118–1127.

Watson, S. J., Khachaturian, S., Lewis, M. E., & Akil, H. (1986). Chemical neuroanatomy as a basis for biological psychiatry. In P. A. Berger & K. H. Brodie (Eds.), *Biological psychiatry* (2nd ed., Vol. 8, pp. 3–33). New York: Basic Books.

Weiss, J. M., & Simson, P. G. (1986). Depression in an animal model: Focus on the locus ceruleus. *Ciba Foundation Symposium, 123,* 191–215.

Willis, W. D., & Westlund, K. N. (1997). Neuroanatomy of the pain system and of the pathways that modulate pain. *Journal of Clinical Neurophysiology, 14,* 2–31.

4

Social Influences and the Communication of Pain

Thomas Hadjistavropoulos
Department of Psychology,
University of Regina

Kenneth D. Craig
Department of Psychology,
University of British Columbia

Shannon Fuchs-Lacelle
Department of Psychology,
University of Regina

THE FUNCTIONS OF PAIN COMMUNICATION

Pain is commonly described as emerging in the course of evolution as a biological system for signaling real or impending tissue damage and motivating withdrawal or escape from physical danger. These functions undoubtedly are essential to the safety and survival of all animal species, including humans, but do not address many uniquely human needs and capabilities that emerged in our societies. Evolution of the human brain, with its extensive capacities for those psychological computations associated with social interdependencies, complex problem solving, language, and speech, introduced novel features that must be understood if the complexities of human pain are to be appreciated. Reconsideration of the nature of pain from the broader perspective of human biological functioning necessitates consideration of the social ramifications of pain.

The uniquely human adaptations were superimposed on the biological and behavioral capabilities of nonhuman species for escape from physical danger. The ability to engage in reflexive withdrawal from noxious insult is readily demonstrated in nonhuman progenitor species. This aspect of pain is evident even in invertebrates and is emphasized in the animal research that has provided the basis for neuroscience approaches to the study of pain. The immediate reflexive reaction remains conspicuous in humans, allowing study of nociceptive reflexes even in newborns (Andrews & Fitzgerald, 2002), and nonverbal behavior through the life span. Emergence of the capacity to recognize and react to events signaling imminent physical trauma, evident in Pavlovian classical conditioning, permitted the opportunity to learn to fear and avoid potentially damaging situations. Fear of pain remains a powerful phenomenon for humans (Asmundson, Norton, & Norton, 1999). But neither of these behavioral reaction patterns (i.e., fear and avoidance) necessitates a capacity for the complexities of the human subjective experience of pain. Both reflexive withdrawal and an ability to associate cues with risk of harm require minimal cognitive capabilities.

It seems likely that the capacity to subjectively experience pain as humans know it would have been one of the first primordial conscious experiences demanding problem solving. Somewhere in the course of evolution, the ability to reflect on self-interest, risks, and how they could be avoided emerged, permitting flexibility in adaptive responding. Humans benefit substantially from the ability to understand the significance of the pain experience, their ability to plan strategies for establishing control, and the sophisticated skills people use to engage others in providing assistance. These skills free humans, to some extent, from the strong biological predispositions that govern pain behavior in other species, and permit substantially greater participation in social networks for support and care.

Others' Pain Reactions as Signs of Danger

Numerous adaptive advantages emerged when a capacity to recognize and react to the pain of others appeared in the course of evolution. Acute sensitivity to the reactions of others may have represented the first social or communicative feature of pain. Social alarms would warn of personal threat and could enhance vigilance and protective behavior, including escape from threat. This is relatively obvious in domesticated animals; for example, humans breed dogs for watch purposes, and use them to guard from threat. Language is not always needed, as alert observers can respond to evidence of physical damage, withdrawal reflexes, reflexive vocalizations, guarded postures, facial expressions, or evidence of destabilized homeostasis in breathing, skin pallor, and so on. These primordial reactions would not necessarily have had interpersonal functions in the first instance, but they could have been captured for social purposes, because sensitivity to them would have enhanced survival prospects and other adaptive advantages (Darwin, 1965; Fridlund, 1994). The beneficial social consequences could have contributed to their persistence as species characteristics, through either genetic inheritance or cultural inheritance. It may be useful to characterize persistence of the capacity to engage in certain behaviors as inherited, with their realization in social action as dependent on socialization in familial/cultural contexts.

Pain as an Instigator of Altruistic Behavior

The safety benefits conferred on observers by sensitivity to the experiences of others would be reciprocated if the observers were motivated to provide care for the individual in distress. Care for kin and conspecifics characterizes many species. The case is clearest with newborns and infants. Different species can be characterized as precocial or altricial. Precocial species are born capable of independent survival. They are not dependent on parents or other species for food, shelter, or protection. In contrast, members of altricial species are wholly dependent on the care provided by others. In the case of humans, newborns are remarkably fragile and vulnerable, requiring care for years following birth. Throughout this span of time, parents and other caretaking adults must be sensitive to the details of children's needs, as this ensures specific care and conserves resources. Hunger, fatigue, the impact of injury or disease, and other states require the particular ministrations of others. Most often, the adult response must be specific to the infant's state. Although there are some fascinating exceptions (Blass & Watt, 1999), food does not serve to palliate pain, nor do analgesics diminish hunger. Evidence of pain often signifies great urgency. On the other hand, for at least a brief period of time, ignoring fatigue or hunger can be accomplished without cost to the child. In contrast, pain reactions can alert to serious tissue trauma and the presence of danger that may be prevented by immediate intervention. There is evidence that children's cries are particularly salient and commanding of parental attention and feelings of urgency (Murray, 1979).

Despite the importance of accurate judgments to the well-being of the child, it is clear that parents and other adults often have considerable difficulty identifying an infant's needs. Witness parents' frustration when unable to settle a child who has awakened in distress in the middle of the night. Caring for infants often is a matter of parents anticipating needs as a result of prior experience, and trial and error when their anticipation is unsuccessful. Parents come to sequence through known and experimental methods for palliating an upset child.

It is noteworthy that the human capacity for altruistic behavior has its limits. Persistent crying can lead to deterioration of the attachment bond between infants and parents, and increases the risk of physical abuse (Blackman, 2000). Limits on what seem biological imperatives to minimize children's pain and distress are evident in use of corporal punishment, infanticide, and willingness to disregard pain when it is incidental to procedures of known prophylactic, diagnostic, or treatment value to the child. There also is evidence of pervasive underestimation of pain in children, perhaps the basis for systematic underassessment and undermanagement of children's pain (Bauchner, 1991). The case is well illustrated in parents' proxy estimates of their children's pain. When these are contrasted with available children's self-reports, they almost always, but not invariably, are underestimates (Chambers, Giesbrecht, Craig, Bennett, & Hunstman, 1999; Chambers, Reid, Craig, McGrath, & Finley, 1999). Many health professionals seem to underestimate pain to an even greater degree (Chambers, Giesbrecht, Craig, Bennett, & Hunstman, 1999; Chambers, Reid, Craig, McGrath, & Finley, 1999; Lander, 1990).

Similar cases can be developed concerning the care provided to other vulnerable populations where communication of painful distress is even more difficult or there is a tendency to ignore the needs of the individual. The argument can be generated for children and adults with intellectual disabilities, brain damage leading to cognitive or neuromotor impairment, and older adults suffering from dementia, among other possibilities (Hadjistavropoulos, von Baeyer, & Craig, 2001).

Pain Expression as a Determinant of Social Bonding and Relationships

Pain also has important implications for social relationships among people. Again there is considerable evidence of continuity with nonhuman animal species. This can be observed clearly in nonhuman primates when painful conditions impact on hierarchical power structures (De Waal, 1988). Indeed, dominance among rivals often is established when one successfully inflicts through violent aggression injury and pain upon another. Many illustrations in human society are also available. As noted earlier, the normally positive emotional attachment between infants and their mothers or fathers may be affected by prolonged distress in the child. Persistent pain in school-aged children can influence social relationships. Chronic abdominal pain relates to school avoidance (Walker, 1999) and can partly be exacerbated by aversions to social demands in school and overprotective parenting. Children suffering from chronic conditions may become estranged from peers. People suffering chronic pain often find their interpersonal relationships deteriorating. This may reflect inability to participate in usual activities at home, work, or in recreational pursuits and irritability associated with persistent pain, but there may be a broader phenomenon analogous to the interpersonal difficulties experienced by people suffering from chronic depression.

There is also widespread suspicion of people suffering chronic pain from the community at large, and from health care practitioners and providers. Pain cannot be directly observed, and insurance providers frequently deny benefits to patients who suffer chronic pain without a medical explanation. Elderly people are often acutely sensitive to the implications of their complaining about pain. They may suppress pain complaints because they fear unattractive labels, such as "old crock" or "whiner," and may believe that they need to reserve their complaints until they experience something "serious." They also may fear the effects of complaining (e.g., being deprived of their independence or given potent analgesics with possible negative effects). Numerous other illustrations could be generated demonstrating the impact of painful conditions on how others react to the person in pain.

Also, the nature and quality of social support made available to the person in pain have an impact on pain, suffering, and pain disability. Social support can enhance psychological wellness and quality of life for patients with chronic pain (Burckhardt, 1985; Faucett & Levine, 1991; Murphy, Creed, & Jayson, 1988; Schultz & Decker, 1985; Turner & Noh, 1988). In contrast, conflict and problems with social relationships seem to increase depression and somatization (Feuerstein, Sult, & Houle, 1985; Fiore, Becker, & Coppel, 1983; Goldberg, Kerns, & Rosenberg, 1993).

A COMMUNICATIONS MODEL
OF PAIN EXPRESSION

It seems clear that a comprehensive model of pain must include the interpersonal domain. In several papers, we have developed a communications model of pain. This model can be used, for example, to examine facial expression of pain (Prkachin & Craig, 1995), to overcome social barriers to optimal care of infants and children (Craig, Lilley, & Gilbert, 1996), and to differentiate the usefulness and functions of self-report and observational measures of pain (Hadjistavropoulos & Craig, 2002). The model is based on an earlier formulation by Rosenthal (1982). In this model, the experience of pain may be encoded in particular features of expressive behavior (reflexes, cry, self-report) that can then be decoded by observers who draw inferences about the sender's experience. The model is depicted on Fig. 4.1.

The central row depicts the sequence already described wherein tissue stress or trauma would ordinarily instigate the acute pain experience. Behavioral reactions may or may not be evident to observers or caregivers who may or may not deliver aid. The row above describes intrapersonal determinants of the responses and actions of person in pain and the potential caregiver. The bottom row depicts environmental and social con-

92

The Sociocommunications Model of Pain

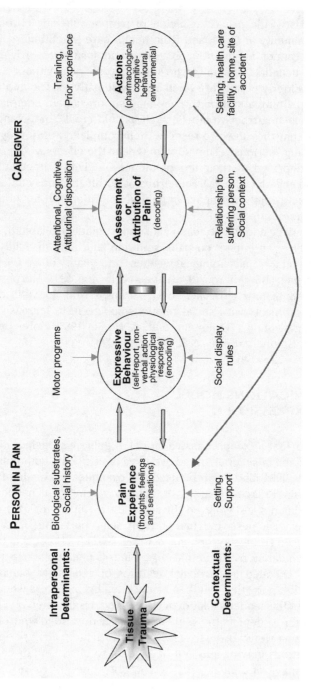

FIG. 4.1. The sociocommunications model of pain: components of a comprehensive model of pain. Care can be provided only if the caregiver can decode the expressive behavior of the person reacting to a source of pain and provide safe and effective care. Both the experience and expression of the person in pain and judgments and decisions of the caregiver will be influenced by complex intrapersonal dispositions and the context where pain is being experienced.

textual factors that determine the subjective experience and behavior of the person in pain, as well as the judgments and action dispositions of the observer.

The subjective pain experience represents the biological systems that provide its corporeal basis. The physiological processes have complex determinants in genetics, nutrition, and experience, including the social history of the individual. Central motor programs responsible for self-report and nonverbal behavioral reactions are also the product of both the biological and social history of the individual (Prkachin & Craig, 1995). The motor programs would reflect both biological capabilities and learning of social display rules—the specifics of how one should behave to optimize the care of others and not violate normative social standards.

Observer inferences of pain and the actions they instigate also have complex, multiple determinants. Caregivers not only integrate indications of pain evident in self-report, nonverbal behavior, or physiological reactivity, but they may also attend to evidence of injury, characteristics of the person in pain, and their understanding of the nature of pain. The assessment will reflect attentional and attitudinal dispositions of the observer as well as the context in which pain is being assessed. For example, someone who has a close personal relationship with the person being assessed might provide a different assessment than an aloof health professional. Care provided to the person in pain would be expected to reflect the background and training of the person treating the pain, as well as the setting where the person in pain was encountered. Caring for the person in pain is a complex process, with numerous intra- and interpersonal factors determining whether appropriate care is delivered. The following considers various features of this social communications model of pain, illustrating how the relatively unique social capabilities of humans require consideration, and are not ordinarily included in neuroscience-based models of pain.

Pain Experience

Pain in competent and mature humans can be characterized as a synthesis of thoughts and feelings, as well as sensory input. Sensory input and its modulation are the primary focus of most neuroscience approaches to pain. The most notable exemptions would be psychophysiological approaches to the study of pain that have attempted to help us understand the nature of pain in humans through use of external physiological monitoring (e.g., the study of autonomic reactivity; Sternbach, 1968), electroencephalography, and evoked potential recordings (Chen, Niddam, Crawfor, Oostenveld, & Arendt-Nielsen, 2002), culminating in the exciting advances current techniques of brain imaging (e.g., fMRI, PET scans) have generated (Casey & Bushnell, 2000). These approaches have permitted detailed understanding of the biological substrates of those cognitive and affective features of pain that are well described using self-report and observational behavior methodologies (Hadjistavropoulos & Craig, 2002).

Fundamental to the social communications model of pain is the proposition that the focus on pain as a private, internal experience neglects its fundamental social features. The arguments outlined earlier lead to the conclusion that the experience itself is shaped by the evolution of the human brain. For example, humans use language to evaluate the meaning and significance of painful events. In other words, both the biological structures and social processes leading to language acquisition will have an indelible impact on how individuals experience pain in terms of both cognitive appraisal and emotional reaction. Similarly, the adaptive significance of painful expression as a warning to conspecifics and instigators of care demands an appreciation of pain as a type of social behavior of which the form cannot be appreciated without consideration of interpersonal factors.

Fundamental to the communications model of pain is recognition of the striking plasticity of the pain experience, with the social context and interpersonal interventions serving as powerful determinants that often account for the lack of one-to-one correspondence between the severity of physical insult and the severity of pain suffered by the individual. This lack of one-to-one correspondence represents the most serious limitation of traditional biophysical models of pain. It dictates provision of care that goes beyond traditional medical models that focus exclusively on physical pathology.

Social Influences on the Experience of Pain. Although it is often difficult to determine whether social influences and context affect the experience of pain or simply the report of pain, there is both anthropological and experimental evidence in support of their importance. With respect to anthropological evidence there are well-documented rituals that involve substantial tissue damage with little manifest evidence that the persons affected experience much pain. Practices involving the intentional self-infliction of pain can include self-flagellation, barefoot pilgrimages, extreme fasting, sleepless nights in prayer vigils, piercing the body, wearing coarse and irritating garments, and others (Glucklich, 2000). They can be legitimized through religious explanation as serving constructive religious and social purposes. The Hindu ritual of Thaipusam is celebrated annually in Singapore and Malaysia (although banned in India) as an expression of faith and penance. On the day of the festival, thousands of celebrants march several kilometers from one temple to another carrying substantial metal and wooden frames decorated with peacock feathers, paper, and fruit. The frames are suspended by metal rods that pierce the celebrants' flesh. Others pull weighty trailers with metal hooks skewered through the flesh of their backs. One of the most cited rituals of this kind involves a hook swinging ceremony practiced in remote Indian villages (e.g., Kosambi, 1967; Melzack & Wall, 1965). The ritual involves steel hooks that are attached to ropes that are inserted in the back of the celebrant who later, during the ceremony, swings freely suspended only by the hooks. The celebrant shows no sign of pain. Explanations for the effect vary. The celebrants are likely to refer to divine intervention. Others believe hypnosis induces altered states of consciousness, and some choose social psychological explanations that refer to social learning of coping skills and pain behavior (Craig, 1986).

The medical use of both placebos and hypnosis for analgesic purposes effectively illustrate well-documented, powerful forms of social influence on pain. Placebos are commonly used in evaluations of pharmaceutical interventions because even inert substances can have a major impact on physical symptoms. In the case of pain, inert substances frequently induce reports of analgesia when their impact is compared with no intervention controls. For this reason, the gold standard research design for pharmaceutical evaluations is the double-blind randomized control design. The recommended use of double-blind procedures (where neither the patient nor the experimenter is aware of who is receiving the placebo or the active chemical) provides further evidence of the impact of social influence on physical symptoms. Double-blind procedures control for patient expectancy and implicit experimenter influence that could bias the outcome of clinical trials.

Research also demonstrates the social impact of the expression and experience of pain. Craig and Weiss (1975), for example, showed that research participants who observe people modeling high levels of pain tolerance reported less pain in response to electric shock than research participants who were not exposed to these models. Similarly, observing models with low pain tolerance produced comparable changes in the pain tolerance of observers. A succession of related studies in this and other research centers have replicated the finding and explored features of the phenomenon (cf. Craig, 1986). Central to the subsequent research were findings indicating that the impact of the models was not only upon the willingness of the research participant to report pain, but there also was an impact on a variety of measures of pain experience (psychophysiological measures of autonomic reactivity, derived psychophysical measures of experience, nonverbal measures that are not usually subject to self-monitoring and self-control for the purposes of impression management) (see Craig, 1986). Other forms of social influence can have a substantial impact on measures of pain experience. Levine and De Simon (1991) found that males report less pain in response to a cold pressor stimulus (i.e., holding one's hand in very cold water) in the presence of an attractive female experimenter than in the presence of a male one. Moreover, a dental procedure administered in a dental clinic is associated with greater reports of pain than the same procedure administered in a research laboratory (Dworkin & Chen, 1982). A recent focus upon the importance of controlling pain in infants and neonates has demonstrated the value of systematically simulating the techniques mothers and other caregivers spontaneously use to control pain in these fragile infants (Johnston, Stremler, Stevens, & Horton, 1997). It seems clear that social contexts and interventions have a potent impact on pain experience; their inclusion in programs of pain intervention have considerable positive potential.

Modes of Pain Expression

Pain communication can be intentional (e.g., in response to a query) or unintentional (e.g., reflexive pain reactions), with verbal and nonverbal measures (e.g., body and limb movements, facial expressions and paralinguistic vocalizations) providing some differentiation. Self-report of pain normally requires some self-awareness and attention to the task, whereas nonverbal indices of pain largely occur spontaneously without commanding prior attention, although the person may monitor the action. Although some nonhuman species appear capable of intentionality and can use vocalizations to communicate (Dennett, 1988), they do not have the remarkable capacity for self-expression exercised by humans. This uniquely human form of pain communication is subject to conscious control and the influence of a variety of factors including, but not limited to, social desirability.

Verbal Communication and Other Forms of Self-Report. Although the most common forms of self-reported pain rely on the use of spoken or written language, other forms of self-reported communication also exist. This includes intentional gestures that indicate that someone is in pain, the use of sign language, and the use of nonverbal self-report measures of pain (e.g., pain faces scales; Chambers & Craig, 2001; Frank, Moll, & Hort, 1982; von Baeyer & Hicks, 2000).

Self-report includes any deliberate act to communicate pain to another person (Champion, Goodenough, von Baeyer, & Thomas, 1998). When people are asked for descriptions of pain severity, their accounts represent integrated summations and often retrospective accounts of the complexities of their subjective experiences. Verbal communication and self-report are often described as representing the "gold standard" for understanding the subjective state of pain (Craig, 1992). Unquestionably, self-report can provide a means for describing subjective experiences and it is methodologically convenient, but it should only be used if it is recognized that pain is a complex experience not readily reduced to language, and with awareness of the possibilities for response biases, situational demand, and the risks of conscious distortion (e.g., malingering). Failure to recognize these limitations could mean that self-report was a form of "fool's gold."

The ideal would be to have well-validated systematic measures. It is now recognized that subtle variations in psychometric questionnaires for assessing any internal state can elicit very different responses. For example, Schwartz (1999) has shown that even minor changes in wording can affect the responses obtained. In an illustrative study (Schwartz, Knauper, Hippler, Noelle-Newman, & Clark, 1991), participants were asked to respond to a question about life success using two types of 11-point scales (i.e., 0 to 10 vs. +5 to 5) with the anchors being kept constant (i.e., "not successful" to "extremely successful"). The researchers found that 34% of the participants endorsed a value between +5 and 5 whereas only 13% endorsed the equivalent values (i.e., between 0 and 5) in the 0–10 scale. It is noteworthy that pain clinicians adopt self-report scales that vary widely with respect to the metric used (e.g., 0–10, 1–5, 0–100) (von Baeyer & Hicks, 2000). Thus, it is difficult to compare pain levels reported by different patient populations. Additional factors such as content of adjacent scales and research affiliation of the researcher/clinician also affect responses to self-report scales (Schwartz, 1999; Strack, Schwartz, & Wanke, 1991). Chambers and colleagues have observed that self-report and proxy judgments of children's pain using the very popular faces scales vary systematically as a function of whether the lower end of the scale is anchored by a neutral face or a smiling face. When a smiling face is used, children tend to endorse faces indicating more severe pain (Chambers, Giesbrecht, Craig, McGrath, & Finley, 1999; Chambers & Craig, 2001). Thus, estimates of children's pain, and potentially the use of potent analgesics, is influenced by biases built into the scale. Greater effort should be devoted to developing accurate and useful self-report measures.

Nonverbal Communication. Hadjistavropoulos and Craig (2002) observed that nonverbal expressions of pain that do not fall in the self-report category are likely to be less subject to distortion than verbal report because their relatively more automatic and reflexive nature reduces their dependence on conscious processes and executive cognitive mediation. Nonverbal pain expression includes facial reactions, paralinguistic vocalizations, body and limb movements, visible physiological activity (e.g., muscle tension, sweating), and other nonverbal qualities of speech such as volume and timbre (Craig, Prkachin, & Grunau, 2001). These manifestations of pain always play an important role in pain communication, but become most vital where self-report is unavailable (e.g., in infants and persons with severe cognitive impairments).

Facial expression is recognized as being particularly important, because it plays a crucial role in normal social interchanges and can convey a remarkable amount of information. Faces are extremely plastic, tend to change rapidly, and can represent a dramatic range of states. The Facial Action Coding System (FACS; Ekman & Friesen, 1978) provides an atheoretical, anatomically based system designed for thorough description of facial movements that create facial expressions. A number of investigators have studied expressions of pain in adults of all ages (e.g., Craig et al., 2001; Hadjistavropoulos, LaChapelle, Hadjistavropoulos, Green, & Asmundson, 2002). Although some variability exists across individuals in identified features of the facial expression of pain, lowering of the brows, narrowing of the eyes, raising of the cheeks, blinking or closing of the eyes, raising the upper lip, dropping of the jaw, and parting of the lips are commonly found pain-related actions. This "fuzzy prototype" of a facial display appears relatively sensitive and specific to pain, accounting for its usefulness in clinical settings. There is much support for the argument that the display is relatively reflexive and automatic in nature. Evidence shows that there are real differences in the specific facial actions and their timing between spontaneous and faked displays of pain, and findings indicate that people cannot fully suppress facial reactions to painful physical insult. Some evidence indicates, for example, that observers can discriminate between genuine, suppressed, and exaggerated pain expressions (Hadjistavropoulos, Craig, Hadjistavropoulos, & Poole, 1996; Hill & Craig, 2002), although the number of false positives and false negatives presently is too high for application to the individual case (Hill & Craig, 2002). Training observers to attend to specific features of the facial expression can help improve accuracy rates (see Hill & Craig, in press).

Nonverbal behavior represents the only form of pain expression available for the assessment of pain in populations that do not have language available as a medium of communication. This is the case for infants and very young children, many children and adults with cognitive and serious psychological disabilities, people suffering traumatic brain damage, and seniors suffering from severe dementia. When the total number of people with communication impairments is considered, it represents a substantial proportion of the public at large (Hadjistavropoulos et al., 2001) and special consideration of their needs is required. This was recognized by the International Association for the Study of Pain in 2001 when it modified its widely endorsed definition of pain as "An unpleasant sensory and emotional experience associated with actual or potential tissue damage, or described in terms of such damage." It added the note, "The inability to communicate verbally in no way negates the possibility that an individual is experiencing pain and is in need of appropriate pain relieving treatment" (see http://www.iasp-pain.org/terms-p.html). The note reflects a concern for people who are unable to articulate their distress. Fortunately, people with communication limitations usually are quite capable of letting others know about their distress through nonverbal communication channels.

Nonverbal communication of pain has been explored substantially in young infants, who express distress primarily through cry, facial expression, and body and limb movements. Because the facial display appears the most sensitive and specific modality of nonverbal expression, the Neonatal Facial Coding System has been developed as a measure of infant pain (Craig, 1998; Grunau & Craig, 1987, 1990). The characteristic pattern of infant pain display includes lowered brows, eyes squeezed shut, opened mouth, and deepened nasolabial furrow (the fold that extends down and beyond the lip corners). Often these displays are accompanied by a taut cupped tongue that has also been associated with other stressful states (Grunau & Craig, 1990). Infant facial expressions of pain show a greater degree of consistency than do adult expressions, are central to adult judgments of infant pain, provide outcome measures for analgesic trials, and demonstrate long-term impact of severe neonatal pain (Craig et al., 2001).

Vocalizations, other than those with linguistic meaning, also are often present. Patients can scream, moan, or otherwise vocally express their distress when they are in pain. In infants, cry powerfully elicits parental attention from afar and effectively encodes the severity of distress, although the specific source of distress may not be readily identified (e.g., Craig, Gilbert-McLeod, & Lilley, 2000). Consequentially, parents usually seek other evidence, including the other behavioral signs noted earlier, and use contextual information (e.g., evidence of injury or knowledge about infant need states such as fatigue, hunger, etc.) in order to determine whether pain is present.

Other nonverbal pain signals are available (Keefe, Williams, & Smith, 2001). Various studies have examined the validity of a series of behaviors that are associated with pain (e.g., guarding, bracing, rubbing the affected area) (Keefe & Block, 1982), finding them to be valid indices of pain, including low back pain, osteoarthritis, and postoperative pain (e.g., Hadjistavropoulos, LaChapelle, Hadjistavropoulos, Green, & Asmundson, 2002; Hadjistavropoulos, LaChapelle, MacLeod, Snider, & Craig, 2000). Keefe and Block (1982) asked patients with low back pain to engage in a series of standardized activities (e.g., walking, standing, reclining) and validated an observational system designed to measure motor pain behaviors. The method showed concurrent validity and excellent reliability. This system, which has been used in a variety of studies (Keefe et al., 2001), has helped demonstrate the usefulness of nonverbal pain signals that are not limited to facial expressions.

Factors Affecting the Communication of Pain. A variety of social, psychological, and dispositional variables influence both the expression and experience of pain. Pain expression is often predicted better by psychological rather than physical or medical factors (e.g., Difede, Jaffe, Musngi, Perry, & Yurt, 1997). A perfect relationship between experience and expression would not be expected, as activation thresholds vary as a function of expressive modality, cognitive modulation of expression, and situational determinants. In fact, studies have shown that nonverbal pain expressions often do not correlate with self-report (Craig et al., 2001). Expression of pain can be extremely sensitive to contextual factors. Even the simple task of asking people to provide self-report measures of pain could draw attention to the pain state and exacerbate it. Alternatively, completing a questionnaire could be a distracting and palliating event. Several studies have confirmed the presence of reactive effects of measurement in studies of experimental pain, postoperative pain, and labor pain (Leventhal, Leventhal, Shacham, & Easterling, 1989; Mikail, VanDeursen, & von Baeyer, 1986), although one study of persistent pain (von Baeyer, 1994) failed to find an impact of self-report on the experience of pain.

Deliberate attempts to misrepresent whether one is in pain or not can affect both self-report and nonverbal expression. Incentives exist for deceiving others (e.g., to manipulate the emotions of others). Moreover, people may malinger because of financial incentives. Because these actions are inherently dishonest and detection could lead to shame or punishment, it is difficult to know how often they occur, but estimates are usually quite low (5%; Craig, Hill, & McMurtry, 1999). Perhaps more common are efforts to conceal pain for a variety of reasons, including the desire to conform to social ideals of stoicism, or the fear of the consequences of being diagnosed, such as loss of privileged positions, loss of independence, or exposure to fearsome drugs, dependency, or addiction.

Gender differences in pain expression are present from infancy (Guinsburg et al., 2000), before any learned reaction patterns could appear. This suggests the presence of constitutional differences in pain expression. Acculturation also has an impact on pain expression. Men are often socialized to downplay pain reports in order to meet social, religious and cultural expectations (Otto & Dougher, 1985). Fearon, McGrath, and Achat (1996) found that among school-age children and preschoolers, girls were much more likely to react to pain by crying, screaming, and displaying other signs of anger. Men who scored high on masculinity measures were found to display a higher pain tolerance (Otto & Dougher, 1985). Unruh (1996) has reported that females show increased emotional responses to pain compared to men. In a recent study, Keefe et al. (2000) found that women with osteoarthritis expressed more pain (both in a self-report measure and behaviorally) than men, but this sex difference was eliminated after controlling for catastrophizing. This mediating effect of catastrophizing was maintained even after controlling for levels of depression. The authors postulated that sex differences in catastrophizing may be a function of social learning. Some gender differences in the meaning of pain appear to exist. But there is also evidence in support of the presence of biological and hormonal mechanisms that could account for some of the gender differences in pain experience and expression (see Introduction, this volume). A variety of other intraindividual factors (e.g., beliefs) may also affect pain expressiveness (e.g., Manstead, 1991; Wagner, Lewis, Ramsey, & Krediet, 1992). Rollman considers cross-cultural influences in chapter 6 of this volume.

Relationships Between Self-Report and Nonverbal Indices of Pain. Given that nonverbal pain expression and self-report differ with respect to the extent to which they are subject to self-control, and represent different features of the complex pain reaction, it is not surprising that studies have varied in whether these separate measures of pain are correlated. A number of studies report nonsignificant correlations (Hadjistavropoulos, La-Chapelle, MacLeod, Hale, O'Rourke, & Craig, 1998; Hadjistavropoulos et al., 2002; LeResche & Dworkin, 1988; Prkachin, 1992), whereas others have reported significant correlations (e.g., Patrick, Craig, & Prkachin, 1986). Facial displays appear to best reflect the immediate onset of pain or exacerbations of pain. For example, Craig and Patrick (1985) observed that the most vigorous facial displays of pain occurred at the onset of immersion of the hand and forearm in ice cold water, and dissipated thereafter, whereas self-report of pain increased with time. Contextual factors are also likely crucial determinants of discrepancies between self-report and nonverbal displays of pain. Nonverbal expression taps the more immediate, reflexive aspects of the pain experience, whereas self-report measures can often be construed as retrospective and more likely to be affected by anticipation of consequences and social desirability (Craig et al., 2001). The neurophysiological systems responsible for self-report and nonverbal expression also appear to differ (Hadjistavropoulos & Craig, 2002). Self-report requires higher neocortical operations to control the executive cognitive functions engaged. In contrast, the reflexive, involuntary nature of nonverbal expression operates without intention and outside awareness. It is noteworthy that nonverbal measures of pain are less likely than self-report measures to be correlated with patient mood and depression (Green, Hadjistavropoulos, & LaChapelle, 2000).

Decoding Pain

The pain message has to be decoded and understood by observers if they are to provide care and assistance. There appear to be powerful inherent dispositions to attend and react emotionally to the distress of others, reflecting the adaptive evolutionary value of this sensitivity. However, specific understanding appears to require the ability to process information about the nature of the individual's distress. Relatively little is known about the specific mechanisms and processes that allow the integration of information and formation of judgments. The multiple cues available to trigger one's inferences or attributions of pain require the observer to be attentive, to appreciate their significance, to ignore irrelevant information, and to interpret information from the person in pain in the context of other salient, contextual information. The presence of injury or disease is often heavily weighted by clinicians, to the disadvantage of patients for whom there is no pathophysiological basis for their complaints (e.g., many patients with persistent back pain, fibromyalgia, or chronic fatigue). It is generally believed that self-report is more likely to reflect the subjective experience of pain. Clearly, it is methodologically more convenient. But observers tend to attach greater credibility to nonverbal expression and appear to have little difficulty integrating observations in order to decide the nature and severity of another person's distress and the credibility they should attach to the observation (Craig et al., 2001).

Stereotypes and Other Important Influences in the Decoding of Pain. There is considerable potential for some patients' individual characteristics, not related to the pain experience itself, to elicit erroneous judgments of pain. Hadjistavropoulos, Ross, and von Baeyer (1990) found that physicians were inclined to attribute lower levels of pain, distress, and need for help and higher ratings of health when people in pain were attractive rather than unattractive. Hadjistavropoulos, McMurtry, and Craig (1996) similarly found that the physically attractive and male patients were perceived as experiencing less pain intensity and disability than less attractive and female patients. Physically attractive patients were also perceived as being less likely to catastrophize and less likely to receive compensation than were unattractive patients. Finally, attractive patients were judged as being more likely to use cognitive and behavioral coping strategies than less attractive patients. These impressions were unrelated to actual patient functioning (as assessed using psychometrically valid instruments). The finding that men were viewed as having less pain and disability than women is especially interesting given that, in at least one study (Cleeland et al., 1994), women were found to be more likely to be undermedicated for pain than men. In another study, Hadjistavropoulos, LaChapelle, Hale, and MacLeod (2000) investigated observers' perceptions of patients who differed with respect to age and who were undergoing a painful medical procedure (after controlling for actual levels of patient pain expressiveness). The observers viewed the patients on film. Results showed that older and less physically attractive patients were perceived as experiencing more pain and having lower overall functioning.

The coping style of the patient may also interfere with the ability to make accurate judgments about pain and disability. For example, does the individual who reacts with stoicism to pain receive as much attention as another who reacts in a melodramatic fashion? MacLeod, LaChapelle, Hadjistavropoulos, and Pfeifer (2001) asked undergraduate students to make judgments about pain patients who claimed disability compensation. The patients were described in short fictitious vignettes that highlighted different approaches of coping with pain. Despite keeping the patients' self-reported level of pain constant across all vignettes, claimants who were described as catastrophizing or coping with pain largely by hoping for divine intervention were more likely than other claimants to be perceived as disabled and as deserving compensation. A further study (von Baeyer, Johnson, & Macmillan, 1984) was consistent with the proposition that vigorous complaints led to more sympathetic reactions. High nonverbal expressiveness yielded significantly higher ratings of patients' pain and distress, and observer concern. However, in another vignette study, Chibnall and Tait (1999) did not find any evidence that ethnicity (Caucasian vs. African American) affected symptom evaluations by employees of a university health center. Nonetheless, involvement of social psychological factors in judgments of pain make the task more complex than it might appear on the surface.

Actions to Assist Persons Who Are in Pain

Pain interventions stem directly from the observer's understanding of the patient's experience of pain. Compassionate observers can be expected to intervene. Family members and health care practitioners typically attempt to provide relief, although exceptions are inevitable. Family members might believe that the pain suffered by kin is desirable—for example, when necessary medical procedures are used, or when cultural or religious rituals are followed. The following examples illustrate special contexts in which pain communication assumes particular importance.

Pain Communication in Couples and Families. The onset of painful conditions, whether as a result of physical injury or disease, ordinarily provokes sympathy and support from family members. Usually, these conditions are self-limiting or responsive to treatment. Therefore, the length of time the sick role elicits responsive behavior from family members is limited. However, many people suffer from chronic pain, either recurrent or unremitting. In this case, special demands are made of family members who are unexpectedly committed to intense relationships with patients whose lives are often transformed by chronic pain. The relationship between the person in pain and the other family member has the potential to have an impact on both pain and pain-related disability.

The operant model of chronic pain emphasizes the potential of social reinforcement to perpetuate pain and disability (Block, Kremer, & Gaylor, 1980a; Fordyce, 1976). This model has been supported by studies that demonstrated a relationship between pain-relevant interactions, particularly solicitous attention from the spouse, and pain reports, pain behaviors frequency, and disability ratings (Kerns, Haythornthwaite, Southwick, & Giller, 1990; Kerns, Haythornthwaite, Rosenburg, Southwick, Giller, & Jacob, 1991; Flor, Kerns, & Turk, 1987; Flor, Turk, & Rudy, 1989; Romano et al., 1992; Turk, Kerns, & Rosenberg, 1992). For example, pain patients with spouses who are excessively solicitous may report considerably more pain when in the presence of the spouse than when in the presence of a neutral observer (Block, Kremer, & Gaylor, 1980b). Moreover, pain-contingent spousal responses have been found to reinforce overt expressions of pain in partners who have chronic pain conditions.

The operant model of chronic pain has been challenged by studies that demonstrate a much more complex interaction between spousal feedback and pain behavior. Though pain-contingent spousal responses have been found to reinforce overt expressions of pain in partners who have chronic pain condition, this seems to be mediated by attributions. Specifically, patients who made relationship-enhancing attributions about their spouse's behavior were less depressed than patients who made destructive attributions, even when responding negatively to the partner's pain (Weiss, 1996). For example, a chronic pain patient's perception of social support from spouses may moderate the pain experience and associated depression (Goldberg, Kerns, & Rosenburg, 1993). The perceived spousal support can act as a buffer and protect the person with chronic pain from depression.

Marital conflict in couples in which one suffers chronic pain is associated with increases in subsequent display of pain behaviors, which, in turn, are associated with greater negative affective responses and more punitive behaviors by the spouse (Schwartz, Slater, & Birchler, 1996). Punitive spouse behaviors were also associated with patient physical and psychosocial impairment. Conflict in the family and lack of social support in the workplace also contribute to increases in pain severity (Feuerstein et al., 1985). Lane and Hobfoll (1992) and Schwartz, Slater, Birchler, and Atkinson (1991) found that anger in patients with chronic pain adversely affects the mood of their spouse. Anger and hostility may affect the amount of spousal support given, which influences the adjustment to chronic pain (Burns, Johnson, Mahoney, Devine, & Pawl, 1996; Fernandez & Turk, 1995).

The type of social support (e.g., perceived vs. enacted) affects patient displays of pain. For example, Paulsen and Altmaier (1995) found that patients who reported higher levels of enacted spouse social support displayed a greater number of pain behaviors, regardless of whether the spouse was present, as compared to chronic pain patients who reported lower levels of enacted spousal support. When a measure of perceived support was utilized, the pain behavior displayed differed depending on spouse presence/absence and on the level of support.

Pain Communication and the Health Care System. Physician–patient communication is important for proper pain assessment and management (Feldt, Warne, & Ryden, 1998; McDonald & Sterling, 1998; Zalon, 1997). An estimated 42% of cancer patients do not get sufficient relief from pain, partly because of patient–physician communication barriers (Oliver, Kravitz, Kaplan, & Meyers, 2001). These barriers may include the patients not knowing their options and fear of addiction to drugs (Oliver et al., 2001). Older adults represent a further challenge to physician–patient communication regarding pain. For example, nearly half of a sample of older adults who were interviewed preoperatively indicated that they would not ask for analgesics, and only 13.3% planned on discussing their pain with health care providers (McDonald & Sterling, 1998). Improving patient communication can help eliminate some of these barriers. Older adults who participated in a communication training program reported less postoperative pain over the course of their hospital stay than older adults who were not trained in communication (McDonald, Freeland, Thomas, & Moore, 2001). Communication between patient and physician can be challenging when there are cultural and linguistic diversities (Johnson, Noble, Matthews, & Aguilar, 1999).

Persons With Limited Ability to Communicate. A large number of persons are affected by conditions that limit their ability to communicate pain (Hadjistavropoulos et al., 2001). This group includes persons with severe intellectual and neurological disabilities, persons who have sustained severe head injuries, and seniors in the advanced stages of dementia. This is a topic of great concern as self-report of pain tends to decrease as the level of cognitive impairment increases. This inverse relationship is maintained even after controlling for the number of health problems (Parmelee, Smith, & Katz, 1993). Moreover, physicians often miss pain problems among patients with severe neurological impairments (Sengstaken & King, 1993). The existing evidence suggests that such neurological impairments do not tend to spare sufferers from the vast array of pain-related conditions that could affect anyone (e.g., Proctor & Hirdes, 2001). There is also evidence that such persons may be more likely to die and develop serious health problems, partly due to pain problems going undetected because caretakers are often unable to appropriately decode pain messages (Biersdorff, 1991; Roy & Simon, 1987). Moreover, research suggests that seniors with dementia tend to be undertreated for pain problems as compared to their cognitively intact counterparts (Kaasalainen et al., 1998; Marzinski, 1991). Elderly persons suffering from dementia do not seem to differ with respect to pain thresholds from their cognitively intact age-related peers (Gibson, Voukelatos, Ames, Flicker, & Helme, 2001), although they may be less reliable in reporting these. Moreover, facial reactions to acute phasic pain do not vary as a function of cognitive status and do not correlate with intelligence quotients (Hadjistavropoulos et al., 1998; LaChapelle, Hadjistavropoulos, & Craig, 1999).

Recent work, based on systematic behavioral observation, has begun to address communication challenges with people with cognitive impairment (Breau, Camfield, McGrath, Rosmus, & Finley, 2000, 2001; Hadjistavropoulos, von Baeyer, & Craig, 2001). For example, seniors with dementia seem to display pain reactions (e.g., facial reactions, guarding) that are similar to seniors without cognitive impairments (Hadjistavropoulos et al., 1998; Hadjistavropoulos, LaChapelle, MacLeod, Snider, & Craig, 2000). LaChapelle et al. (1999) found that reaction to acute, phasic pain can be identified among young adults with severe intellectual disabilities using the Facial Action Coding System. Breau et al. (2000, 2001) validated a caregiver-administered checklist of pain behaviors suitable for persons with developmental disabilities. The checklist seems to be sensitive and specific to pain. That is, using the checklist, pain reactions can be discriminated from reactions to distressing but nonpainful events and calm, nonpainful event. More recently, Fuchs, Hadjistavropoulos, and McGrath (2002) and Fuchs and Hadjistavropoulos (2002) have developed a similar instrument for seniors with dementia and reported good initial psychometric properties. These studies taken together have begun to address serious decoding challenges and pave the way for more effective and thus more systematic treatment of pain among such persons.

CONCLUSIONS

This chapter provided an overview of important functions of pain communication within the context of a communications model of pain. Given that pain is a subjective and private experience, its communication is of vital importance both where systematic study and clinical care are involved. This places psychology, with its focus on behavioral expression and subjective states, in a very important position within the multidisciplinary study of pain.

Like any form of interpersonal communication, the communication of pain—and especially the self-report of pain—is subject to conscious distortion. Moreover, it is subject to contextual and social influences that affect both those producing the pain message and those trying to decode it. Findings that suggest pain messages are not perfectly consistent across communication modalities complicate this issue further, and indicate that clinicians and caretakers should give careful consideration to all modes of pain expression.

ACKNOWLEDGMENTS

The preparation of this chapter was supported in part by a Canadian Institutes of Health Research Investigator Award to Thomas Hadjistavropoulos and by a Canadian Institutes of Health Research Senior Investigator Award to Kenneth D. Craig. Direct correspondence to Thomas Hadjistavropoulos.

REFERENCES

Andrews, K., & Fitzgerald, M. (2002). Wound sensitivity as a measure of analgesic effects following surgery in human neonates and infants. *Pain, 99,* 185–196.

Asmundson, G. J. G., Norton, P. J., & Norton, G. R. (1999). Beyond pain: The role of fear and avoidance in chronicity. *Clinical Psychology Review, 19,* 97–119.

Bauchner, H. (1991). Procedures, pain and patients. *Pediatrics, 87,* 563–565.

Biersdorff, K. K. (1991). Incidence of significantly altered pain experience among individuals with developmental disabilities. *American Journal on Mental Retardation, 98,* 619–631.

Blackman, J. A. (2000). Crying in the child with a disability: The special challenge of crying as a signal. In R. G. Barr, B. Hopkins, & J. A. Green (Eds.), *Crying as a sign, a symptom & a signal* (pp. 106–120). London: MacKeith Press.

Blass, E. M., & Watt, L. (1999). Suckling and sucrose-induced analgesia in human newborns. *Pain, 83,* 611–623.

Block, A. R., Kremer, E. F., & Gaylor, M. (1980a). Behavioral treatment of chronic pain: Variable affecting treatment efficacy. *Pain, 8,* 367–371.

Block, A. R., Kremer, E. F., & Gaylor, M. (1980b). Behavioral treatment of chronic pain: The spouse as a discriminative cue for pain behavior. *Pain, 9,* 243–252.

Breau, L. M., Camfield, C., McGrath, P. J., Rosmus, C., & Finley, G. A. (2001). Measuring pain accurately in children with cognitive impairments: Refinement of a caregiver scale. *Journal of Pediatrics, 138,* 721–727.

Breau, L. M., McGrath, P. J., Camfield, C., Rosmus, C., & Finley, G. A. (2000). Preliminary validation of an observational pain checklist for cognitively impaired, non-verbal persons. *Developmental Medicine and Child Neurology, 42,* 609–616.

Burckhardt, C. S. (1985). The impact of arthritis on quality of life. *Nursing Research, 34,* 11–16.

Burns, J. W., Johnson, B. J., Mahoney, N., Devine, J., & Pawl, R. (1996). Anger management style, hostility and spouse responses: Gender difference in predictors of adjustment among chronic pain patients. *Pain, 64,* 445–453.

Casey, K. L., & Bushnell, M. C. (2000). *Pain imaging: Progress in pain research management* (Vol. 18). Seattle, WA: IASP Press.

Chambers, C. T., & Craig, K. D. (2001). Smiling face as anchor for pain intensity scales: Reply to D. Wong and C. Baker (letter to the editor concerning Chambers, C. T. et al. (1999). A comparison of faces scales for the measurement of pediatric pain: Children's and parents' ratings. *Pain, 83,* 25–35). *Pain, 89,* 297–300.

108   HADJISTAVROPOULOS, CRAIG, FUCHS-LACELLE

Chambers, C. T., Giesbrecht, K., Craig, K. D., Bennett, S. M., & Huntsman, E. (1999). A comparison of faces scales for the measurement of pediatric pain: Children's and parents' ratings. *Pain, 83*, 25–35.

Chambers, C. T., Reid, G. J., Craig, K. D., McGrath, P. J., & Finley, G. A. (1999). Agreement between child and parent reports of pain. *Clinical Journal of Pain, 14*, 336–342.

Champion, G. D., Goodenough, B., von Baeyer, C. L., & Thomas, W. (1998). Measurement of pain by self-report. In G. A. Finley & P. J. McGrath (Eds.), *Measurement of pain in infants and children* (pp. 123–160). Seattle, WA: IASP Press.

Chen, A. C. N., Niddam, D. M., Crawford, H. J., Oostenveld, R., & Arendt-Nielsen, L. (2002). Spatial summations of pain processing in the human brain as assessed by cerebral event related potentials. *Neuroscience Letters, 328*, 190–194.

Chibnall, J. T., & Tait, R. C. (1999). Social and medical influences on attributions and evaluations of chronic pain. *Psychology and Health, 14*, 719–729.

Cleeland, C., Gonin, R., Hatfield, A. K., Edmonson, J. H., Blum, R. H., Stewart, J. A., & Pandya, K. J. (1994). Pain and its treatment in outpatients with metastatic cancer. *New England Journal of Medicine, 330*, 592–596.

Craig, K. D. (1986). Social modelling influences: Pain in context. In R. A. Sternbach (Ed.), *The psychology of pain* (2nd ed., pp. 67–96). New York: Raven Press.

Craig, K. D. (1992). The facial expression of pain: Better than a thousand words? *American Pain Society Journal, 1*, 153–162.

Craig, K. D., Gilbert-McLeod, C. A., & Lilley, C. M. (2000). Cry as an indicator of pain in infants. In R. G. Barr, B. Hopkins, & J. Green (Eds.), *Crying as a signal, a sign, and a symptom* (pp. 23–40). London: MacKeith Press.

Craig, K. D., Hill, M. L., & McMurtry, B. (1999). Detecting deception and malingering. In A. R. Block, E. F. Kremer, & E. Fernandez (Eds.), *Handbook of chronic pain syndromes: Biopsychosocial perspectives* (pp. 41–58). Mahwah, NJ: Lawrence Erlbaum Associates.

Craig, K. D., Lilley, C. M., & Gilbert, C. A. (1996). Social barriers to optimal pain management in infants and children. *Clinical Journal of Pain, 12*, 232–242.

Craig, K. D., & Patrick, C. J. (1985). Facial expression during induced pain. *Journal of Personality and Social Psychology, 44*, 1080–1091.

Craig, K. D., Prkachin, K. M., & Grunau, R. V. E. (2001). The facial expression of pain. In D. C. Turk & R. Melzack (Eds.), *Handbook of pain assessment* (2nd ed., pp. 153–169). New York: Guilford Press.

Craig, K. D., & Weiss, S. M. (1975). Verbal reports of pain without noxious stimulation. *Perceptual and Motor Skills, 34*, 943–948.

Darwin, C. (1965). *The expression of emotions in man and animals.* Chicago: University of Chicago Press. (Original work published 1872)

Dennett, D. C. (1988). The intentional stance in theory and practice. In R. Byrne & A. Whiten (Eds.), *Machiavellian intelligence* (pp. 180–202). Oxford: Clarendon Press.

De Waal, F. (1988). Chimpanzee politics. In R. Byrne & A. Whiten (Eds.), *Machiavellian intelligence* (p. 123). Oxford: Clarendon Press.

Difede, J., Jaffe, A. B., Musngi, G., Perry, S., & Yurt, R. (1997). Determinants of pain expression in hospitalized burn patients. *Pain, 72*, 245–251.

Dworkin, S. F., & Chen, A. C. (1982). Pain in clinical and laboratory contexts. *Journal of Dental Research, 61*, 772–774.

Ekman, P., & Friesen, W. V. (1978). *Facial action coding system.* Palo Alto, CA: Consulting Psychologists Press.

Faucett, J. A., & Levine, J. D. (1991). The contributions of interpersonal conflict to chronic pain in the presence or absence of organic pathology. *Pain, 44*, 35–43.

Fearon, I., McGrath, P. J., & Achat, C. (1996). "Booboos": The study of everyday pain among young children. *Pain, 68*, 55–62.

Feldt, K., Warne, M., & Ryden, M. (1998). Examining pain in aggressive cognitively impaired older adults. *Journal of Gerontological Nursing, 24*, 14–22.

Fernandez, E., & Turk, D. C. (1995). The scope and significance of anger in the experience of chronic pain. *Pain, 61*, 165–175.

Feuerstein, M., Sult, S., & Houle, M. (1985). Environmental stressors and chronic low back pain: Life events, family and work environment. *Pain, 22*, 295–307.

Fiore, J., Becker, J., & Coppel, D. (1983). Social network interactions: A buffer or a stress. *American Journal of Community Psychology, 11*, 423–439.

Flor, H., Kerns, R. D., & Turk, D. C. (1987). The role of spouse reinforcement, perceived pain, and activity levels of chronic pain patient. *Journal of Psychosomatic Research, 31*, 251–259.

Flor, H., Turk, D. C., & Rudy, T. E. (1989). Relationship of pain impact and significant other reinforcement of pain behaviors: The mediating role of gender, marital status and marital satisfaction. *Pain, 38*, 45–50.

Fordyce, W. E. (1976). *Behavioral methods for chronic pain and illness.* St. Louis, MO: C. V. Mosby.

Frank, A. J., Moll, J. M., & Hort, J. F. (1982). A comparison of three ways of measuring pain. *Rheumatology Rehabilitation, 21*, 211–217.

Fridlund, A. J. (1994). *Human facial expressions: An evolutionary view.* San Diego, CA: Academic Press.

Fuchs, S., & Hadjistavropoulos, T. (2002). Validation of a pain assessment scale for seniors with severe dementia. In *Aging and society: Taking charge of the future, Official program book of the 31st Annual Scientific and Educational Meeting of the Canadian Association on Gerontology* (p. 79). Ottawa: Canadian Association on Gerontology.

Fuchs, S., Hadjistavropoulos, T., & McGrath, P. J. (2002). Psychometric development of a pain assessment scale for older adults with severe dementia: A report on the first two studies. *Abstracts, 10th World Congress on Pain* (p. 559). Seattle, WA: IASP Press.

Gibson, S. J., Voukelatos, X., Ames, D., Flicker, L., & Helme R. D. (2001). An examination of pain perception and cerebral event-related potentials following carbon dioxide laser stimulation in patients with Alzheimer's disease and age-matched control volunteers. *Pain Research Management, 6*, 126–132.

Glucklich, A. (2000). *Sacred pain.* Oxford: Oxford University Press.

Goldberg, G. M., Kerns, R. D., & Rosenberg, R. (1993). Pain-relevant support as a buffer from depression among chronic pain patients low in instrumental activity. *Clinical Journal of Pain, 9*, 34–40.

Green, S. M., Hadjistavropoulos, T., & LaChapelle, D. (2000). Using behavioral and self-report measures to assess pain in seniors. *Pain Research and Management, 5*(Suppl. A, abstr. 95).

Grunau, R. V. E., & Craig, K. D. (1987). Pain expression in neonates: Facial action and cry. *Pain, 28*, 395–410.

Grunau, R. V. E., & Craig, K. D. (1990). Facial activity as a measure of neonatal pain perception. In D. C. Tyler & E. J. Krane (Eds.), *Advances in pain research and therapy. Proceedings of the 1st International Symposium on Pediatric Pain* (pp. 147–155). New York: Raven Press.

Guinsburg, R., de Araujo Peres, C., Branco de Almeida, M. F., de Cassia Xavier Balda, R., Cassia Berenguel, R., Tonelotto, J., & Kopelman, B. I. (2000). Differences in pain expression between male and female newborn infants. *Pain, 85*, 127–133.

Hadjistavropoulos, H. D., Craig, K. D., Hadjistavropoulos, T., & Poole, G. (1996). Subjective judgments of deception in pain expression: Accuracy and errors. *Pain, 65*, 251–258.

Hadjistavropoulos, H. D., Ross, M., & von Baeyer, C. (1990). Are physicians' ratings of pain affected by patients' physical attractiveness? *Social Science and Medicine, 31*, 69–72.

Hadjistavropoulos, T., & Craig, K. D. (2002). A theoretical framework for understanding self-report and observational measures of pain: A communications model. *Behavior Research and Therapy, 40*, 551–570.

Hadjistavropoulos, T., LaChapelle, D., Hadjistavropoulos, H. D., Green, S., & Asmundson, G. J. G. (2002). Using facial expressions to assess musculoskeletal pain in older persons. *European Journal of Pain, 6*, 179–187.

Hadjistavropoulos, T., LaChapelle, D., Hale, C., & MacLeod, F. K. (2000). Age- and appearance-related stereotypes about patients undergoing a painful medical procedure. *Pain Clinic, 12,* 25–33.

Hadjistavropoulos, T., LaChapelle, D., MacLeod, F., Hale, C., O'Rourke, N., & Craig, K. D. (1998). Cognitive functioning and pain reactions in hospitalized elders. *Pain Research and Management, 3,* 145–151.

Hadjistavropoulos, T., LaChapelle, D., MacLeod, F. K., Snider, B., & Craig, K. D. (2000). Measuring movement exacerbated pain in cognitively impaired frail elders. *Clinical Journal of Pain, 16,* 54–63.

Hadjistavropoulos, T., McMurtry, B., & Craig, K. D. (1996). Beautiful faces in pain: Biases and accuracy in the perception of pain. *Psychology and Health, 11,* 411–420.

Hadjistavropoulos, T., von Baeyer, C., & Craig, K. D. (2001). Pain assessment in persons with limited ability to communicate. In D. C. Turk & R. Melzack (Eds.), *Handbook of pain assessment* (2nd ed., pp. 134–149). New York: Guilford Press.

Hill, M., & Craig, K. D. (2002). Detecting deception in pain expressions: The structure of genuine and deceptive facial displays. *Pain, 98,* 135–144.

Hill, M., & Craig, K. D. (in press). Detecting voluntary misrepresentation in facial expression. In P. Firestone & W. L. Marshall (Eds.), *Pain in infants, children and adolescents* (2nd ed.). Baltimore: Williams & Wilkins.

Johnson, M., Noble, C., Matthews, C., & Aguilar, N. (1999). Bilingual communicators within the health care setting. *Qualitative Health Research, 9,* 329–343.

Johnston, C. C., Stremler, R. L., Stevens, B. J., & Horton, L. J. (1997). Effectiveness of oral sucrose and simulated rocking on pain response in preterm neonates. *Pain, 72,* 193–199.

Kaasalainen, S., Middleton, J., Knezacek, S., Hartely, T., Stewart, N., Ife, C., & Robinson, L. (1998). Pain and cognitive status in the institutionalized elderly: Perceptions and interventions. *Journal of Gerontological Nursing, 24,* 24–31.

Keefe, F. J., & Block, A. R. (1982). Development of an observation method for assessing pain behavior in chronic low back pain patients. *Behavior Therapy, 13,* 363–375.

Keefe, F. J., Lefebvre, J. C., Egert, J. R., Affleck, G., Sullivan, M., & Caldwell, D. (2000). The relationship of gender to pain, pain behavior and disability in osteoarthritis patients: The role of catastrophizing. *Pain, 87,* 325–334.

Keefe, F. J., Williams, D. A., & Smith, S. J. (2001). Assessment of pain behaviors. In D. C. Turk & R. Melzack (Eds.), *Handbook of pain assessment* (2nd ed., pp. 170–187). New York: Guilford Press.

Kerns, R. D., Haythornthwaite, J., Rosenberg, R., Southwick, S., Giller, E. L., & Jacob, M. C. (1991). The Pain Behavior Check List (PBCL): Factor structure and psychometric properties. *Journal of Behavioral Medicine, 14,* 155–167.

Kerns, R. D., Haythornthwaite, J., Southwick, S., & Giller, E. L., Jr. (1990). The role of marital interaction in chronic pain and depressive symptom severity. *Journal of Psychosomatic Research, 34,* 401–408.

Kerns, R. D., & Turk, D. (1987). Depression and chronic pain: The mediating role of the spouse. *Journal of Marriage and Family, 46,* 845–852.

Kosambi, D. D. (1967). Living prehistory in India. *Scientific American, 216,* 105–114.

LaChapelle, D., Hadjistavropoulos, T., & Craig, K. D. (1999). Pain measurement in persons with intellectual disabilities. *Clinical Journal of Pain, 15,* 13–23.

Lander, J. (1990). Clinical judgements in pain management. *Pain, 42,* 15–22.

Lane, C., & Hobfoll, S. E. (1992). How loss affects anger and alienates potential supporters. *Journal of Consulting and Clinical Psychology, 60,* 935–942.

LeResche, L., & Dworkin, S. (1988). Facial expressions of pain and emotion in chronic TMD patients. *Pain, 35,* 71–78.

Leventhal, E. A., Leventhal, H., Shacham, S., & Easterling, D. V. (1989). Active coping reduces reports of pain from childbirth. *Journal of Consulting and Clinical Psychology, 57,* 365–371.

Levine, F. M., & De Simon, L. L. (1991). The effects of experimenter gender on pain report in male and female subjects. *Pain, 44,* 69–72.

MacLeod, F., LaChapelle, D. L., Hadjistavropoulos, T., & Pfeifer, J. E. (2002). The effect of disability claimants' coping styles on judgements of pain, disability and compensation: A vignette study. *Rehabilitation Psychology, 46,* 417–435.

Manstead, A. S. R. (1991). Expressiveness as an individual difference. In R. B. Feldman & B. Rime (Eds.), *Fundamental of nonverbal behavior: Studies in emotion and social interaction* (pp. 285–328). New York: Cambridge University Press.

Marzinski, L. R. (1991). The tragedy of dementia: Clinically assessing pain in the confused, nonverbal elderly. *Journal of Gerontological Nursing, 17,* 25–28.

McDonald, D. D., Freeland, M., Thomas, G., & Moore, J. (2001). Testing a preoperative pain management intervention for elders. *Research in Nursing & Health, 24,* 402–409.

McDonald, D., & Sterling, R. (1998). Acute pain reduction strategies used by well older adults. *International Journal of Nursing Studies, 35,* 265–270.

Melzack, R., & Wall, P. D. (1965). Pain mechanisms: A new theory. *Science, 50,* 971–979.

Mikail, R., VanDeursen, J., & von Baeyer, C. L. (1986). Rating pain or rating serenity: Effects of cold pressor pain tolerance. *Canadian Journal of Behavioral Science, 18,* 126–132.

Murray, A. D. (1979). Infant crying as an elictor of parental behavior: An examination of two models. *Psychological Bulletin, 86,* 191–215.

Murphy, S., Creed, F., & Jayson, M. (1988). Psychiatric disorders and illness behavior in rheumatoid arthritis. *British Journal of Rheumatology, 27,* 357–363.

Oliver, J. W., Kravitz, R. L., Kaplan, S. H., & Meyers, F. J. (2001). Individualized patient education and coaching to improve pain control among cancer outpatients. *Journal of Clinical Oncology, 15,* 2206–2212.

Otto, M. W., & Dougher, M. J. (1985). Sex differences and personality factors in responsivity to pain. *Perceptual and Motor Skills, 61,* 383–390.

Parmelee, P. A., Smith, B., & Katz, I. R. (1993). Pain complaints and cognitive status among elderly institution residents. *Journal of the American Geriatrics Society, 41,* 517–522.

Patrick, C. M., Craig, K. D., & Prkachin, K. M. (1986). Observer judgments of acute pain: Facial action determinants. *Journal of Personality and Social Psychology, 50,* 1291–1298.

Paulsen, J. S., & Altmaier, E. M. (1995). The effects of perceived versus enacted social support on the discriminative cue function of spouses for pain behaviors. *Pain, 60,* 103–110.

Prkachin, K. M. (1992). The consistency of facial expressions of pain: A comparison across modalities. *Pain, 51,* 297–306.

Prkachin, K. M., & Craig, K. D. (1995). Expressing pain: The communication and interpretation of facial pain signals. *Journal of Nonverbal Behavior, 19,* 191–205.

Proctor, W. R., & Hirdes, J. P. (2001). Pain and cognitive status among nursing home residents in Canada. *Pain Research and Management, 6,* 119–125.

Romano, J. M., Turner, J. A., Friedman, L. S., Bulcroft, R. A., Jensne, M. P., Hops, H., & Wright, S. F. (1992). Sequential analysis of chronic pain behaviors and spouse responses. *Journal of Consulting and Clinical Psychology, 60,* 777–782.

Rosenthal, R. (1982). Conducting judgement studies. In K. Scherer & D. Ekman (Eds.), *Handbook of methods in nonverbal behavior research* (pp. 287–361). New York: Cambridge University Press.

Roy, A., & Simon, G. B. (1987). Intestinal obstruction as a cause of death in the mentally handicapped. *Journal of Mental Deficiency Research, 31,* 193–197.

Schultz, R., & Decker, S. (1985). Long-term adjustment to physical disability: The role of social support, perceived control, and self-blame. *Journal of Personality and Social Psychology, 48,* 1162–1172.

Schwartz, N. (1999). Self-reports: How the questions shape the answers. *American Psychologist, 54,* 93–105.

Schwartz, N., Knauper, B., Hippler, H. J., Noelle-Neuman, E., & Clark, F. (1991). Rating scales: Numeric values may change the meaning of scale labels. *Public Opinion Quarterly, 55,* 570–582.

Schwartz, L., Slater, M. A., & Birchler, B. (1996). The role of pain behaviors in the modulation of marital conflict in chronic pain couples. *Pain, 65,* 227–233.

Schwartz, L., Slater, M. A., Birchler, G. R., & Atkinson, J. H. (1991). Depression in spouses of chronic pain patients: The role of patient pain and anger, and marital satisfaction. *Pain, 44,* 61–67.

Sengstaken, E., & King, S. (1993). The problems of pain and its detection among geriatric nursing home residents. *Journal of the American Geriatrics Society, 41,* 541–544.

Sternbach, R. A. (1968). *Pain: A psychophysiological analysis.* New York: Academic Press.

Strack, F., Schwartz, N., & Wanke, M. (1991). Semantic and pragmatic aspects of context effects in social and psychological research. *Social Cognition, 9,* 111–125.

Turk, D. C., Kerns, R. D., & Rosenberg, R. (1992). Effects of marital interaction on chronic pain and disability: Examining the down side of social support. *Rehabilitation Psychology, 37,* 259–274.

Turner, R. J., & Noh, S. (1988). Physical disability and depression: A longitudinal analysis. *Journal of Health and Social Behavior, 29,* 23–37.

Unruh, A. M. (1996). Gender variations in clinical pain experience. *Pain, 65,* 123–167.

von Baeyer, C. L. (1994). Social and pain behavior in the first three minutes of a pain clinic medical interview. *Pain Clinic, 7*(3), 169–177.

von Baeyer, C. L., & Hicks, C. L. (2000). Support for a common metric for pediatric pain intensity scales. *Pain Research and Management, 5,* 157–160.

von Baeyer, C. L., Johnson, M. E., & MacMillan, M. J. (1984). Consequences of nonverbal expression of pain: Patient distress and observer concern. *Social Science & Medicine, 19,* 1319–1324.

Wagner, H. L., Lewis, H., Ramsay, S., & Krediet, I. (1992). Prediction of facial displays from knowledge of norms of emotional expressiveness. *Motivation and Emotion, 16,* 347–362.

Walker, L. (1999). The evolution of research on recurrent abdominal pain: History, assumptions, and a conceptual model. In P. J. McGrath & G. A. Finley (Eds.), *Chronic and recurrent pain in children and adolescents* (pp. 141–172). Seattle, WA: IASP Press.

Weiss, L. H. (1996). From a cognitive-behavioral perspective an examination of pain-relevant marital communication in chronic pain patients. *Dissertation Abstracts International: Section B: Sciences & Engineering, 56,* 4596.

Zalon, M. (1997). Pain in frail, elderly women after surgery. *Image: Journal of Nursing Scholarship, 29,* 21–26.

Pain Over the Life Span:
A Developmental Perspective

Stephen J. Gibson
National Ageing Research Institute, Parkville,
and Department of Medicine, University of Melbourne

Christine T. Chambers
Department of Pediatrics, University of British Columbia,
and Centre for Community Child Health Research, Vancouver

Pain is a complex phenomenon that consists of interacting biological, psychological, and social components (Merskey & Bogduk, 1994). For many years, the study of pain was focused primarily on young and middle-aged adult populations; however, as research in the area of pain expanded, so did consideration of the importance of developmental factors in pain experience and expression, including pain in infants, children, and seniors. Life-span developmental psychology involves the study of constancy and change in behavior through the life course (Baltes, 1987). This approach can be helpful in gaining knowledge about the pain experience across the life span and furthering understanding about interindividual differences and similarity in pain responses.

The present chapter provides a broad overview of developmental perspectives in pain across various life stages, including infancy, childhood, adolescence, adulthood, and seniors. Research pertaining to age differences in pain experience and report and psychosocial and physiological factors that impact on pain for each of these developmental periods are reviewed. Further, developmental factors that relate to pain assessment and management are discussed. An appreciation of the unique challenges faced by individuals at various stages of life is critical to furthering understanding about the developmental progression of pain across the life span.

INTRODUCTION TO CHILDHOOD SEGMENTS
OF THE LIFE SPAN

For the purposes of this chapter, child development is segmented into the following periods (Berk, 2000):

1. Infancy and toddlerhood (from birth to 2 years). This period is characterized by dramatic changes to the body and brain and the emergence of a wide array of cognitive capacities, including language and the capability to engage in social relationships with others.
2. Early to middle childhood (3 to 11 years). These years are characterized by further refinements in motor skills and cognitive functioning. Advances in understanding of the self and others are evident during this phase.
3. Adolescence (from 11 to 18 years). These years form the bridge between childhood and adulthood. Cognitive abilities become more abstract and puberty leads to physical and sexual maturity.

A broad spectrum of pain experiences is evident across these developmental periods. Throughout the sections that follow, the terms *children* or *childhood* are used to refer to the entire range from 0 to 18 years and particular developmental periods are specified as appropriate.

Age Differences in Pain Experience
and Report During Childhood

In comparison to the extensive literature among adult populations, little is known about the epidemiology of pain in children and adolescents (Goodman & McGrath, 1991). Investigations of pain prevalence have traditionally focused on specific pain conditions restricted to particular developmental periods, rather than providing a more comprehensive description of pain problems across childhood. Headache is the pain condition among children that has been most broadly explored (Goodman & McGrath, 1991), with prevalence rates ranging anywhere from 2% (Bille, 1962) to 27% (Abu-Arefeh & Russell, 1994), depending on the type of diagnostic criteria used and the age and gender of the child. Prevalence of headache generally increases with age of the child, and higher prevalence rates are frequently reported for girls as compared to boys (Andrasik, Holroyd, & Abell, 1980; Bille, 1962; Linet, Stewart, Celentano, Ziegler, & Sprecher, 1989).

Other pain conditions commonly reported in childhood include recurrent abdominal pain (Apley & Naish, 1958), recurrent limb pain (Naish & Apley, 1951), and back pain (Balaque, Dutoit, & Waldburger, 1988; Taimela,

Kujala, Salminen, & Viljanen, 1997). It appears that recurrent abdominal pain peaks in prevalence among children aged 5–6 years (with an estimated prevalence of 25%) (Faull & Nicol, 1985), but declines with age from that point on (Davison, Faull, & Nicol, 1986). Limb pain and back pain, on the other hand, have been more commonly reported among older children and adolescents.

A recent study by Perquin, Hazebroek-Kampschreur, Hunfeld, Bohnen, van Suijlekom-Smit, Passchier, and van der Wouden (2000) provided a comprehensive examination of pain prevalence among a sample of 5,424 Dutch children aged 0 to 18 years. A questionnaire regarding pain experiences in the previous 3 months was completed by either the parents (for children aged 0 to 7 years) or the children themselves (for ages 8 to 18 years). Results of this survey indicated that pain was a common experience for children, with 54% of respondents reporting pain within the previous 3 months and 25% of respondents reporting a recurrent or continuous pain that had persisted for more than 3 months. The results of this study also indicated that the prevalence of pain increased with age. For example, chronic pain was reported among 11.8% of 0–3-year-olds, 19.3% of 4–7-year-olds, 23.7% of 8–11-year-olds, 35.7% of 12–15-year-olds, and 31.2% of 16–18-year-olds. Gender differences in pain reports also varied as a function of the age of the child, with girls reporting more pain than boys in all age groups but the youngest (0–3 years). Gender differences were particularly marked among 12- to 18-year-olds, with girls reporting a pain prevalence that was approximately twice that of boys. The most commonly reported pains by children were headache (23%), abdominal pain (22%), and limb pain (22%). Recurrent abdominal pain was most prevalent among children up to age 8, whereas limb and head pains were more common among children aged 8 years and older. Multiple pains were reported by more than half of the children, with the prevalence of multiple pains increasing with child age. The results of this study clearly indicate that chronic pain is a common experience among children and provides important information regarding age-related patterns of pain prevalence in a pediatric sample.

There has been a dearth of epidemiological research documenting patterns of pain prevalence from childhood into adulthood. As a result, conclusions regarding how the pain experiences of children and adolescents compare to those of adults are limited. A study by Blyth and colleagues (2001) examined chronic pain prevalence among a sample of 17,543 Australian individuals. The study focused primarily on the pain experiences of adults up to the age of 84 years; however, the youngest age group included in the study was a group of adolescents aged 15 to 19 years. Results of the study indicated that, overall, chronic pain was reported by approximately 17% of males and 20% of females. Prevalence of pain was lowest among the adolescent group, with less than 10% of males and approximately 12% of females aged 15 to 19 years reporting chronic pain. Pain prevalence increased steadily until a peak of 27% among 65–69-year-old males and 31% among 80–84-year-old females. The adolescent group contained a relatively small number of respondents suggesting caution, but this research does provide preliminary data regarding the continuum of pain experiences from adolescence into adulthood.

In addition to documenting pain prevalence among children, researchers have begun to explore pain-related disability among children and adolescents (Palermo, 2000). Compared to research conducted in this area among adults, specific data regarding the impact of pain on children's lives is scant. However, it is presumed that pain results in disruptions in school functioning, peer and social functioning, sleep disturbance, parental burden, and burden on the health care system (Palermo, 2000). Initial attempts to document pain-related disability among school-aged children and adolescents have failed to reveal any age-related differences (Walker & Greene, 1991). Research documenting physician consultation and medication use among children and adolescents aged 0 to 18 years experiencing chronic pain has revealed that parents of children aged 0 to 3 years were the most likely to consult a physician and use medication for pain in their children (Perquin, Hazebroek-Kampschreur, Hunfeld, van Suijlekom-Smit, Passchier, & van der Wouden, 2000). The authors indicate that this finding could be explained by anxiety or inexperience on the part of parents, rather than being indicative of higher levels of pain-related interference or disability among this age group (Perquin, Hazebroek-Kampschreur, Hunfeld, van Suijlekom-Smit, Passchier, & van der Wouden, 2000). Interestingly, the study by Blyth et al. (2001) found that although the prevalence of pain was lowest among the adolescents aged 15 to 19 years in their sample, interference of daily activities caused by pain was highest in this group. Future research is needed to document and explore age-related differences in interference and disability due to pain in children.

Beyond the realm of chronic pain in children, considerable research has examined developmental differences in children's responses to acute stimuli, such as medical procedures. For many years, it was believed that infants did not feel or remember pain that resulted from procedures (Schechter, 1989). These myths frequently led to substandard pain management for young children (Craig, Lilley, & Gilbert, 1996). However, advances in our ability to assess pain in infants have led to the acknowledgment that infants are indeed capable of experiencing pain from birth onwards (Stevens & Franck, 2001). Although infants are not capable of providing a self-report of their pain, substantial empirical evidence collected over the last 20 years supports that infants do show an acute pain response through both behavioral (e.g., facial activity, cry, gross motor movement) and physiological (e.g., heart rate, palmar sweating) means (Anand, Sippell, & Aynsley-Green, 1987; Stevens, Johnston, & Gibbins, 2000). Remarkable changes in all areas of functioning are evident during the first 2 years of life known as infancy and toddlerhood. Developmental changes in children's acute pain responses during this period have also been explored. Using measures of facial expression and cry, Lewis and Thomas (1990) found that 6-month-old infants quieted more quickly than did 2- or 4-month-olds following routine immunization injections. Similar studies have found that infants under 4 months of age evidenced a longer duration of pain responses (measured by facial expression, cry, and body movement) compared to infants over 4 months of age (Maikler, 1991) and that infants under 12 months of age showed more generalized responses to pain following immunization whereas infants aged 13–24 months demonstrated more coordinated, goal-directed behavior in response to pain (Craig, Hadjistavropoulos, Grunau, & Whitfield, 1994).

A study conducted by Lilley, Craig, and Grunau (1997) examined age-related changes in facial expression of pain during routine immunization over the first 18 months of life (2-, 4-, 6-, 12-, and 18-month age groups). Although there were some age-related differences in the magnitude of the infants' pain reactions, there was remarkable continuity in the infants' pain expression. Johnston, Stevens, Craig, and Grunau (1993) conducted the only study examining age-related changes in pain expression to include a comparison group of premature infants. They compared the pain responses (measured by cry and facial expression) of premature infants undergoing heel stick, full-term infants receiving an intramuscular injection, and 2- and 4-month-old infants receiving subcutaneous injection. Results showed that all groups of children displayed a pain response; however, the premature infants' ability to communicate pain via facial actions was not as well developed as in the full-term children. Additional research has suggested that age differences in infant pain responses are linked to social context and parenting style (Sweet, McGrath, & Symons, 1999).

In brief, research examining age-related changes in children's pain expression within the infancy and toddler period indicates that these children demonstrate a pain response. Although some modes of pain expression may not be fully formed in preterm infants (e.g., facial activity), there is considerable consistency in pain responses evidenced from birth to 18 months of age. However, age-related changes in children's abilities to suppress or control their pain expression do appear to emerge over this developmental period. Unfortunately, in part due to issues related to the complexities of measuring pain in a uniform way across developmental periods, no research has compared the intensity and quality of infants' acute pain experiences to those of older children and adolescents.

Research has explored age-related differences in older children's pain experiences using both behavioral measures and self-reports of pain. Two early laboratory-based studies examined pain threshold in children using pressure pain (Haslam, 1969) and pinpoint heat stimulus (Schludermann & Zubek, 1962). The study by Haslam (1969) explored pain perception in children aged 5 to 18 years, whereas the study by Schludermann and Zubek (1962) compared a sample of adolescents aged 12 years and up to a sample of adults up to the age of 83 years. Haslam (1969) reported that children's pain threshold increased between the ages of 5 and 18 years. Similarly, Schuldermann and Zubek (1962) reported increased levels of pain threshold from adolescence through to adulthood. These findings would indicate that sensitivity to acute pain appears to decline with age; however, it is noted that the measures used in this research may confound pain experience and pain expression and that the results of this research should be viewed as suggestive rather than conclusive.

Research examining children's distress behaviors in response to painful medical procedures has typically shown that young children exhibit more distress behaviors than older children (Jay, Ozolins, Elliott, & Caldwell, 1983; Katz, Kellerman, & Siegel, 1980). For example, Katz and colleagues examined behavioral distress among a sample of 115 children with cancer, aged 8 months to 18 years, undergoing painful medical procedures. A significant relationship was found between age and quantity and type of anxious behavior, with younger children showing a greater variety of anxious behaviors over a longer period of time than older children. However, research using behavioral measures more specific to pain has failed to confirm the presence of age-related differences in children's longer term, postoperative pain expression (Chambers, Reid, McGrath, & Finley, 1996).

Older children are capable of using validated measures to provide self-reports of pain and there currently exist a number of tools designed to elicit self-reports from children (Champion, Goodenough, von Baeyer, & Thomas, 1998). Using these measures, there are well-documented findings indicating that younger children report more pain from medical procedures (e.g., venipuncture, immunization) than older children (Arts et al., 1994; Fowler-Kerry & Lander, 1987; Fradet, McGrath, Kay, Adams, & Luke, 1990; Lander & Fowler-Kerry, 1991; Manne, Redd, Jacobsen, Gorfinkle, & Schorr, 1990; Palermo & Drotar, 1996). For example, a study by Goodenough and colleagues (1997) compared needle pain ratings of children aged 3 to 7 years, 8 to 11 years, and 12 to 17 years. Results confirmed that younger children gave significantly higher ratings of pain severity than did older children. Additional research by this group has indicated that age effects in children's self-reports of pain are predominantly manifested in ratings of sensory intensity, rather than its affective qualities (Goodenough et al., 1999).

A few studies have provided observational assessments of children's "everyday" pain experiences outside of the clinical realm (Fearon, McGrath, & Achat, 1996; von Baeyer, Baskerville, & McGrath, 1998). Results of this research have indicated that young children experience an "everyday" pain event (e.g., falling down and hurting themselves) approximately once every 3 hours (Fearon et al., 1996; von Baeyer et al., 1998). Using a sample of children aged 3 to 7 years, this research has failed to establish any age-related differences in children's intensity or duration of pain responses, although increasing age was found to be associated with decreasing help-seeking behaviors as a result of pain (Fearon et al., 1996).

Discordance among multiple measures of acute pain in children is not uncommon (Beyer, McGrath, & Berde, 1990), with recent research demonstrating age-related differences in the relationships among different measures of pain in children. Goodenough, Champion, Laubreaux, Tabah, and Kampel (1998) reported that correlations between behavioral and self-report measures were strongest for the 3–7-year-olds in their sample and weakest for the 12–17-year-olds. Evidence from research based on both behavioral and self-report measures appears to indicate that younger children express and report more pain than older children and adolescents, who are occasionally included in these studies.

In summary, data regarding age-related patterns in both chronic pain and acute pain experiences of children are available. Although conclusions regarding age-related differences are sometimes limited due to restrictions in the age range examined, the evidence generally supports that, as children grow older, prevalence of chronic pain increases. Conversely, research examining acute pain reactions indicates that increasing child age is associated with decreased pain and distress. To date, no research has explored potential mechanisms that might account for these contrasting patterns; however, it is likely that various complex psychological (e.g., coping strategies), social (e.g., family influence), and biological factors (e.g., pubertal status) interact to contribute to these findings. Research examining the developmental progression of pain experiences and pain-related disability across childhood and into adulthood is needed.

Psychosocial Influences on the Experience and Expression of Pain During Childhood

McGrath (1994) described a model depicting psychosocial factors that affect a child's pain perception. The model includes consideration of cognitive, behavioral/social, and emotional factors. Individual child characteristics, including age, are thought to be related to each of these factors, which in turn can influence children's pain experiences (McGrath, 1994).

Although additional research is needed to provide empirical evidence supporting certain components of this model, it is useful in the consideration of a broad range of psychosocial factors that could be related to children's pain.

Cognitive factors include children's understanding of the cause of their pain, expectations regarding continuing pain and treatment efficacy, the relevance or meaning of the pain, and coping strategies (McGrath, 1994). Considerable research has examined children's concepts of general illness from a developmental perspective (Bibace & Walsh, 1980; Burbach & Peterson, 1986), with most data suggesting that children's concepts of illness evolve in a systematic, age-related sequence, consistent with Piagetian theory of cognitive development. Far less research has examined the developmental course of children's specific understanding of pain. Harbeck and Peterson (1992) found, among a sample of children and youth aged 3 to 23 years, that older children and youth had more complex and precise understandings of pain than younger children. For example, children in the preoperational stage of development were unlikely to be able to offer an explanation for the value of pain, whereas children in the formal operations stage were able to acknowledge that pain often carries a preventative or diagnostic value (Harbeck & Peterson, 1992). Ability to understand the cause and value of pain is likely related to pain perception, although no research has explored the links between children's understanding of pain and subsequent pain responses. Research has also confirmed the presence of age-related differences in children's predictions of pain intensity, with younger children making less accurate predictions than older children (von Baeyer, Carlson, & Webb, 1997).

Children's coping strategies for dealing with pain are an area that has received considerable research attention (Bennett-Branson & Craig, 1993; Reid, Gilbert, & McGrath, 1998). Reid and colleagues (1998) detailed the development of a measure of pain coping in children that assessed coping in three broad areas: approach (e.g., information seeking, seeking social support), problem-focused avoidance (e.g., behavioral distraction, cognitive distraction), and emotion-focused avoidance (e.g., internalizing, catastrophizing). Use of this measure among a sample of children aged 8 to 18 years revealed that adolescents (13–18 years) reported higher levels of emotion-focused avoidance than children aged 8 to 12 years (Reid et al., 1998). The authors attributed this finding to increased frequency of pain among adolescents for which they may experience difficulties managing and consequently resort to more emotion-focused avoidant approaches. Other research has examined children's coping with postoperative pain (Bennett-Branson & Craig, 1993). Results of this research showed that older children (aged 10 to 16 years) spontaneously reported a higher frequency of cognitive coping strategies for dealing with postoperative pain when compared to younger children (aged 7 to 9 years). The family is a common social factor that is related to children's pain experiences (McGrath, 1994). Studies of the aggregation of pain complaints in families have highlighted the important context of the family in childhood pain (Goodman, McGrath, & Forward, 1997). For example, studies have shown that children with recurrent abdominal pain are more likely to have parents who report similar pain problems (Apley, 1975; Apley & Naish, 1958; Zuckerman, Stevenson, & Bailey, 1987), and that persons with recurrent pain often come from families with a positive family history for pain (Ehde, Holm, & Metzger, 1991; Turkat, Kuczmierczyk, & Adams, 1984). Goodman et al. (1997) conducted a prospective community-based study of over 500 families and found that children whose parents reported a large number of painful incidents during the 1-week study period were more likely to also report a large number of painful incidents themselves. Parental modeling and reinforcement of pain are often hypothesized to be important mechanisms that could contribute to transmission of pain within families (Craig, 1986). Recent research has shown that parental behavior can have a strong direct effect on children's pain experiences (Chambers, Craig, & Bennett, 2002); however, to date, no research has examined family influences on children's pain experiences as a function of age of the child. It seems probable that parental influences might be most salient among younger children.

Similar to adult populations, emotional factors, such as anxiety, fear, frustration, and anger, are also related to children's pain expression in important ways (Craig, 1989; McGrath, 1994). For example, in a study of children aged 7 to 17 years undergoing surgery, anticipatory anxiety emerged as a significant predictor of children's postoperative pain experiences (Palermo & Drotar, 1996). Further, research has shown age-related effects in children's decisions to control or express emotions (Zeman & Garber, 1996). Results of this research, which compared children aged 6 to 10 years, showed that younger children were more willing to express emotions such as anger and sadness than older children (Zeman & Garber, 1996). It is likely that age-related differences in children's emotional displays are associated with developmental changes in children's pain expression.

In summary, a variety of psychosocial factors can impact on children's pain experiences. The majority of research has been conducted in the early to middle childhood periods. Additional research focusing on age-related differences in psychosocial factors that influence pain among infants and adolescents is needed. Regardless, existing data appear to support the notion that developmental differences in psychosocial factors likely contribute to children's pain experiences and expression.

Age Differences in Neurophysiological Mechanisms and Correlates of Pain During Childhood

Relatively little research has examined age-related variation in physiological systems that control pain in children. It is noted that, due to its complex nature, physiological and psychological factors likely interact to contribute to a child's pain. Age-related differences are noted on a number of physiological variables frequently associated with pain in children. For example, heart rate generally decreases with age (Izard et al., 1991). Bournaki (1997) studied the physiological pain responses of 8- to 12-year-old children and found a greater deviation in heart rate from venipuncture to baseline compared to older children.

Although the pain systems required for detection, transmission, and reaction to noxious stimuli are present in the neonate, a number of developmental changes in pain processing have been described. For example, in terms of peripheral transmission of pain, C-fibers are slow to make final synaptic contacts among neonates (Fitzgerald, 1985, 1987). It is also understood that excitatory neurotransmitters and their receptors within the dorsal horn undergo marked changes in the postnatal period (Fitzgerald, 1993). Further, the nervous system of neonates is more plastic than that of adults, and alteration in typical activity patterns in development can permanently change patterns of connections within the CNS (Dickenson & Rahman, 1999). A more comprehensive review of the development of the pain system in infants is available elsewhere (Fitzgerald & de Lima, 2001).

Increasingly, researchers have become interested in the long-term effects of pain in infants (Taddio, 1999). Animal studies have indicated that early pain experience may alter the subsequent development of pain pathways (for a review, see Schellinck & Anand, 1999). Research with human infants examining the effects of single medical procedures and prolonged hospitalization indicates that these factors can contribute to alterations in infants' pain behaviors and clinical outcomes (Anand, Phil, & Hickey, 1992; Taddio, Katz, Ilersich, & Koren, 1997; Taddio, Nulman, Goldbach, Ipp, & Koren, 1994; Taddio, Stevens, Craig, Rastogi, Ben David, Shennan, Mulligan, & Koren, 1997). For example, Taddio, Nulman, Goldbach, Ipp, and Koren (1997) compared the pain responses to inoculation at age 4 or 6 months of three groups of boys: uncircumcised, circumcised with topical anesthetic cream, and circumcised with placebo cream. Results showed that the uncircumcised boys responded less to inoculation, measured by observer reports using a visual analogue scale (VAS) and recordings of infant cry and facial activity, when compared to the other two groups. The group treated with the topical anesthetic differed significantly from the group treated with placebo on the VAS measure, but not in cry or facial activity. Research has also examined the long-term consequences of pain at developmental stages beyond the infancy period. For example, Grunau and her colleagues have conducted a series of studies comparing the pain responses of former preterm and full-term children postinfancy. This research has shown lower levels of reactivity in response to everyday pain at age 18 months among the low birthweight children (Grunau, Whitfield, & Petrie, 1994), a higher incidence of somatization among 4.5-year-old preterm children (Grunau, Whitfield, Petrie, & Fryer, 1994), and higher ratings of pain in response to vignettes depicting medical events at age 8–10 years among former preterm children (Grunau, Whitfield, & Petrie, 1998), when compared to full-term peers.

Another biological factor that is thought to contribute to age-related differences in children's pain experiences is body surface area (BSA). In their study of needle pain ratings of children between the ages of 3 and 17 years, Goodenough et al. (1997) found that self-reported pain intensity scores were predicted equally well by the BSA of the child, an anatomical metric, as by chronological age. The authors hypothesized that developmental anatomical differences may form a component of age-related responses to pain in children (Goodenough et al., 1997). Future research is needed to explore age differences in physiological factors that may relate to pain across infancy, childhood, and adolescence.

Age Differences in Pain Assessment During Childhood

There exist a variety of measures to assess pain in children, including self-report, behavioral, and physiological measures. Comprehensive reviews of these measures are available elsewhere (Finley & McGrath, 1998; McGrath & Gillespie, 2001). Due to its subjective nature, self-reports are generally considered to be the gold standard in pediatric pain assessment, where possible (Merskey & Bogduk, 1994). Examples of self-report tools include numeric ratings scales, faces scales, and colored analogue scales (Champion, Goodenough, von Baeyer, & Thomas, 1998). Assessment measures designed specifically for adolescents are also available (Savedra, Tesler, Holzemer, Wilkie, & Ward, 1990) as are more comprehensive chronic pain inventories (Varni, Thompson, & Hanson, 1987). However, cognitive and emotional limitations may hinder the appropriateness of use of self-report measures with some children. Although researchers have employed self-report measures with children as young as 3 years of age (Goodenough et al., 1997), recent research has indicated that children younger than approximately 7 years of age may not possess the cognitive abilities to appropriately use these measures (Chambers & Johnston, 2002). For example, young children tend to rely on the extremes of ratings scales (Chambers & Johnston, 2002; von Baeyer et al., 1997). Future research is needed to examine cognitive skills necessary for providing accurate self-reports of pain, methods to estimate the age at which these skills emerge, and ways to train young children to more appropriately use self-report measures.

A variety of behavioral measures also exist to assess pain in children. These range from detailed coding of facial expressions (Craig, 1998) to quantification of broad band behaviors (McGrath, 1998), such as screaming or flailing. Behavioral measures have typically been developed for a particular developmental period. For example, specific behavioral measures exist for assessment of premature infants (e.g., the Premature Infant Pain Profile; Stevens, Johnston, Petryshen, & Taddio, 1996) and toddlers and preschoolers (e.g., the Toddler–Preschooler Postoperative Pain Scale; Tarbell, Cohen, & Marsh, 1992). Behavioral measures are especially valuable in the case where self-reports of pain are not possible (e.g., in infants, children with developmental disabilities). Observer (e.g., parent, nurse) ratings are often employed to provide a global assessment of children's pain. Research has generally indicated that observer ratings underestimate children's pain intensity (Chambers, Reid, Craig, McGrath, & Finley, 1998), although no research has documented age-dependent differences in agreement between observer and child reports of pain.

Physiological measures are also employed in the assessment of pain in children (Sweet & McGrath, 1998). These include heart rate, respiratory rate, and skin blood flow, among others. Research has generally shown that such physiological responses tend to habituate over time and are not specific to pain, although they can be useful in providing complementary information regarding a child's pain experience (Sweet & McGrath, 1998). As indicated earlier, age-related differences in children's physiological responsiveness to pain have been reported (Bournaki, 1997).

Regardless of the specific type of pain measure of interest, it is of importance to give consideration to the unique developmental features of the measure and its appropriateness for use with children of particular ages. Although it is helpful that available measures have been tailored to children of specific ages, this approach may, in part, hinder our ability to conduct comparisons of children's pain responses across developmental periods.

Treatment Considerations During Various Stages of Childhood

Developmental factors must also be taken into account when considering pain management in children. Pain management techniques can be broadly classified into either pharmacological or cognitive/behavioral approaches. Specific guidelines for the management of children's acute pain have been established by the American Academy of Pediatrics and the American Pain Society and are beyond the scope of this chapter (AAP, 2001). Research has shown that the efficacy of certain pharmacological interventions may vary depending on the age of the child. For example, Arts et al. (1994) compared the efficacy of a local anesthetic cream and music distraction in reducing pain from intravenous cannulation in children aged 4 to 16 years. Using children's self-reports of pain, the results showed a superiority of the local anesthetic cream in the youngest age group (4 to 6 years) when compared to the older children and adolescents in their sample. Characteristics of newborn physiology and the pharmacology of opioids and local anesthetics within the infancy period may also contribute to age-related differences in responsiveness to pharmacological interventions for pain (Houck, 1998).

Similarly, the appropriateness of certain psychological interventions, such as hypnosis, muscle relaxation, and control of negative thoughts, may also vary depending on the age of the child. A recent systematic review of randomized controlled trials of psychological therapy for pediatric chronic pain has revealed strong evidence in support of relaxation and cognitive behavioral therapy as effective treatments for reducing the severity and frequency of chronic pain in children (Eccleston, Morley, Williams, Yorke, & Mastroyannopoulou, 2002). The authors indicate that there is insufficient evidence to permit conclusions regarding the effectiveness of these treatments in reducing pain-related mood disturbance and disability. Of note, the age of the youngest children included in these trials was 9 years (Sanders & Morrison, 1990; Sanders et al., 1989). As a result, data regarding the effectiveness of these approaches for treating chronic pain in younger children are not available. Indeed, children less than 8 or 9 years of age may have difficulties engaging in these interventions and require the in vivo assistance of a parent or other coach (McGrath, 1995). In contrast, a recent review of psychological treatments for procedure-related pain (e.g., breathing exercises, behavioral rehearsal) has documented the overall efficacy of these approaches in children as young as 3 years of age (Powers, 1999). Additional research is needed to provide data regarding the relative efficacy of different psychological approaches to pain management among children of varying ages. This information, in turn, could be used to inform psychological treatment of chronic pain among young children.

PAIN DURING THE ADULT YEARS

As previously noted, the developmental pain literature has emphasized notions of order change, growth, and maturation when dealing with neonatal and pediatric samples. In marked contrast, the adult phase of the life span has been characterized by concepts of stability, invariance and eventual senescence or decline. An important implication of this general view has been the decided lack of interest in developmental processes over the adult years. In fact, the conceptualization of a life-span approach has been a very recent innovation in the adult pain literature (Gagliese & Melzack, 2000; Riley, Wade, Robinson, & Price, 2000; Walco & Harkins, 1999) and developmental concepts have been largely ignored. This situation must change if we are to develop a more comprehensive understanding of the pain experience in all persons, both young and old, who suffer severe or unremitting pain and seek our clinical care.

From a developmental perspective it is clear that biological, psychological, and social factors all alter over the life cycle, and these influences have been used to help define stage of life during the adult years. However, social transitions, biological processes, and even chronological life stage can vary as a function of gender, culture, and individual experience. As a result, chronological age has become the de facto gold standard in most research settings, and it is argued to provide the best overall surrogate of life stage (Birren & Schaie, 1996). Demographic and epidemiological convention has often divided the adult population into two broad age cohorts: 18–65 and 65 plus, which presumably reflects the official retirement age in most Western societies. Others have added further age subdivisions in describing the population as being young adult, mid-aged, the "young" old (65–74), the "old" old (75–85), and more recently the "oldest" old (85+; Suzman & Riley, 1985) and the "very oldest" old (95+). Although these age categories can help account for specific differences in physical, social, mental, and functional abilities particularly during the later years of life, they have rarely been used in the study of pain. In fact, the working adult population (18–65) has attracted the overwhelming majority of interest in pain research studies and has formed the customary comparison group for studies on children or the aged. For this reason, discussions are focused around the broad categories of adulthood and the aged with appropriate demarcations into finer age cohorts where possible.

Age Differences in Pain Experience and Report During the Adulthood

Recent reviews of the epidemiologic literature reveal a marked age-related increase in the prevalence of persistent pain up until the seventh decade of life and then a plateau or decline (Helme & Gibson, 2001; Verhaak, Kerssens, Dekker, Sorbi, & Bensing, 1998). In contrast, the point prevalence of acute pain appears to remain relatively constant at approximately 5% regardless of age (Crook, Rideout, & Browne, 1984; Kendig, Helme, & Teshuva, 1996). The absolute prevalence figures of persistent pain vary widely between cross-sectional studies and probably reflect differences in the time sample under consideration (e.g., pain in the last week, 6-month or 12-month period, etc.) and the method of survey (postal, telephone, interview), as well as the type and sites of pain included in the survey (Helme & Gibson, 1999).

Nonetheless, with one exception (Crook et al., 1984), epidemiologic studies show a progressive increase in pain prevalence throughout early adulthood (10–40%) with a peak prevalence during late middle age (50–65; 20–80%) followed by a plateau or decline in the "old" old (75–85) and "oldest" old (85+; 15–70%) adults (Andersson, Ejlertsson, Leden, & Rosenberg, 1993; Bassols, Bosch, Campillo, Cannelas, & Banos, 1999; Blyth et al., 2001; Brattberg, Parker, & Thorslund, 1997; Brattberg, Thorslund, & Wikman, 1989; Kendig et al., 1996; Kind, Dolan, Gudex, & Williams, 1998; Magni, Marchetti, Moreschi, Merskey, & Luchini, 1993; Mobily, Herr, Clark, & Wallace, 1994). These findings of reduced pain in very advanced age are perhaps surprising given that disease prevalence and pain associated pathology continues to rise throughout the entire life span.

If one examines pain at specific anatomical sites, a slightly different picture emerges. The prevalence of articular joint pain more than doubles in adults over 65 years (Barberger-Gateau et al., 1992; Bergman et al., 2001; Harkins, Price, & Bush, 1994; Sternbach, 1986; von Korff, Dworkin, & Le Resche, 1990). Foot and leg pain have also been reported to increase with advancing age well into the ninth decade of life (Benvenuti, Ferrucci, Guralnik, Gagnermi, & Baroni, 1995; Herr, Mobily, Wallace, & Chung, 1991; Leveille, Gurlanik, Ferrucci, Hirsch, Simonsick, & Hochberg, 1998). Conversely, the prevalence of headache (Andersson et al., 1993; D'Allesandro et al., 1988; Kay, Jorgensen, & Schultz-Larsen, 1992; Sternbach, 1986), abdominal pain (Kay et al., 1992; LaVasky-Shulan et al., 1985) and chest pain (Andersson et al., 1993; Sternbach, 1986; Tibblin, Bengtsson, Furness, & Lapidus, 1990; von Korff, Dworkin, Le Resche, & Kruger, 1988) all peak during later middle age (45–55) and then decline thereafter. Studies of age-specific rates of back pain are more mixed with some reports of a progressive increase over the life span (Harkins et al., 1994; von Korff et al., 1988), whereas others have reported the reverse trend after a peak prevalence at 40–50 years (Andersson et al., 1993; Borenstein, 2001; Perez, 2000; Sternbach, 1986; Tibblin et al., 1990).

Another useful source of information on age differences in the pain experience involves a review of symptom presentation in those clinical disease states that are known to have pain as a usual component. The majority of studies in this area focused on visceral pain complaints and particularly myocardial pain, abdominal pain associated with acute infection, and different forms of malignancy. Variations in the classic presentations of "crushing" myocardial pain in the chest, left arm, and jaw are known to be much more common in older adults. Remarkably, approximately 35–42% of adults over the age of 65 years experience apparently silent or painless heart attack (Konu, 1977; MacDonald, Baillie, & Williams, 1983). This represents a striking example of tissue damage without pain signaling the obvious threat, although the level of nociceptive input is seldom known with clinical pain states. Nonetheless, attempts to address this issue by using more controlled and quantitative examples of cardiac pain have been recently undertaken. For many patients with coronary artery disease, strenuous physical exercise will induce myocardial ischemia as indexed by a 1-mm drop in the ST segment of the electrocardiogram. By comparing the onset and degree of exertion-induced ischemia with subjective pain report, it is possible to provide an experimentally controlled evaluation of myocardial pain across the adult life span. Several studies have documented a significant age-related delay between the onset of ischemia and the report of chest pain (Ambepitiya, Iyengar, & Roberts, 1993; Ambepitiya, Roberts, & Ranjadayalan, 1994; Miller, Sheps, & Bragdon, 1990). Adults over 70 years take almost 3 times as long as young adults to first report the presence of pain (Ambepitiya et al., 1993, 1994). Moreover, the severity of pain report is reduced even after controlling for variations in the extent of ischemia. Collectively, these findings provide strong support for the view that myocardial pain may be somewhat muted in adults of advanced age.

The presentation of clinical pain associated with abdominal complaints such as peritonitis, peptic ulcer, and intestinal obstruction show a similar pattern of age-related change. Pain symptoms become more occult after the age of 60 years and in marked contrast to young adults, the collection of clinical symptoms (nausea, fever, tachycardia) with the highest diagnostic accuracy does not even include abdominal pain (Albano, Zielinski, & Organ, 1975; Wroblewski & Mikulowski, 1991). With regard to pain associated with various types of malignancy, a recent retrospective review of more than 1,500 cases revealed a marked difference in the incidence of pain between younger adults (55% with pain), middle-aged adults (35% with pain), and older adults (26% with pain). With one exception (Vigano, Bruera, & Suarex-Almazor, 1998), most studies also note a significant decline in the intensity of cancer pain symptoms in adults of advanced age (70+ years; Brescia, Portenoy, Ryan, Krasnoff, & Gray, 1992; Caraceni & Portenoy, 1999; McMillan, 1989). It remains somewhat unclear as to whether the apparent decline in pain reflects some age difference in disease severity, in the willingness to report pain as a symptom, or an actual age-related change in the pain experience itself.

Other reports of atypical pain presentation have been documented for pneumonia, pneumothorax, and postoperative pain. For instance, several studies suggest that older adults report a lower intensity of pain in the postoperative recovery period even after matching for the type of surgical procedure and the extent of tissue damage (Gagliese, Wowk, Sandler, & Katz, 1999; Meier, Morrison, & Ahronheim, 1996; Oberle, Paul, & Wry, 1990; Thomas, Robinson, & Champion, 1998). This change is thought to be clinically significant and is on the order of a 10–20% reduction per decade after the age of 60 years (Meier et al., 1996; Thomas et al., 1998). Recent studies of chronic musculoskeletal pain have also started to address the issue of age differences. This is of considerable importance given that more than three-fourths of persistent pain states are of musculoskeletal origin. Unfortunately, the findings are quite equivocal with reports of increased arthritic pain in older adults (Harkins et al., 1994; Wilkinson, Madhok, & Hunter, 1993), decreased pain severity (Lichtenberg, Skehan, & Swensen, 1984; Parker et al., 1988), and no change (Gagliese & Melzack, 1997b; Yunus, Holt, Masi, & Aldag, 1998). Studies on patients with predominantly musculo-skeletal pain attending multidisciplinary pain management centers show similar variable findings and appear to depend on the type of pain assessment scale used for measurement. Studies using a unidimensional scale such as visual analogue of pain intensity or a simple word descriptor have typically found no age difference (Benbow, Cossins, & Wiles, 1996; Corran, Gibson, Farrell, & Helme, 1994; Middaugh, Levin, Kee, Barchiesi, & Roberts, 1988; Riley et al., 2000; Sorkin, Rudy, Hanlon, Turk, & Stieg, 1990), whereas reports based on multidimensional measures or composite scores have reported an age-related decline in pain intensity and unpleasantness (Corran, Farrell, Helme, & Gibson, 1997; Gagliese & Melzack, 1997b; Gibson & Helme, 2001; Mosley, McCracken, Gross, Penzien, & Plaud, 1993; Turk, Okifuji, & Scharff, 1995). In explaining this apparent disparity it may be that VAS scales are less appropriate for use in older persons (see section on pain assessment), or it could be that only the quality of chronic pain sensation changes rather than the intensity per se (Gagliese & Melzack, 1997b). This would be more likely if there were diagnostic differences in the cause of pain between younger and older adult patients attending multidisciplinary pain management centers.

A full understanding of changes in the chronic pain experience over the life span requires some consideration of pain-related impacts, such as the occurrence of emotional distress and functional disability. There have been fewer studies of age differences in the mood and function of chronic pain patients, but some relatively consistent trends have emerged. Despite one or two exceptions (Corran et al., 1997; Riley et al., 2000), there is now good evidence for no age difference in the number of self-reported depressive symptoms (Cossins, Benbow, & Wiles, 1999; Gagliese & Melzack, 1997b; Herr, Mobily, & Smith, 1993; Middaugh et al., 1988; Mosley et al., 1993; Sorkin et al., 1990; Turk et al., 1995) or in the percentage of patients diagnosed with a depressive disorder (Benbow et al., 1996; Corran et al., 1994; Herr et al., 1993; Wijeratne et al., 2001). Pain-related anxiety, on the other hand, may be less pervasive and intense in adults over the age of 60 years. Results are not universal (Cossins et al., 1999), but several studies have shown an obvious decline in the reported symptoms of anxiety (Benbow, Cossins, & Bowsher,

1995; Cook & Chastain, 2001; Corran et al., 1994; Cossins et al., 1999; Mosley et al., 1993; Parmelee, 1997; Riley et al., 2000) for older chronic pain patients and the magnitude of change (approximately 25% reduction) is likely to be of clinical significance.

With regard to pain-related disability or impact on the level of general activity, there have been five reports of age differences (Corran et al., 1994; Cutler, Fishbain, Rosomoff, & Rosomoff, 1994; Mosley et al., 1993; Riley et al., 2000; Wijeratne et al., 2001) and seven studies that found no change over the adult life span (Benbow et al., 1995; Cook & Chastain, 2001; Corran et al., 1997; Cossins et al., 1999; Middaugh et al., 1988; Sorkin et al., 1990; Turk et al., 1995). Moreover, the direction of any age difference is unclear with three studies noting a decrease in self-rated disability for older adult patients (Cutler et al., 1994; Riley et al., 2000; Wijeratne et al., 2001), one study noting higher levels of disability (Mosley et al., 1993), and the final report indicating an age-related increase in functional impact on physical activities but a decrease on psychosocial impact (Corran et al., 1994). At this stage it would seem unwise to draw any firm conclusions, although a focus on measurement issues and the age range of the sample under study may provide useful topics for future research.

In summary, the findings from numerous large-sample epidemiologic studies suggest that pain is most common during the late middle-aged phase of life, and this is true regardless of the anatomical site or the pathogenic cause of pain. The one exception appears to be degenerative joint disease (e.g., osteoarthritis), which shows an exponential increase up until at least 90 years of age. Studies of clinical disease and injury would suggest a relative absence of pain, often atypical presentation, and a reduction in the intensity of pain symptoms with advancing age. Changes in myocardial chest pain and abdominal pain have been most frequently documented, but age differences in postoperative pain, cancer pain, and musculoskeletal pain conditions have also been reported. It is important to note that most studies in this area have relied on retrospective review of medical records rather than direct patient report. Much of the information comes from hospital admission data, and this may underestimate the prevalence of painless disease or injury seen in the community setting. On the other hand, a lack of age differences in disease presentation is unlikely to be reported or published and this could overemphasize age differences in clinical pain presentation. Studies of clinical pain have usually defined adult groups as being either young or old and there has been little recognition of finer nuances in life stage (e.g., young adult, middle-aged, old, "old" old, and "oldest" old). Indeed, very few studies have included adults over the age of 80 years. Nonetheless, a consensus view would be that there are clinically significant changes in the pain experience over the adult life span and that such changes are most obvious in late middle age and the very old age cohorts.

Psychosocial Influences on the Experience and Expression of Pain Over the Adult Life Span

Pain is a complex perceptual experience that combines sensory, affective, and cognitive dimensions. The context in which noxious input is processed, the cognitive beliefs of the individual, and the meanings attributed to pain symptoms are known to be important factors in shaping the overall pain experience. A number of recent studies have examined psychological components of pain over the adult life span, and there is now clear evidence for some important age differences in cognitive beliefs and coping mechanisms.

It has been suggested that older adults perceive pain as something to be expected and just a normal companion of advancing age (Hofland, 1992). A number of empirical studies provide clear support for this view (Harkins et al., 1984; Liddell & Locker, 1997; Ruzicka, 1998; Weiner & Rudy, 2000), although there are some exceptions (Gagliese & Melzack, 1997b; McCracken, 1998). Stoller (1993) examined causal attributions in 667 community dwelling adults aged 65 plus and found that 43% of the sample attributed joint or muscle pain to the normal aging process. Conversely, in a sample of 396 adults only 21% of the elderly aged 60-plus attributed aching to a specific disease, whereas 36% of young adults aged 20–39 perceived this symptom as a warning sign of disease (Leventhal & Prohaska, 1986; Prohaska, Leventhal, Leventhal, & Keller, 1985). One exception may occur in the presence of severe or persistent pain. Under such circumstances older adults may be more likely to interpret pain as a sign of serious illness and seek more rapid medical treatment than their young counterparts (Stoller, 1993; Leventhal, Leventhal, Schaefer, & Easterling, 1993). There are also a number of studies that demonstrate that mild pain symptoms do not affect self-rated perceptions of health in older adults, but do so in the young (Ebrahim, Brittis, & Wu, 1991; Mangione et al., 1993). On the basis of these findings, it is clear that older adults underreport pain as a symptom of illness. Seniors are very aware of the increasing prevalence of disease with advancing age, and this is thought to contribute to the widespread misattribution of pain symptoms. However, attributing mild aches and pains to the normal aging process greatly reduces the importance of this symptom and alters the fundamental meaning of pain itself.

Other types of pain beliefs and attitudes have also started to attract increasing attention from the pain research community. Gagliese and Melzack (1997b) reported a lack of age differences in both pain-free individuals and chronic pain patients when using the pain beliefs questionnaire (Williams & Thorn, 1989). This instrument monitors beliefs about psychological influences over pain (i.e., that depression makes pain seem worse) as well as physiological causes of pain (i.e., pain is a result of tissue damage). Regardless of age, patients with chronic pain were more likely to endorse psychological beliefs than organic causes of pain. In contrast, others have noted that chronic pain patients show significant age differences in most of the beliefs as assessed by the cognitive risks profile (Cook, DeGood, & Chastain, 1999). Older adults (60–90) were found to have a lower cognitive risk of helplessness, self-blame, and absence of emotional support, but an increased desire for a medical treatment breakthrough and a greater denial of pain-related mood disturbance. In a recent study, the locus of control scale was used to examine cognitive factors and the experience of pain and suffering in older adults (Gibson & Helme, 2000). Chronic pain patients aged over 80 years were shown to have a greater belief in pain severity being controlled by factors of chance or fate (Gibson & Helme, 2000). This contrasts with younger pain patients, who endorse their own behaviors and actions as a strongest determinant of pain severity. In agreement with previous studies (see Melding, 1995, for review), a belief in chance factors was also shown to be associated with increased pain, depression, functional impact, and choice of maladaptive coping strategies. Finally, using a newly developed psychometric measure of pain attitudes, Yong, Gibson, Horne, and Helme (2001) found that older persons living in the community exhibited a greater belief in the need for stoic reticence and an increased cautious reluctance and self-doubt when making a report of pain. These findings are in agreement with early psychophysical studies that show that older persons adopt a more stringent response criterion for the threshold report of pain and are less willing to label a sensation as painful (Clark & Mehl, 1971; Harkins & Chapman, 1976, 1977). The finding is also consistent with other recent studies of stoic attitudes in older pain patients (Klinger & Spaulding, 1998; Machin & Williams, 1998; Morley, Doyle, & Beese, 2000) and provides strong empirical support for the widely held view that older cohorts are generally more stoic in response to pain.

Another potentially important psychological influence relates to possible age differences in self-efficacy and the use of pain coping strategies. Self-efficacy in being able to use coping strategies to effectively reduce the severity of pain does not appear to change between early adulthood and older age (Corran et al., 1994; Gagliese, Jackson, Ritvo, Wowk, & Katz, 2000; Harkins, 1988; Keefe & Williams, 1990; Keefe et al., 1991), although adolescents may have slightly poorer self-efficacy than other segments of the adult population (Burckhart, Clark, & Bennett, 2001; Goyen & Anshell, 1998). These findings would seem to challenge the commonly held view that older persons have less self-efficacy and instead show a stability and resilience in beliefs of personal competence across the major portion of the adult life span. The literature on coping strategy use is less clear-cut. Studies by Keefe and colleagues (1990, 1991) showed no age differences in the frequency of coping strategy use, although there was a strong trend for older adults to use more praying and hoping than their younger counterparts.

Conversely, older people with chronic pain have been found to report fewer cognitive coping strategies and an increased use of physical methods of pain control when compared to young adults (Sorkin et al., 1990). Corran et al. (1994) examined a large sample of outpatients attending a multidisciplinary pain treatment center, aged from 18 to 92 years. Consistent with others (Gardner, Garland, Workman, & Mendelson, 2001; Mosley et al., 1993), they found a significantly higher use of praying and hoping as well as less frequent use of ignoring pain in adults aged greater than 60 years. Such differences are thought to be more likely due to sociocultural cohort effects rather than to some maturational change per se (Corran et al., 1994).

Corran et al. (1994) also reported some age differences in the relationship between coping strategy use and self-reported levels of pain, depression, anxiety, and disability. The use of catastrophizing as a cognitive coping strategy was found to be the strongest predictor of negative clinical presentation in both young and older adults (accounting for 20–30% of the variation in outcome scores). This finding is consistent with many earlier studies in young adult chronic pain patients (see Jensen, Turner, Romano, & Karoly, 1991, for review) and has since been confirmed in older populations as well (Bishop, Ferraro, & Borowiak, 2001). It is in the use of other coping strategies, however, that age differences start to emerge. In the elderly cohort, self-coping statements and diverting attention were shown to be significant predictors of clinical outcome measures, whereas ignoring pain and reinterpretation of pain sensations were of more importance in young chronic pain patients. As these coping strategies were secondary to catastrophizing and only account for between 5 and 10% of the variation in reports of pain, mood disturbance, and disability, the observed age difference probably represents a subtle shift in the interaction between coping and clinical presentation rather than some major change.

In summary, these findings document some clear age-related differences in many types of pain beliefs, coping mechanisms, attribution of pain symptoms, and attitudes towards pain. These psychological influences are likely to shape the overall pain experience, but observed age differences may be very dependent on the intensity of painful symptoms. If a pain symptom is mild or transient in older adults, it is likely to be attributed to the normal aging process, be more readily accepted, and be accompanied by a different choice of strategy to cope with pain. These factors are likely to diminish the importance of mild aches and pains, and actually alter the fundamental meaning of pain symptoms. More stoic attitudes to mild pain and a stronger belief in chance factors as the major determinant of pain onset and severity are likely to lead to the underreporting of pain symptoms by older segments of the adult population. However, many of the age differences in coping, misattribution, and beliefs disappear if pain is persistent or severe.

Age Differences in Neurophysiologic Mechanisms and Correlates of Pain During Adulthood

Any age-related change in the function of nociceptive pathways would be expected to alter pain sensitivity and therefore alter the perception of noxious events and the prevalence of pain complaints over the adult life span. There is some limited evidence of an age-related decline in the physiologic function of peripheral, spinal, and central nervous system nociceptive mechanisms. For instance, a marked decrease in the density of myelinated and unmyelinated nerve fibers has been found in older adults (Ochoa & Mair, 1969). Moreover, the neuronal content of the pain-related neuropeptides substance P and calcitonin gene-related peptide (CGRP) are known to fall with advancing age (Helme & McKernan, 1984; Li & Duckles, 1993). Nerve conduction studies indicate a prolonged latency and decreased amplitude of sensory nerve action potentials in apparently healthy older adults (Adler & Nacimiento, 1988; Buchthal & Rosenfalck, 1966). Studies of the perceptual experience associated with activation of nociceptive fibers indicate a selective age-related impairment in A fiber function and a greater reliance on C-fiber information for the report of pain in older adults (Chakour, Gibson, Bradbeer, & Helme, 1996). Given that A fibers subserve the epicritic, first warning aspects of pain, while C-fiber sensation is more prolonged, dull, and diffuse, one might reasonably expect some changes in pain quality and intensity in older adults. Spinal mechanisms of nociception also appear to change with age. Three recent studies have shown that the temporal summation of noxious input may be altered in older persons (Edwards & Fillingim, 2001; Gibson, Chang, & Farrell, 2002; Harkins, Davis, Bush, & Price, 1996). Temporal summation refers to the enhancement of pain sensation associated with repeated stimulation. It results from a transient sensitization of dorsal horn neurons in the spinal cord and is thought to play an important role in the development and expression of postinjury tenderness and hyperalgesia. Zheng, Gibson, Khalil, McMeeken, and Helme (2000) extended these observations by comparing the intensity and time course of postinjury hyperalgesia in young (20–40) and older (73–88) adults. Although the intensity and area of hyperalgesia were similar in both groups, the state of mechanical tenderness persisted for a much longer duration in the older group. As mechanical tenderness is known to be mediated by sensitized spinal neurons, these findings may indicate a reduced capacity of the aged CNS to reverse the sensitization process once it has been initiated. The clinical implication is that postinjury pain and tenderness will resolve more slowly in older persons. However, in combination with the studies of temporal summation, these findings provide strong evidence for an age-related reduction in the functional plasticity of spinal nociceptive neurons following an acute noxious event.

Variations in pain sensitivity depend not only on activity in the afferent nociceptive pathways but also endogenous pain inhibitory control mechanisms that descend from the cortex and midbrain onto spinal cord neurons. A recent study has shown that the analgesic efficacy of this endogenous inhibitory system may decline with advancing age (Washington, Gibson, & Helme, 2000). Following activation of the endogenous analgesic system, young adults showed an increase in pain threshold of up to 150% whereas the apparently healthy older adult group increased pain threshold by approximately 40%. Such age differences in the efficiency of endogenous analgesic modulation are consistent with many earlier animal studies (see Bodnar, Romero, & Kramer, 1988, for review) and would be expected to reduce the ability of older adults to cope with severe or persistent pain states.

There are widespread morphological and neurochemical changes to the central nervous system with advancing age, although few studies have examined those areas specifically related to the processing of nociceptive information (see Gibson & Helme, 1995, for review). An investigation of the cortical response to painful stimulation has documented some changes in adults over 60 years. Using the pain-related encephalographic response in order to index the central nervous system processing of noxious input, older adults were found to display a significant reduction in peak amplitude and an increased latency of response (Gibson, Gorman, & Helme, 1990). These findings might suggest an age-related slowing in the cognitive processing of noxious information and a reduced cortical activation. There has also been one report of a more diffuse topographic spread in the poststimulus electroencephalogram (Gibson, Helme, & Gorman, 1993). Although this finding could indicate a wider recruitment of CNS neurons during the cortical processing of noxious input, more recent neuroimaging techniques, with better temporal and spatial resolution, would be needed to confirm this suggestion.

Age Differences in Pain Assessment During the Adult Years

Three main approaches have been used to assess clinical pain in the adult population: self-report psychometric measures, behavioral–observational methods, and third-party proxy ratings. The vast majority of research into pain measurement has been conducted on young and middle-aged adults and there is a huge literature on this topic (for review see Katz & Melzack, 1999; Lee, 2001; Williams, 2001). In order to consider pain measurement from a developmental perspective there need to be direct comparative studies between young and older adults. There is no literature on age differences in pain assessment, although issues of measurement reliability and validity have been investigated within specific age segments of the adult population.

Evidence from a variety of sources would suggest that any measurement approach found to be useful in young adult populations, also has a potential for use with most older persons (Helme & Gibson, 1998; Parmelee, 1994). Single-item scales of self-reported pain intensity, such as verbal descriptor scales, numeric rating scales, colored analogue scales, and the pictorial pain faces scale, have all been shown to possess some attributes of validity and reliability when used with healthy older adults and even in those with mild cognitive impairment (Benesh, Szigeti, & Ferraro, 1997; Chibnall & Tait, 2001; Cook, Niven, & Downs, 1999; Corran, Helme, & Gibson, 1991; Ferrell, 1995; Gloth, 2000; Helme et al., 1989; Herr & Mobily, 1993; Herr, Mobily, Koout, & Wagenaar, 1998; Weiner, Pieper, McConnell, Martinez, & Keefe, 1996; Weiner, Peterson, Logue, & Keefe, 1998). Visual analogue scales (VAS) also have some evidence of validity (Scherder & Bouma, 2000), although several others have raised concerns about the suitability of this measure for use with older patients (Benesh et al., 1997; Ferrell, 1995; Herr et al., 1993; Tiplady, Jackson, Maskrey, & Swift, 1998). In particular, it has been suggested that older persons may have difficulties with the more abstract nature of the visual analogue scale scaling properties (Herr et al., 1993; Jensen & Karoly, 1992; Kremer, Atkinson, & Ignelzi, 1981). Multidimensional word descriptor inventories (e.g., the McGill Pain Questionnaire) have also been questioned due to complexity and the need for advanced language skills (Herr & Mobily, 1991). However, most data would support the use of such instruments in older adults with and without cognitive impairment (Corran et al., 1991; Ferrell et al., 1995; Gagliese, 2002; Gagliese & Melzack, 1997a; Helme et al., 1989; Weiner, Peterson, Logue, & Keefe, 1998), although completion rates may drop somewhat (Ferrell, 1995; Hadjistavropoulos, Craig, Martin, Hadjistavropoulos, & McMurtry, 1997; Parmelee, 1994).

Some older persons will suffer from multiple comorbid medical illnesses, physical impairments in vision or hearing, severe cognitive impairment, or difficulties with verbal communication skills, all of which may complicate routine psychometric pain assessment. Behavioral–observational measures of pain can bypass many of these difficulties and have been examined for use in frail older populations (e.g., nursing home residents, demented elderly). Standardized protocols have been developed (e.g., Keefe & Block, 1982) to monitor the frequency of pain-related behaviors (i.e., guarding, bracing, rubbing, grimace, sighing). Interrater reliability and concurrent validity appear to be adequate in older nursing home residents, including those with mild to moderate cognitive impairment (Kovach, Griffie, Matson, & Muchka, 1999; Simons & Malabar, 1995; Weiner et al., 1996, 1998; Weiner,

Peterson, & Keefe, 1999). However, the level of agreement between resident and staff perceptions of pain as indexed by behavioral markers has been shown to be relatively poor (kappa   .3; Weiner et al., 1999). A related approach involves measurement of discrete facial expressions as nonverbal indicators of pain (Craig, Prkachin, & Grunau, 2001). A characteristic pain face has been noted (including lowered eyebrows, raised cheeks, closed eyes, parting or tightening of lips), and despite some individual differences, this expression is instantly recognizable by other third-party observers. The complexity and speed of facial gestures can lead to errors of judgment, but a facial action coding system (Ekman & Friesen, 1969) has been developed to systematically analyze facial expressions from videotaped recordings. When using this technique in frail older adults, interrater reliability has been shown to be excellent and there is good validity evidence (Hadjistavropoulos et al., 1997; Hadjistavropoulos, LaChapelle, MacLeod, Snider, & Craig, 1998; Hadjistavropoulos, LaChapelle, Hadjistavropoulos, Green, & Asmundson, 2002). It is noted, however, that self-report measures of pain and nonverbal indices do not always correspond (e.g., Hadjistavropoulos et al., 2000) and there may be some age differences in the correspondence between pain self-report and the intensity of facial reactions (Matheson, 1997). Nonetheless, these findings are encouraging and may offer another method of pain measurement that is sensitive to differences in functional capacity and can capitalize on the available communication repertoire of persons at the end stage of the life span.

The final class of measures involves third-party proxy ratings of pain by medical staff, carers, or others who know the individual well. Given that pain is a latent and subjective experience, which is really only accessible to the individual who is suffering, this method cannot be recommended for routine pain assessment. However, such measures may be of some value when no other method is available. For instance, some studies of older patients with dementia have shown a reasonable level of agreement (70%) between nursing staff and patient ratings when identifying the presence of pain (Krulwitch et al., 2000; Weiner, Peterson, Logue, & Keefe, 1998; Werner, Cohen-Mansfield, Watson, & Pasis, 1998). On the other hand, staff often underestimate the presence of pain, there is often poor interrater reliability, and estimates of pain intensity may vary widely between patient and proxy ratings (Krulwitch et al., 2000; Weiner, Peterson, & Keefe, 1998).

In summary, there are several different methods by which pain can be assessed although the utility, validity, and reliability may vary as a function of life stage due to the inherent strengths and weaknesses of each approach. Self-report measures represent the de facto gold standard and can be used in most segments of the adult population, although nonverbal behavioral methods may be particularly useful in frail older samples.

Treatment Considerations Across the Adult Life Span

There are a myriad of pharmacological, surgical, psychological, behavioral, and physical therapies that have demonstrated efficacy for use in those suffering from severe or unremitting pain. The vast majority of treatments have been developed in young adult populations and there have been very few investigations of age differences in the treatment response over the adult life span. In the absence of adequate data, most pain clinicians simply extrapolate treatment guidelines from younger patients, tempering their judgments with prudence appropriate for the frailities of the aged (Portenoy & Farkash, 1988). It is not entirely clear why there has been a limited interest in pursuing age differences, although recent evidence indicates a substantial age bias against patient referral and prognosis, as well as bias against the perceived effectiveness of many pharmacological and nonpharmacological treatments (Kee, Middaugh, Redpath, & Hargadon, 1998).

Pharmacological approaches, whether self-administered or prescribed, are the most frequently used method of pain management and include simple analgesics (e.g., paracetamol, nonsteroidal anti-inflammatory drugs), opioid medications (e.g., codeine, morphine), and adjuvant analgesic drugs (tricyclic antidepressants, anticonvulsants). Older adults are more likely to experience adverse side effects and are more sensitive to analgesic actions than their younger counterparts (Katz & Helme, 1998; Wall, 1990). This may be due to the well-known age-related changes in drug metabolism and clearance with associated alterations in the pharmacokinetic and pharmacodynamic profile. As a result, drugs with a short half-life are thought to be preferable, commenced at a low dose and titrated upward in a steady but slow regime. Patient-controlled analgesia is one way to help ensure adequate dosage with a tolerable side-effect profile, and a recent study has shown that this method is appropriate for older postsurgical patients (Gagliese, Verma, & Mossey, 2000). Dosing requirements must also take into account any concurrent medications and coexisting disease states that may alter the time course and profile of analgesic action (Helme & Gibson, 1998). For instance, the average 70-year-old is likely to take seven different medications and have three comorbid medical complaints (Gloth, 2000). A more comprehensive discussion of these matters can be found in the clinical practice guidelines on the management of chronic pain from the American Geriatrics Society expert panel (AGS, 2002).

Pharmacological therapy is always more effective when combined with nonpharmacological approaches designed to optimize pain management. The application of heat or cold, massage (Eisenberg et al., 1993), or transcutaneous electrical nerve stimulation (Thorstiensson, 1987) may be useful. Regular physical activity can increase fitness and reverse the physical deconditioning that is often seen in patients with chronic pain problems. A recent randomized control trial demonstrated a significant overall improvement in pain, functional status, and performance measures in elderly veterans with chronic musculoskeletal pain (Ferrell, Josephson, Pollan, Loy, & Ferrell, 1997). Unfortunately, this study did not include a young adult comparison group and there is no other evidence to show whether older persons respond as well, less well, or to the same extent as younger cohorts.

Psychological approaches for the management of pain have been well established in young adult populations (for review see Gatchel & Turk, 1998). Uncontrolled, essentially descriptive studies have also shown that older adults can benefit from relaxation training (Arena, Hannah, Bruno, & Meador, 1991; Arena, Hightower, & Chong, 1988), biofeedback (Nicholson & Blanchard, 1993), behavior therapy (Miller & Le Lieuvre, 1982), and cognitive-behavioral treatment programs (Puder, 1988). Recently there has been one randomized control trial of cognitive-behavioral therapy in nursing home residents (Cook, 1998). Cognitive-behavioral therapy involving 10 weekly sessions of education, reconceptualization of pain and belief structures, and training in coping skills, relaxation, and goal setting was shown to greatly improve self-rated pain and functional disability, but not depressed mood. These effects were maintained at 4-month follow-up. In combination, these findings may help refute the notion that older persons are less accepting of psychological approaches to pain management (Kee, Middaugh, & Pawlick, 1996), but without formal age comparative data, it is impossible to evaluate the relative treatment efficacy within different age segments of the adult population.

Multidisciplinary pain management facilities are thought to offer state-of-the-art treatment for more complex chronic pain problems, particularly when conventional management strategies have failed (Flor, Fydrich, & Turk, 1992; Guzman et al., 2001). Several authors have noted the importance of modifying standard treatment protocols in order to accommodate the special needs of older patients (Arena et al., 1988; Gibson, Farrell, Katz, & Helme, 1996; Portenoy & Farkash, 1988). Such factors may include ensuring age-relevant treatment goals, a recognition of comorbid disease and its influence on treatment decisions, allowing greater time for assessment and treatment instructions, and ensuring that the older person takes an active role in the treatment process and has good self-efficacy for the recommended treatment approach (Gibson et al., 1996). It may also be important to ensure that the social milieu of the clinic is appropriate for older persons, as group therapy is more effective if members share similar life experience, have similar aspirations, and face similar problems. Nonetheless, the available literature on treatment outcome for older adults provides strong support for multidisciplinary treatment (see Gibson et al., 1996, for review). With few exceptions (Aronoff & Evans, 1982; Guck, Meilman, Skultety, & Dowd, 1986; Painter, Seres, & Newman, 1980), it appears that older adults can show substantial posttreatment benefits (e.g., Cutler et al., 1994; Farrell & Gibson, 1993; Groves, Garland, Mendelson, & Gibson, 2002; Hallet & Pilowsky, 1982; Helme et al., 1989, 1996; Hodgson, Suda, Bruce, & Rome, 1993; Kolter-Cope & Gerber, 1993; Middaugh et al., 1988; Ysla, Rosomoff, & Rosomoff, 1986). Although these findings are encouraging, it is worth noting that there has yet to be a randomized control trial of multidisciplinary treatment in older adults and many studies have not even included a control group. The choice of outcome measures may also be questioned in some cases and the sample size of the older segment of the population is often small. Despite these limitations, it is apparent that the vast majority of studies suggest clear benefits from multidisciplinary treatment across the entire adult life span.

CONCLUDING REMARKS

As is evident from the research reviewed in this chapter, pain experiences of individuals across the life span are characterized by both patterns of similarities and idiosyncratic features unique to particular developmental periods. Awareness of the impact of developmental factors on clinical pain assessment and management across the life span is needed. Our understanding of pain could be enhanced greatly by more directly applying developmental methodologies and extending research across developmental periods and a broader age range of individuals.

REFERENCES

Abu-Arefeh, I., & Russell, G. (1994). Prevalence of headache and migraine in school children. *British Medical Journal, 309*, 765–769.

Adler, G., & Nacimiento, A. C. (1988). Age-dependent changes of short-latency somatosensory evoked potentials in healthy adults. *Applied Neurophysiology, 51*(1), 55–59.

AGS Panel on Persistent Pain in Older Persons. (2002). The management of persistent pain in older persons. *Journal of the American Geriatric Society, 50*(Suppl. 6), S205–S224.

Albano, W., Zielinski, C. M., & Organ, C. H. (1975). Is appendicitis in the aged really different? *Geriatrics, 30*, 81–88.

Ambepitiya, G. B., Iyengar, E. N., & Roberts, M. E. (1993). Silent exertional myocardial ischaemia and perception of angina in elderly people. *Age Ageing, 22*, 302–307.

Ambepitiya, G. B., Roberts, M. E., & Ranjadayalan, K. (1994). Silent exertional myocardial ischemia in the elderly: A quantitative analysis of anginal perceptual threshold and the influence of autonomic function. *Journal of the American Geriatrics Society, 42*, 732–737.

American Academy of Pediatrics Committee on Psychosocial Aspects of Child and Family Health & American Pain Society Task Force on Pain in Infants, Children and Adolescents. (2001). The assessment and management of acute pain in infants, children, and adolescents. *Pediatrics, 108*, 793–797.

Anand, K. J. S., Phil, D., & Hickey, P. R. (1992). Halothane-morphine compared with high-dose sufentanil for anesthesia and postoperative analgesia in neonatal cardiac surgery. *New England Journal of Medicine, 326*, 1–9.

Anand, K. J. S., Sippell, W. G., & Aynsley-Green, A. (1987). Randomized trial of fentanyl anaesthesia in preterm babies undergoing surgery: Effects on stress response. *Lancet, 1*, 243–248.

Andersson, H. I., Ejlertsson, G., Leden, I., & Rosenberg, C. (1993). Chronic pain in a geographically defined general population: Studies of differences in age, gender, social class, and pain localization. *Clinical Journal of Pain, 9*, 174–182.

Andrasik, F., Holroyd, K. A., & Abell, T. (1980). Prevalence of headache within a college student population: A preliminary analysis. *Headache, 19*, 384–387.

Apley, J. (1975). *The child with abdominal pains* (2nd ed.). Oxford: Blackwell.

Apley, J., & Naish, N. (1958). Recurrent abdominal pains: A field survey of 1,000 school children. *Archives of Disease in Childhood, 33*, 165–170.

Arena, J. G., Hannah, S. L., Bruno, G. M., & Meador, K. J. (1991). Electromyographic biofeedback training for tension headache in the elderly: A prospective study. *Biofeedback Self Regulation, 16*(4), 379–390.

Arena, J. G., Hightower, N. E., & Chong, G. C. (1988). Relaxation therapy for tension headache in the elderly: A prospective study. *Psychology Aging, 3*(1), 96–98.

Aronoff, G. M., & Evans, W. O. (1982). The prediction of treatment outcome at a multidisciplinary pain center. *Pain, 14*(1), 67–73.

Arts, S. E., Abu-Saad, H. H., Champion, G. D., Crawford, M. R., Fisher, R. J., Juniper, K. H., & Ziegler, J. B. (1994). Age-related response to lidocaine-prilocaine (EMLA) emulsion and effect of music distraction on the pain of intravenous cannulation. *Pediatrics, 93*, 797–801.

Balaque, F., Dutoit, G., & Waldburger, M. (1988). Low back pain in school children: An epidemiological study. *Scandinavian Journal of Rehabilitation Medicine, 20*, 175–179.

Baltes, P. B. (1987). Theoretical propositions of life-span developmental psychology: On the dynamics between growth and decline. *Developmental Psychology, 23*, 611–626.

Barberger-Gateau, P., Chaslerie, A., Dartigues, J., Commenges, D., Gagnon, M., & Salamon, R. (1992). Health measures correlates in a French elderly community population: The PAQUID study. *Journals of Gerontology, 472*, S88–S95.

Bassols, A., Bosch, F., Campillo, M., Cannelas, M., & Banos, J. E. (1999). An epidemiologic comparison of pain complaints in the general population of Catalonia (Spain). *Pain, 83*, 9–16.

Benbow, S., Cossins, L., & Wiles, J. R. (1996). A comparative study of disability, depression and pain severity in young and elderly chronic pain patients. *8th World Congress on Pain*, 1996, Abstract No. 238a.

Benbow, S. J., Cossins, L., & Bowsher, D. (1995). A comparison of young and elderly patients attending a regional pain centre. *Pain Clinic, 8*, 323–332.

Benesch, L. S., Szigeti, E., & Ferraro, F. R. (1997). Tools for assessing chronic pain in rural elderly women. *Home HealthCare Nurse, 15*, 207–212.

Bennett-Branson, S. M., & Craig, K. D. (1993). Postoperative pain in children—Developmental and family influences on spontaneous coping strategies. *Canadian Journal of Behavioural Science, 25*, 355–383.

Benvenuti, F., Ferrucci, L., Guralnik, J. M., Gagnermi, S., & Baroni, A. (1995). Foot pain and disability in older persons. *Journal of the American Geriatrics Society, 43*, 479–484.

Bergman, S., Herrstrom, P., Hogstrom, K., Petersson, I. F., Svensson, B., & Jacobsson, L. T. (2001). Chronic musculoskeletal pain, prevalence rates, and sociodemographic associations in a Swedish population study. *Journal of Rheumatology, 28*, 1369–1377.

Berk, L. E. (2000). *Child development* (5th ed.). Boston: Allyn & Bacon.

Beyer, J. E., McGrath, P. J., & Berde, C. B. (1990). Discordance between self-report and behavioral pain measures in children aged 3–7 years after surgery. *Journal of Pain and Symptom Management, 5*, 350–356.

Bibace, R., & Walsh, M. E. (1980). Development of children's concepts of illness. *Pediatrics, 66,* 912–917.

Bille, B. (1962). Migraine in schoolchildren. *Acta Paediatrica Scandinavia, 51*(Suppl. 136), 1–151.

Bishop, K. L., Ferraro, F. R., & Borowiak, D. M. (2001). Pain management in older adults: Role of fear avoidance. *Clinical Gerontologist, 23*(1–2), 33–42.

Birren, J. E., & Schaie, K. W. (1996). *Handbook of the psychology of aging* (4th ed.). San Diego, CA: Academic Press.

Blyth, F. M., March, L. M., Brnabic, A. J. M., Jorm, L. R., Williamson, M., & Cousins, M. J. (2001). Chronic pain in Australia: A prevalence study. *Pain, 89,* 127–134.

Bodnar, R. J., Romero, M. T., & Kramer, E. (1988). Organismic variables and pain inhibition: Roles of gender and aging. *Brain Research Bulletin, 21*(6), 947–953.

Borenstein, D. G. (2001). Epidemiology, etiology, diagnostic evaluation, and treatment of low back pain. *Current Opinions in Rheumatology, 13,* 128–134.

Bournaki, M. (1997). Correlates of pain-related responses to venipunctures in school-age children. *Nursing Research, 46,* 147–154.

Brattberg, G., Thorslund, M., & Wikman, A. (1989). The prevalence of pain in the general community: The results of a postal survey in a county of Sweden. *Pain, 37,* 21–32.

Brattberg, G., Parker, M. G., & Thorslund, M. (1997). A longitudinal study of pain: Reported pain from middle age to old age. *Clinical Journal of Pain, 13,* 144–149.

Brescia, F. J., Portenoy, R. K., Ryan, M., Krasnoff, L., & Gray, G. (1992). Pain, opioid use, and survival in hospitalized patients with advanced cancer. *Journal of Clinical Oncology, 10,* 149–155.

Buchthal, F., & Rosenfalck, P. (1966). Evoked action potentials and conduction velocity in human sensory nerves. *Brain Research, 3,* 1–22.

Burbach, D. J., & Peterson, L. (1986). Children's concepts of physical illness: A review and critique of the cognitive-developmental literature. *Health Psychology, 5,* 307–325.

Burckhardt, C. S., Clark, S. R., & Bennett, R. M. (2001). Pain coping strategies and quality of life in women with fibromyalgia: Does age make a difference? *Journal of Musculoskeletal Pain, Special Issue, 9,* 5–18.

Caraceni, A., & Portenoy, R. K. (1999). An international survey of cancer pain characteristics and syndromes. *Pain, 82,* 263–274.

Chakour, M. C., Gibson, S. J., Bradbeer, M., & Helme, R. D. (1996). The effect of age on A-delta and C-fibre thermal pain perception. *Pain, 64,* 143–152.

Chambers, C. T., & Craig, K. D. (1998). An intrusive impact of anchors in children's faces pain scales. *Pain, 78,* 27–37.

Chambers, C. T., Craig, K. D., & Bennett, S. M. (2002). The impact of maternal behavior on children's pain experiences. *Journal Pediatric Psychology, 27,* 293–301.

Chambers, C. T., & Johnston, C. (2002). Developmental differences in children's use of rating scales. *Journal of Pediatric Psychology, 27,* 27–36.

Chambers, C. T., Reid, G. J., Craig, K. D., McGrath, P. J., & Finley, G. A. (1998). Agreement between child and parent reports of pain. *Clinical Journal of Pain, 14,* 336–342.

Chambers, C. T., Reid, G. J., McGrath, P. J., & Finley, G. A. (1996). Development and preliminary validation of a postoperative pain measure for parents. *Pain, 68,* 307–313.

Champion, G. D., Goodenough, B., von Baeyer, C. L., & Thomas, W. (1998). Measurement of pain by self-report. In G. A. Finley & P. J. McGrath (Eds.), *Measurement of pain in infants and children, Progress in pain research and management* (Vol. 10, pp. 123–160). Seattle, WA: IASP Press.

Chibnall, J. T., & Tait, R. C. (2001). Pain assessment in cognitively impaired and unimpaired older adults: A comparison of four scales. *Pain, 92,* 173–186.

Clark, W. C., & Mehl, L. (1971). Thermal pain: A sensory decision theory analysis of the effect of age and sex on d , various response criteria, and 50% pain threshold. *Journal of Abnormal Psychology, 78,* 202–212.

Cook, A. J. (1998). Cognitive-behavioral pain management for elderly nursing home residents. *Journals of Gerontology, 53B*, P51–P59.

Cook, A. J., & Chastain, D. C. (2001). The classification of patients with chronic pain: Age and sex differences. *Pain Research Management, 6*, 142–151.

Cook, A. J., DeGood, D. E., & Chastain, D. C. (1999, August). Age differences in pain beliefs. *9th World Congress on Pain*, 1999, Abstract No. 182, p. 557.

Cook, A. K., Niven, C. A., & Downs, M. G. (1999). Assessing the pain of people with cognitive impairment. *International Journal Geriatric Psychiatry, 14*, 421–425.

Corran, T. M., Farrell, M. J., Helme, R. D., & Gibson, S. J. (1997). The classification of patients with chronic pain: Age as a contributing factor. *Clinical Journal of Pain, 13*, 207–214.

Corran, T. M., Gibson, S. J., Farrell, M. J., & Helme, R. D. (1994). Comparison of chronic pain experience between young and elderly patients. In G. F. Gebhart, D. L. Hammond, & T. S. Jensen (Eds.), *Progress in pain research and management* (pp. 895–906). Seattle, WA: IASP Press.

Corran, T. M., Helme, R. D., & Gibson, S. J. (1991). An assessment of psychometric instruments used in a geriatric outpatient pain clinic. *Australian Psychologist, 26*, 128–131.

Cossins, L., Benbow, S., & Wiles, J. R. (1999, August). A comparison of outcome in young and elderly patients attending a pain clinic. *9th World Congress on Pain*, 1999, Abstract No. 299, p. 90.

Craig, K. D. (1986). Social modelling influence: Pain in context. In R. A. Sternbach (Ed.), *The psychology of pain* (2nd ed., pp. 67–95). New York: Raven Press.

Craig, K. D. (1989). Emotional aspects of pain. In P. D. Wall & R. Melzack (Eds.), *Textbook of pain* (2nd ed., pp. 220–230). Oxford: University Printing House.

Craig, K. D. (1998). The facial display of pain. In G. A. Finley & P. J. McGrath (Eds.), *Measurement of pain in infants and children* (pp. 103–122). Seattle, WA: IASP Press.

Craig, K. D., Prkachin, K. M., & Grunau, R. V. E. (2001). The facial expression of pain. In D. C. Turk & R. Melzack (Eds.), *Handbook of pain assessment* (2nd ed., pp. 153–169). New York: Guilford Press.

Craig, K. D., Hadjistavropoulos, H. D., Grunau, R. V. E., & Whitfield, M. F. (1994). A comparison of 2 measures of facial activity during pain in the newborn child. *Journal of Pediatric Psychology, 19*, 305–318.

Craig, K. D., Lilley, C. M., & Gilbert, C. A. (1996). Social barriers to optimal pain management in infants and children. *Clinical Journal of Pain, 12*, 232–242.

Crook, J., Rideout, E., & Browne, G. (1984). The prevalence of pain complaints in a general population. *Pain, 18*, 299–305.

Cutler, R. B., Fishbain, D. A., Rosomoff, R. S., & Rosomoff, H. L. (1994). Outcomes in treatment of pain in geriatric and younger groups. *Archives Physical Medicine Rehabilitation, 75*, 457–464.

D'Alessandro, R., Benassi, G., Lenzi, P. L., Gamberini, G., DeCarolis, P., & Lugaseri, E. (1988). Epidemiology of headache in the republic of San Marino. *Journal Neurology Neurosurgery Psychiatry, 51*, 21–27.

Davison, I. S., Faull, C., & Nicol, A. R. (1986). Research note. Temperament and behaviour in six-year-olds with recurrent abdominal pain: A follow-up. *Journal of Child Psychology and Psychiatry and Allied Disciplines, 27*, 539–544.

Dickenson, A. H., & Rahman, W. (1999). Mechanisms of chronic pain and the developing nervous system. In P. J. McGrath & G. A. Finley (Eds.), *Chronic and recurrent pain in children and adolescents, Progress in pain research and management* (Vol. 13, pp. 5–38). Seattle, WA: IASP Press.

Ebrahim, S., Brittis, S., & Wu, A. (1991). The valuation of states of ill-health: The impact of age and disability. *Age and Ageing, 20*, 37–40.

Eccleston, C., Morley, S., Williams, A., Yorke, L., & Mastroyannopoulou, K. (2002). Systematic review of randomised controlled trials of psychological therapy for chronic pain in children and adolescents, with a subset meta-analysis of pain relief. *Pain, 99*, 157–165.

Ekman, P., & Friesen, W. (1969). The repertoire of nonverbal behavior: Categories, origins, usage and coding. *Semiotica, 1*, 49–98.

Edwards, R. R., & Fillingim, R. B. (2001). The effects of age on temporal summation and habituation of thermal pain: Clinical relevance in healthy older and younger adults. *Journal of Pain, 6*(2), 307–317.

Ehde, D. M., Holm, J. E., & Metzger, D. L. (1991). The role of family structure, functioning, and pain modeling in headache. *Headache, 31*, 35–40.

Eisenberg, D. M., Kessler, R. C., Foster, C., Norlock, F. E., Calkins, D. R., & Delbanco, T. L. (1993). Unconventional medicine in the United States. Prevalence, costs, and patterns of use. *New England Journal Medicine, 328*(4), 246–252.

Farrell, M. J., & Gibson, S. J. (1993, February). Outcomes for geriatric pain clinic patients. *14th Scientific Meeting of the Australian Pain Society*, p. 48. Melbourne, Australia.

Faull, C., & Nicol, A. (1985). Abdominal pain in six-year-olds: An epidemiological study in a new town. *Journal of Child Psychology and Psychiatry, 27*, 251–260.

Fearon, I., McGrath, P. J., & Achat, H. (1996). "Booboos": The study of everyday pain among young children. *Pain, 68*, 55–62.

Ferrell, B. A. (1995). Pain evaluation and management in the nursing home. *Annals of Internal Medicine, 123*, 681–695.

Ferrell, B. A., Josephson, K. R., Pollan, A. M., Loy, S., & Ferrell, B. R. (1997). A randomized trial of walking versus physical methods for chronic pain management. *Aging (Milano), 9*(1–2), 99–105.

Finley, G. A., & McGrath, P. J. (Eds.). (1998). *Measurement of pain in infants and children* (Progress in Pain Research and Management, Vol. 10). Seattle, WA: IASP Press.

Fitzgerald, M. (1985). The postnatal development of cutaneous afferent fibre input and receptive field organization in the rat dorsal horn. *Journal of Physiology, 364*, 1–18.

Fitzgerald, M. (1987). The prenatal growth of fine diameter afferents into the rat spinal cord—A transganglionic study. *Journal of Comprehensive Neurology, 261*, 98–104.

Fitzgerald, M. (1993). The developmental neuroanatomy and neurophysiology of pain. In N. Schechter, C. Berde, & M. Yaster (Eds.), *Pain management in infants, children and adolescents* (pp. 11–32). Baltimore, MD: Williams & Wilkins.

Fitzgerald, M., & de Lima, J. (2001). Hyperalgesia and allodynia in infants. In G. A. Finley & P. J. McGrath (Eds.), *Acute and procedure pain in infants and children* (pp. 1–12). Seattle, WA: IASP Press.

Flor, H., Fydrich, T., & Turk, D. C. (1992). Efficacy of multidisciplinary pain treatment centers: A meta-analytic review. *Pain, 49*(2), 221–230.

Fowler-Kerry, S., & Lander, J. R. (1987). Management of injection pain in children. *Pain, 30*, 169–175.

Fradet, C., McGrath, P. J., Kay, J., Adams, S., & Luke, B. (1990). A prospective survey of reactions to blood-tests by children and adolescents. *Pain, 40*, 53–60.

Gagliese, K., Wowk, A., Sandler, A., & Katz, J. (1999, August). Pain and opioid self-administration following prostatectomy in middle-aged and elderly men. *9th World Congress on Pain*, 1999, Abstr. 185, p. 558.

Gagliese, L. (2002). Assessment of pain in elderly people. In D. C. Turk & R. Melzack (Eds.), *Handbook of pain assessment* (pp. 119–133). New York: Guilford Press.

Gagliese, L., Jackson, M., Ritvo, P, Wowk, A., & Katz, J. (2000). Age is not an impediment to effective use of patient-controlled analgesia by surgical patients. *Anesthesiology, 93*, 601–610.

Gagliese, L., & Melzack, R. (1997a). Age differences in the quality of chronic pain: A preliminary study. *Pain Research and Management, 2*, 157–162.

Gagliese, L., & Melzack, R. (1997b). Lack of evidence for age differences in pain beliefs. *Pain Research and Management, 2*, 19–28.

Gagliese, L., & Melzack, R. (2000). Age differences in nociception and pain behaviours in the rat. *Neuroscience & Biobehavioral Reviews, 24*(8), 843–854.

Gallagher, R. M., Verma, S., & Mossey, J. (2000). Chronic pain. Sources of late-life pain and risk factors for disability. *Geriatrics, 55*, 40–44.

Gardner, P., Garland, K., Workman, B., & Mendelson, G. (2001, April). A comparison of the use of coping strategies by older-aged chronic pain patients with a general chronic pain sample using the Coping Strategies Questionnaire (CSQ). *22nd Australian Pain Society Conference*, p. 45.

Gatchel, R. J., & Turk, D. C. (Eds.). (1999). *Psychosocial factors in pain: Critical perspectives*. New York: Guilford Press.

Gibson, S. J., Chang, W. C., & Farrell, M. J. (2002, August). Age interacts with frequency in the temporal summation of painful electrical stimuli. *10th World Congress on Pain*, Abstr. 905, p. 175.

Gibson, S. J., Farrell, M., Katz, B., & Helme, R. D. (1996). Multidisciplinary management of chronic non-malignant pain in older adults. In B. R. Ferrell & B. A. Ferrell (Eds.), *Pain in the elderly* (pp. 91–99). Seattle, WA: IASP Press.

Gibson, S. J., Gorman, M. M., & Helme, R. D. (1990). Assessment of pain in the elderly using event-related cerebral potentials. In M. R. Bond, J. E. Charlton, & C. Woolf (Eds.), *Proceedings of the VIth World Congress on Pain* (pp. 523–529). Amsterdam: Elsevier.

Gibson, S. J., & Helme, R. D. (1995). Age differences in pain perception and report: A review of physiological, psychological, laboratory and clinical studies. *Pain Reviews, 2*, 111–137.

Gibson, S. J., & Helme, R. D. (2000). Cognitive factors and the experience of pain and suffering in older persons. *Pain, 85*, 375–383.

Gibson, S. J., & Helme, R. D. (2001). Age-related differences in pain perception and report. *Clinics in Geriatric Medicine, 17*, 433–456.

Gibson, S. J., Helme, R. D., & Gorman, M. M. (1993, August). Age related changes in the scalp topography of cerebral event related potentials following noxious CO_2 laser stimulation. *7th World Congress on Pain*, 1993, Abstr. 428, p. 159.

Gloth, F. M. (2000). Factors that limit pain relief and increase complications. *Geriatrics, 55*, 46–54.

Goodenough, B., Champion, G. D., Laubreaux, L., Tabah, L., & Kampel, L. (1998). Needle pain severity in children: Does the relationship between self-report and observed behaviour vary as a function of age? *Australian Journal of Psychology, 50*, 1–9.

Goodenough, B., Kampel, L., Champion, G. D., Laubreaux, L., Nicholas, M. K., Ziegler, J. B., & McInerney, M. (1997). An investigation of the placebo effect and age-related factors in the report of needle pain from venipuncture in children. *Pain, 72*, 383–391.

Goodenough, B., Thomas, W., Champion, G. D., Perrott, D., Taplin, J. E., von Baeyer, C. L., & Ziegler, J. B. (1999). Unravelling age effects in needle pain: Ratings of sensory intensity and unpleasantness of venipuncture pain by children and their parents. *Pain, 80*, 179–190.

Goodman, J. E., & McGrath, P. J. (1991). The epidemiology of pain in children and adolescents—A review. *Pain, 46*, 247–264.

Goodman, J. E., McGrath, P. J., & Forward, S. P. (1997). Aggregation of pain complaints and pain-related disability and handicap in a community sample of families. In T. S. Jensen, J. A. Turner, & Z. Wiesenfeld-Hallin (Eds.), *Proceedings of the 8th World Congress on Pain: Progress in pain research and management* (pp. 673–682). Seattle, WA: IASP Press.

Goyen, M. J., & Anshel, M. H. (1998). Sources of acute competitive stress and use of coping strategies as a function of age and gender. *Journal of Applied Developmental Psychology, 19*, 469–486.

Groves, F., Garland, K., Mendelson, G., & Gibson, S. J. (2002, August). Multidisciplinary pain treatment outcome differs as a function of age. *10th World Congress on Pain*, Abstr. 230, p. 226.

Grunau, R. V. E., Whitfield, M. F., & Petrie, J. H. (1994). Pain sensitivity and temperament in extremely-low-birthweight premature toddlers and preterm and full-term controls. *Pain, 58*, 341–346.

Grunau, R. V. E., Whitfield, M. F., Petrie, J. H., & Fryer, E. L. (1994). Early pain experience, child and family factors as precursors of somatization: A prospective study of extremely premature and fullterm children. *Pain, 56*, 353–359.

Grunau, R. V. E., Whitfield, M. F., & Petrie, J. H. (1998). Children's judgments about pain at age 8–10 years: Do extremely low birthweight (1000 g) children differ from full birthweight peers? *Journal of Child Psychology and Psychiatry, 39*, 587–594.

Guck, T. P., Meilman, P. W., Skultety, F. M., & Dowd, E. T. (1986). Prediction of long-term outcome of multidisciplinary pain treatment. *Archives of Physical Medicine Rehabilitation, 67*(5), 293–296.

Guzman, J., Esmail, R., Karjalainen, K., Malmivaara, A., Irvin, E., & Bombardier, C. (2002). Multidisciplinary bio-psycho-social rehabilitation for chronic low back pain. *Cochrane Database Systematic Reviews, 1*, CD000963.

Hadjistavropoulos, T., Craig, K. D., Martin, N., Hadjistavropoulos, H., & McMurtry, B. (1997). Toward a research outcome measure of pain in frail elderly in chronic care. *Pain Clinic, 10*, 71–79.

Hadjistavropoulos, T., LaChapelle, D., MacLeod, F., Hale, C., O'Rourke, N., & Craig, K. D. (1998). Cognitive functioning and pain reactions in hospitalized elders. *Pain Research and Management, 3*, 145–151.

Hadjistavropoulos, T., LaChapelle, D. L., Hadjistavropoulos, H. D., Green, S., & Asmundson, G. J. G. (2002). Using facial expressions to assess musculoskeletal pain in older persons. *European Journal of Pain, 6*, 174–187.

Hadjistavropoulos, T., LaChapelle, D. L., MacLeod, F. K., Snider, B., & Craig, K. D. (2000). Measuring movement-exacerbated pain in cognitively impaired frail elders. *Clinical Journal of Pain, 16*, 54–63.

Hallett, E. C., & Pilowsky, I. (1982). The response to treatment in a multidisciplinary pain clinic. *Pain, 12*(4), 365–374.

Harbeck, C., & Peterson, L. (1992). Elephants dancing in my head: A developmental approach to children's concepts of specific pains. *Child Development, 63*, 138–149.

Harkins, S. W. (1988). Pain in the elderly. In R. Dubner, G. F. Gebhart, & M. R. Bond (Eds.), *Proceedings of the Vth World Congress on Pain* (pp. 355–367). Amsterdam: Elsevier.

Harkins, S. W., & Chapman, C. R. (1976). Detection and decision factors in pain perception in young and elderly men. *Pain, 2*, 253–264.

Harkins, S. W., & Chapman, C. R. (1977). The perception of induced dental pain in young and elderly women. *Journals of Gerontology, 32*, 428–435.

Harkins, S. W., Davis, M. D., Bush, F. M., & Price, D. D. (1996). Suppression of first pain and slow temporal summation of second pain in relation to age. *Journals of Gerontology, 51*, M260–265.

Harkins, S. W., Kwentus, J., & Price, D. D. (1984). Pain and the elderly. In C. Benedetti, C. R. Chapman, & G. Moricca (Eds.), *Advances in pain research and therapy* (Vol. 7, pp. 103–112). New York: Raven Press.

Harkins, S. W., & Price, D. D. (1992). Assessment of pain in the elderly. In R. Melzack & D. C. Turk (Eds.), *Handbook of pain assessment* (pp. 315–331). New York: Guilford Press.

Harkins, S. W., Price, D. D., & Bush, F. M. (1994). Geriatric pain. In P. D. Wall & R. Melzack (Eds.), *Textbook of pain* (pp. 769–787). New York: Churchill Livingstone.

Haslam, D. R. (1969). Age and the perception of pain. *Psychonomic Science, 15*, 86–87.

Helme, R. D., & Gibson, S. J. (1998). Measurement and management of pain in older people. *Australasian Journal on Ageing, 17*, 5–9.

Helme, R. D., & Gibson, S. J. (1999). Pain in older people. In I. K. Crombie (Ed.), *Epidemiology of pain* (pp. 103–112). Seattle, WA: IASP Press.

Helme, R. D., & Gibson, S. J. (2001). The epidemiology of pain in elderly people. *Clinics in Geriatric Medicine, 17*, 417–431.

Helme, R. D., Katz, B., Gibson, S. J., Bradbeer, M., Farrell, M., Neufeld, M., & Corran, T. (1996). Multidisciplinary pain clinics for older people: Do they have a role? *Clinics in Geriatric Medicine, 12*(3), 563–582.

Helme, R. D., Katz, B., Neufeld, M., Lachal, S., Herbert, T., & Corran, T. (1989). The establishment of a geriatric pain clinic: A preliminary report on the first 100 patients. *Australian Journal on Ageing, 8*, 27–30.

Helme, R. D., & McKernan, S. (1985). Neurogenic flare responses following topical application of capsaicin in humans. *Annals of Neurology, 18*, 505–511.

Herr, K. A., & Mobily, P. R. (1991). Pain assessment in the elderly—Clinical considerations. *Journal of Gerontological Nursing, 17*, 12–19.

Herr, K. A., & Mobily, P. R. (1993). Comparison of selected pain assessment tools for use with the elderly. *Applied Nursing Research, 6*, 39–46.

Herr, K. A., Mobily, P. R., Wallace, R. B., & Chung, Y. (1991). Leg pain in the rural Iowa 65+ population: Prevalence, related factors, and association with functional status. *Clinical Journal of Pain, 7*, 114–121.

Herr, K. A., Mobily, P. R., Koout, F. J., & Wagenaar, D. (1998). Evaluation of the Faces Pain Scale for use with the elderly. *Clinical Journal of Pain, 14*, 29–38.

Herr, K. A., Mobily, P. R., & Smith, C. (1993). Depression and the experience of chronic back pain: A study of related variables and age differences. *Clinical Journal of Pain, 9*, 104–114.

Hodgson, J. E., Suda, K. T., Bruce, B. K., & Rome, J. D. (1993, August). Depression in the elderly chronic pain patient. *7th World Congress on Pain*, 1993, Abstr. 287, p. 99.

Hofland, S. L. (1992). Elder beliefs: Blocks to pain management. *Journal of Gerontological Nursing, 18*, 19–24.

Houck, C. S. (1998). The management of acute pain in the child. In M. A. Ashburn & L. J. Rice (Eds.), *The management of pain* (pp. 651–666). New York: Churchill Livingstone.

Izard, C. E., Porges, S. W., Simons, R. F., Haynes, O. M., Hyde, C., Parisi, M., & Cohen, B. (1991). Infant cardiac activity: Developmental changes and relations with attachment. *Developmental Psychology, 27*, 432–439.

Jay, S. M., Ozolins, M., Elliott, C. H., & Caldwell, S. (1983). Assessment of children's distress during painful medical procedures. *Health Psychology, 2*, 133–147.

Jensen, M. P., & Karoly, P. (1992). Self-report scales and procedures for assessing pain in adults. In R. Melzack & D. C. Turk (Eds.), *Handbook of pain assessment* (pp. 135–151). New York: Guilford Press.

Jensen, M. P., Turner, J. A., Romano, J. M., & Karoly, P. (1991). Coping with chronic pain: A critical review of the literature. *Pain, 47*, 249–283.

Johnston, C. C., Stevens, B., Craig, K. D., & Grunau, R. V. E. (1993). Developmental changes in pain expression in premature full-term, 2-month-old and 4-month-old infants. *Pain, 52*, 201–208.

Katz, B., & Helme, R. D. (2001). Pain problems in old age. In J. Brockelhurst (Ed.), *Textbook of geriatric medicine and gerontology* (pp. 1423–1430). Oxford: Cambridge Press.

Katz, E. R., Kellerman, J., & Siegel, S. E. (1980). Behavioral distress in children with cancer undergoing medical procedures: Developmental considerations. *Journal of Consulting and Clinical Psychology, 48*, 356–365.

Katz, J., & Melzack, R. (1999). Measurement of pain. *Surgery Clinics North America, 70*, 231–352.

Kay, L., Jorgensen, T., & Schultz-Larsen, K. (1992). Abdominal pain in a 70-year old Danish population. *Journal Clinical Epidemiology, 45*, 1377–1382.

Kee, W. G., Middaugh, S. J., & Pawlick, K. L. (1996). Persistent pain in older patient. Evaluation and treatment. In R. J. Gatchel & D. C. Turk (Eds.), *Psychosocial factors in pain: Critical perspectives* (pp. 371–402). New York: Guilford Press.

Kee, W. G., Middaugh, S. J., Redpath, S., & Hargadon, R. (1998). Age as a factor in admission to chronic pain rehabilitation. *Clinical Journal of Pain, 14*(2), 121–128.

Keefe, F. J., & Block, A. R. (1982). Development of an observational method for assessing pain behaviour in chronic low back pain patients. *Behavior Therapy, 13*, 363–375.

Keefe, F. J., & Williams, D. A. (1990). A comparison of coping strategies in chronic pain patients in different age groups. *Journal of Gerontology, 45*, P161–165.

Keefe, F. J., Caldwell, D. S., Martinez, S., Nunley, J., Beckham, J., & Williams, D. A. (1991). Analyzing pain in rheumatoid arthritis patients. Pain coping strategies in patients who have had knee replacement surgery. *Pain, 46*, 153–160.

Kendig, H., Helme, R. D., & Teshuva, K. (1996). *Health status of older people project: Data from a survey of the health and lifestyles of older Australians.* Report to the Victorian Health Promotion Foundation, Melbourne, Australia.

Kind, P., Dolan, P., Gudex, C., & Williams, A. (1998). Variations in population health status: Results from a United Kingdom national questionnaire survey. *British Medical Journal, 316*, 736–741.

Klinger, L., & Spaulding, S. J. (1998). Chronic pain in the elderly: Is silence really golden? *Physical and Occupational Therapy in Geriatrics, 15*, 1–17.

Kolter-Cope, S., & Gerber, K. E. (1993, August). Is age related to response to treatment for chronic pain? *7th World Congress on Pain*, Abstr. 290, p. 100.

Konu, V. (1977). Myocardial infarction in the elderly. *Acta Medicine Scandanavia, 604*, 3–68.

Kovach, C. R., Griffie, J., Matson, S., & Muchka, S. (1999). Assessment and treatment of discomfort in people with late-stage dementia. *Journal Pain Symptom Management, 18*, 412–419.

Kremer, E., Atkinson, J. H., & Ignelzi, R. J. (1981). Measurement of pain: Patient preference does not confound pain measurement. *Pain, 10*(2), 241–248.

Krulewitch, H., London, M. R., Skakel, V. J., Lundstedt, G. J., Thomason, H., & Brummel-Smith, K. (2000). Assessment of pain in cognitively impaired older adults: A comparison of pain assessment tools and their use by non-professional caregivers. *Journal of the American Geriatrics Society, 48*, 1607–1622.

Lander, J., & Fowler-Kerry, S. (1991). Age-differences in children's pain. *Perceptual and Motor Skills, 73*, 415–418.

Lavsky-Shulan, M., Wallace, R. B., Kohout, F. J., Lemke, J. H., Morris, M. C., & Smith, I. M. (1985). Prevalence and functional correlates of low in the elderly: The Iowa 65+ rural health study. *Journal of American Geriatrics Society, 33*, 23–28.

Lee, J. S. (2001). Pain measurement: Understanding existing tools and their application in the emergency department. *Emergency Medicine, 13*, 279–287.

Leventhal, E. A., Leventha, H., Schaefer, P., & Easterling, D. (1993). Conservation of energy, uncertainty reduction, and swift utilization of medical care among the elderly. *Journal of Gerontology, 48*, 78–86.

Leventhal, E. A., & Prohaska, T. R. (1986). Age, symptom interpretation, and health behavior. *Journal of the American Geriatrics Society, 34*, 185–191.

Leveille, S. G., Gurlanik, J. M., Ferrucci, L., Simonsick, E., Hirsch, R., & Hochberg, M. C. (1998). Foot pain and disability in older women. *American Journal Epidemiology, 148*, 657–665.

Lewis, M., & Thomas, D. (1990). Cortisol release in infants in response to inoculation. *Child Development, 61*, 50–59.

Li, Y., & Duckles, S. P. (1993). Effect of age on vascular content of calcitonin gene-related peptide and mesenteric vasodilator activity in the rat. *European Journal Pharmacology, 236*(3), 373–378.

Lichtenberg, P. A., Skehan, M. W., & Swensen, C. H. (1984). The role of personality, recent life stress and arthritic severity in predicting pain. *Journal of Psychosomatic Research, 28*, 231–236.

Liddell, A., & Locker, D. (1997). Gender and age differences in attitudes to dental pain and dental control. *Community Dental and Oral Epidemiology, 25*(4), 314–318.

Lilley, C. M., Craig, K. D., & Grunau, R. E. (1997). The expression of pain in infants and toddlers: Developmental changes in facial action. *Pain, 72*, 161–170.

Linet, M. S., Stewart, W. F., Celentano, D. D., Ziegler, D. K., & Sprecher, M. (1989). An epidemiologic study of headache among adolescents and young adults. *Journal of the American Medical Association, 261*, 2211–2216.

MacDonald, J. B., Baillie, J., & Williams, B. O. (1983). Coronary care in the elderly. *Age and Ageing, 12*, 17–20.

Machin, P., & Williams, A. C. de C. (1998). Stiff upper lip: Coping strategies of World War II veterans with phantom limb pain. *Clinical Journal of Pain, 14*, 290–294.

Magni, G., Marchetti, M., Moreschi, C., Merskey, H., & Luchini, S. (1993). Chronic musculoskeletal pain and depression in the National Health and Nutrition Examination. *Pain, 53*, 163–168.

Maikler, V. E. (1991). Effects of a skin refrigerant/anesthetic and age on the pain responses of infants receiving immunizations. *Research Nursing Health, 14*, 397–403.

Mangione, C. M., Marcantonio, E. R., Goldman, L., Cook, E. F., Donaldson, M. C., Sugarbaker, D. J., Poss, R., & Lee, T. H. (1993). Influence of age on measurement of health status in patients undergoing elective surgery. *Journal of the American Geriatrics Society, 41*(4), 377–383.

Manne, S. L., Redd, W. H., Jacobsen, P. B., Gorfinkle, K., & Schorr, O. (1990). Behavioral intervention to reduce child and parent distress during venipuncture. *Journal of Consulting and Clinical Psychology, 58*, 565–572.

Matheson, D. H. (1997). The painful truth: Interpretation of facial expression of pain in older adults. *Journal of Nonverbal Behavior, 21*(3), 223–238.

McCracken, L. M. (1998). Learning to live with the pain: Acceptance of pain predicts adjustment in persons with chronic pain. *Pain, 74*, 21–27.

McGrath, P. A. (1994). Psychological aspects of pain perception. *Archives of Oral Biology, 39*, S55–S62.

McGrath, P. J. (1995). Aspects of pain in children and adolescents. *Journal of Child Psychology and Psychiatry and Allied Disciplines, 36*, 717–730.

McGrath, P. J. (1998). Behavioral measures of pain. In G. A. Finley & P. J. McGrath (Eds.), *Measurement of pain in infants and children* (Progress in Pain Research and Management, Vol. 10) (pp. 83–102). Seattle, WA: IASP Press.

McGrath, P. A., & Gillespie, J. (2001). Pain assessment in children and adolescents. In D. C. Turk & R. Melzack (Eds.), *Handbook of pain assessment* (pp. 97–118). New York: Guilford Press.

McMillan, S. C. (1989). The relationship between age and intensity of cancer related symptoms. *Oncology Nursing Forum, 16*, 237–342.

Meier, D. E., Morrison, R. S., & Ahronheim, J. C. (1996). Quantifying pain and discomfort from procedures in hospitalized patients: Validation of a new tool. *Proceedings of the American Geriatric Society*, Abstr. 123, p. 127.

Melding, P. S. (1995). How do older people respond to chronic pain? A review of coping with pain and illness in elders. *Pain Reviews, 2*, 65–75.

Merskey, H., & Bogduk, N. (1994). *Classification of chronic pain: Descriptions of chronic pain and definition of pain terms* (2nd ed.). Seattle, WA: IASP Press.

Middaugh, S. J., Levin, R. B., Kee, W. G., Barchiesi, F. D., & Roberts, J. M. (1988). Chronic pain: Its treatment in geriatric and younger patients. *Archives Physical Medicine Rehabilitation, 69*, 1021–1026.

Miller, C., & LeLieuvre, R. B. (1982). A method to reduce chronic pain in elderly nursing home residents. *Gerontologist, 22*(3), 314–317.

Miller, P. F., Sheps, D. S., & Bragdon, E. E. (1990). Aging and pain perception in ischemic heart disease. *American Heart Journal, 120*, 22–30.

Mobily, P. R., Herr, K. A., Clark, M. K., & Wallace, R. B. (1994). An epidemiologic analysis of pain in the elderly. *Journal of Ageing Health, 6*, 139–154.

Morley, S., Doyle, K., & Beese, A. (2000). Talking to others about pain: Suffering in silence. In M. Devor, M. C. Rowbotham, & Z. Wiesenfeld-Hallin (Eds.), *Progress in pain research and management* (pp. 1123–1129). Seattle, WA: IASP Press.

Mosley, T. H., McCracken, J. J., Gross, R. T., Penzien, D. B., & Plaud, J. J. (1993, August). Age, pain and impairment: Results from two clinical samples. *7th World Congress on Pain*, Abstr. 286, p. 99.

Naish, J. M., & Apley, J. (1951). "Growing pains": A clinical study of non-arthritis limb pains in children. *Archives of Disease in Childhood, 26*, 134–140.

Nicholson, N. L., & Blanchard, E. B. (1993). A controlled evaluation of behavioral treatment of chronic headache in the elderly. *Behavior Therapy, 24*(3), 395–408.

Ochoa, J., & Mair, W. G. P. (1969). The normal sural nerve in man. II. Changes in the axon and schwann cells due to ageing. *Acta Neuropathology (Berlin), 13*, 217–253.

Oberle, K., Paul, P., & Wry, J. (1990). Pain, anxiety and analgesics: A comparative study of elderly and younger surgical patients. *Canadian Journal of Ageing, 9*, 13–19.

Painter, J. R., Seres, J. L., & Newman, R. I. (1980). Assessing benefits of the pain center: Why some patients regress. *Pain, 8*(1), 101–113.

Palermo, T. M. (2000). Impact of recurrent and chronic pain on child and family daily functioning: A critical review of the literature. *Journal of Developmental and Behavioral Pediatrics, 21*, 58–69.

Palermo, T. M., & Drotar, D. (1996). Prediction of children's postoperative pain: The role of presurgical expectations and anticipatory emotions. *Journal Pediatric Psychology, 21*, 683–698.

Parker, J., Frank, R., Beck, N., Finan, M., Walker, S., Hewett, J. E., Broster, C., Smarr, K., Smith, E., & Kay, D. (1988). Pain in rheumatoid arthritis: Relationship to demographic, medical and psychological factors. *Journal of Rheumatology, 15*, 433–447.

Parmelee, P. (1997). Pain and psychological function in late life. In D. I. Mostofsky & J. Lomranz (Eds.), *Handbook of pain and aging* (pp. 207–227). New York: Plenum Press.

Parmelee, P. A. (1994). Assessment of pain in the elderly. In M. P. Lawton & J. A. Tevesi (Eds.), *Annual Review of Gerontology and Geriatrics, 14*, 281–301.

Perez, C. E. (2000). Chronic back problems among workers. *Health Reports, 12*, 45–60.

Perquin, C. W., Hazebroek-Kampschreur, A. A. J. M., Hunfeld, J. A. M., Bohnen, A. M., van Suijlekom-Smit, L. W. A., Passchier, J., & van der Wouden, J. C. (2000). Pain in children and adolescents: A common experience. *Pain, 87*, 51–58.

Perquin, C. W., Hazebroek-Kampschreur, A. A. J. M., Hunfeld, J. A. M., van Suijlekom-Smit, L. W. A., Passchier, J., & van der Wouden, J. C. (2000). Chronic pain among children and adolescents: Physician consultation and medication use. *Clinical Journal of Pain, 16*, 229–235.

Portenoy, R. K., & Farkash, A. (1988). Practical management of non-malignant pain in the elderly. *Geriatrics, 43*(5), 29–47.

Powers, S. W. (1999). Empirically supported treatments in pediatric psychology: Procedure-related pain. *Journal of Pediatric Psychology, 24*, 131–145.

Prohaska, T. R., Leventhal, E. A., Leventhal, H., & Keller, M. L. (1985). Health practices and illness cognition in young, middle aged, and elderly adults. *Journal of Gerontology, 40*, 569–578.

Puder, R. S. (1988). Age analysis of cognitive-behavioral group therapy for chronic pain outpatients. *Psychology of Aging, 3*(2), 204–207.

Reid, G. J., Gilbert, C. A., & McGrath, P. J. (1998). The Pain Coping Questionnaire: Preliminary validation. *Pain, 76*, 83–96.

Riley, J. L. III, Wade, J. B., Robinson, M. E., & Price, D. D. (2000). The stages of pain processing across the lifespan. *Journal of Pain, 1*(2), 162–170.

Ruzicka, S. A. (1998). Pain beliefs: What do elders believe? *Journal Holistic Nursing, 16*, 369–382.

Sanders, M. R., & Morrison, M. (1990). Behavioral treatment of childhood recurrent abdominal pain: Relationship between pain, children's psychological characteristics and family functioning. *Behavior Change, 7*, 16–24.

Sanders, M. R., Rebgetz, M., Morrison, M., Bor, W., Gordon, A., Dadds, M., & Shepherd, R. (1989). Cognitive-behavioral treatment of recurrent nonspecific abdominal pain in children: An analysis of generalization, maintenance and side-effects. *Journal of Consulting and Clinical Psychology, 57*, 294–300.

Savedra, M. C., Tesler, M. D., Holzemer, W. L., Wilkie, D. J., & Ward, J. A. (1990). Testing a tool to assess postoperative pediatric and adolescent pain. In D. C. Tyler & E. J. Krane (Eds.), *Advances in pain research therapy* (pp. 85–93). New York: Raven Press.

Schechter, N. L. (1989). The undertreatment of pain in children. *Pediatric Pain Clinics of North America, 36*, 781–794.

Schellinck, H. M., & Anand, K. J. S. (1999). Consequences of early experience. Lessons for rodent models of newborn pain. In P. J. McGrath & G. A. Finley (Eds.), *Chronic and recurrent pain in children and adolescents* (Progress in Pain Research and Management, Vol. 13) (pp. 39–55). Seattle, WA: IASP Press.

Scherder, E. J. K., & Bouma, A. (2000). Visual analogue scales for pain assessment in Alzheimer's disease. *Gerontology, 46*, 47–53.

Schludermann, E., & Zubek, J. P. (1962). Effect of age on pain sensitivity. *Perceptual and Motor Skills, 14*, 295–301.

Simons, W., & Malabar, T. (1995). Assessing pain in elderly patients who cannot respond verbally. *Journal of Advanced Nursing, 22*, 663–669.

Sorkin, B. A., Rudy, T. E., Hanlon, R. B., Turk, D. C., & Stieg, R. L. (1990). Chronic pain in old and young patients: Differences appear less important than similarities. *Journal of Gerontology: Psychological Sciences, 45*, 64–68.

Sternbach, R. A. (1986). Survey of pain in the United States: The Nuprin pain report. *Clinical Journal of Pain, 2*, 49–54.

Stevens, B. J., & Franck, L. S. (2001). Assessment and management of pain in neonates. *Paediatric Drugs, 3*, 539–558.

Stevens, B., Johnston, C. C., & Gibbins, S. (2000). Pain assessment in the neonate. In K. J. S. Anand, B. Stevens, & P. J. McGrath (Eds.), *Pain in neonates* (2nd ed., pp. 101–134). Amsterdam: Elsevier.

Stevens, B., Johnston, C., Petryshen, P., & Taddio, A. (1996). Premature Infant Pain Profile: Development and initial validation. *Clinical Journal of Pain, 12*, 13–22.

Stoller, E. P. (1993). Interpretations of symptoms by older people. *Journal of Aging and Health, 5*, 58–81.

Suzman, R., & Riley, M. W. (1985). Introducing the "oldest old." Milbank Members Fund Q. *Health and Society, 63*(2), 177–86.

Sweet, S. D., & McGrath, P. J. (1998). Physiological measures of pain. In G. A. Finley & P. J. McGrath (Eds.), *Measurement of pain in infants and children* (Progress in Pain Research and Management, Vol. 10) (pp. 59–81). Seattle, WA: IASP Press.

Sweet, S. D., McGrath, P. J., & Symons, D. (1999). The roles of child reactivity and parenting context in infant pain response. *Pain, 80*, 655–661.

Taddio, A. (1999). Effects of early pain experience: The human literature. In P. J. McGrath & G. A. Finley (Eds.), *Chronic and recurrent pain in children and adolescents* (Progress in Pain Research and Management, Vol. 13) (pp. 57–74). Seattle, WA: IASP Press.

Taddio, A., Katz, J., Ilersich, A. L., & Koren, G. (1997). Effect of neonatal circumcision on pain response during subsequent routine vaccination. *Lancet, 349*, 599–603.

Taddio, A., Nulman, I., Goldbach, M., Ipp, M., & Koren, G. (1994). Use of lidocaine-prilocaine cream for vaccination pain in infants. *Journal of Pediatrics, 124*, 643–648.

Taddio, A., Stevens, B., Craig, K. D., Rastogi, P., Ben David, S., Shennan, A., Mulligan, P., & Koren, G. (1997). Efficacy and safety of lidocaine-prilocaine cream for pain during circumcision. *New England Journal of Medicine, 336*, 1197–1201.

Taimela, S., Kujala, U., Salminen, J., & Viljanen, T. (1997). The prevalence of low back pain among children and adolescents: A nationwide, cohort-based questionnaire survey in Finland. *Spine, 22*, 1132–1136.

Tarbell, S. E., Cohen, T., & Marsh, J. L. (1992). The Toddler–Preschool Postoperative Pain Scale: An observational scale for measuring postoperative pain in children aged 1–5. Preliminary report. *Pain, 50*, 273–280.

Thomas, T., Robinson, C., & Champion, D. (1998). Prediction and assessment of the severity of post operative pain and of satisfaction with management. *Pain, 75*, 177–185.

Thorsteinsson, G. (1987). Chronic pain: Use of TENS in the elderly. *Gerontology, 42*, 75–82.

Tibblin, G., Bengtsson, C., Furness, B., & Lapidus, L. (1990). Symptoms by age and sex. *Scandinavian Journal Primary Health Care, 8*, 9–17.

Tiplady, B., Jackson, S. H. D., Maskrey, V. M., & Swift, C. G. (1998). Validity and sensitivity of visual analogue scales in young and older healthy subjects. *Age and Ageing, 27*, 63–73.

Turk, D. C., Okifuji, A., & Scharff, L. (1995). Chronic pain and depression: Role of perceived impact and perceived control in different age cohorts. *Pain, 61*, 93–101.

Turkat, I. D., Kuczmierczyk, A. R., & Adams, H. E. (1984). An investigation of the aetiology of chronic headache: The role of headache models. *British Journal of Psychiatry, 145*, 665–666.

Varni, J. W., Thompson, K. L., & Hanson, V. (1987). The Varni/Thompson Pediatric Pain Questionnaire. I. Chronic musculoskeletal pain in juvenile rheumatoid arthritis. *Pain, 28*, 27–38.

Verhaak, P. F., Kerssens, J. J., Dekker, J., Sorbi, M. J., & Bensing, J. M. (1998). Prevalence of chronic benign pain disorder among adults: A review of the literature. *Pain, 77*(3), 231–239.

Vigano, A., Bruera, E., & Suarex-Almazor, M. E. (1998). Age, pain intensity, and opioid dose in patients with advanced cancer. *Cancer, 83*, 1244–1250.

von Baeyer, C. L., Baskerville, S., & McGrath, P. J. (1998). Everyday pain in three- to five-year-old children in day care. *Pain Research and Management, 3*, 111–116.

von Baeyer, C. L., Carlson, G., & Webb, L. (1997). Underprediction of pain in children undergoing ear piercing. *Behaviour Research and Therapy, 35*, 399–404.

von Korff, M., Dworkin, S. F., & Le Resche, L. (1990). Graded chronic pain status: An epidemiologic evaluation. *Pain, 40*, 279–291.

von Korff, M., Dworkin, S. F., Le Resche, L., & Kruger, A. (1988). An epidemiologic comparison of pain complaints. *Pain, 32*, 173–183.

Walco, G. A., & Harkins, S. W. (1999). Lifepan developmental approaches to pain. In R. J. Gatchel & D. C. Turk (Eds.), *Psychosocial factors in pain: Critical perspectives* (pp. 107–117). New York: Guilford Press.

Walker, L. S., & Greene, J. W. (1991). The Functional Disability Inventory: Measuring a neglected dimension of child health status. *Journal of Pediatric Psychology, 16*, 39–58.

Wall, R. T. (1990). Use of analgesics in the elderly. *Clinics in Geriatric Medicine, 6*(2), 345–364.

Washington, L. L., Gibson, S. J., & Helme, R. D. (2000). Age-related differences in the endogenous analgesic response to repeated cold water immersion in human volunteers. *Pain, 89*(1), 89–96.

Weiner, D., Peterson, B., & Keefe, F. (1998). Evaluating persistent pain in long term care residents: What role for pain maps? *Pain, 76*, 249–257.

Weiner, D., Peterson, B., & Keefe, F. (1999). Chronic pain-associated behaviors in the nursing home: Resident versus caregiver perceptions. *Pain, 80*(3), 577–588.

Weiner, D., Pieper, C., McConnell, E., Martinez, S., & Keefe, F. (1996). Pain measurement in elders with chronic low back pain: Traditional and alternative approaches. *Pain, 67*, 461–467.

Weiner, D. K., Peterson, B. L., Logue, P., & Keefe, F. J. (1998). Predictors of pain self-report in nursing home residents. *Aging Clinical and Experimental Research, 10*, 411–420.

Weiner, D. K., & Rudy, T. E. (2000). Attitudinal barriers to effective pain management in the nursing home. In M. Devor, M. C. Rowbotham, & Z. Wiesenfeld-Hallin (Eds.), *Progress in pain research and management* (pp. 1097–2003). Seattle, WA: IASP Press.

Werner, P., Cohen-Mansfield, J., Watson, V., & Pasis, S. (1998). Pain in participants of adult day care centers: Assessment by different raters. *Journal of Pain Symptom Management, 15*, 8–17.

Wijeratne, C., Shome, S., Hickie, I., & Koschera, A. (2001). An age-based comparison of chronic pain clinic patients. *International Journal of Geriatric Psychiatry, 16*, 477–483.

Wilkinson, C. A., Madhok, R., & Hunter, J. A. (1993). Toleration, side-effects and efficacy of sulphasalazine in arthritis patients of different ages. *Quarterly Journal of Medicine, 86*, 501–505.

Williams, A. C. de C. (2001). Outcome assessment in chronic non-cancer pain treatment. *Acta Anaesthesiologica Scandinavia, 45*, 1076–1079.

Williams, D. A., & Thorn, B. E. (1989). An empirical assessment of pain beliefs. *Pain, 36*, 351–358.

Wroblewski, M., & Mikulowski, P. (1991). Peritonitis in geriatric inpatients. *Age and Ageing, 20*, 90–94.

Yong, H.-H., Gibson, S. J., Horne, D. J., & Helme, R. D. (2001). Development of a pain attitudes questionnaire to assess stoicism and cautiousness for possible age differences. *Journal of Gerontology: Psychological Services, 56B*(5), 279–284.

Ysla, R., Rosomoff, R. S., & Rosomoff, H. L. (1986). Functional improvement in geriatric pain patients. *Archives of Physical Medicine Rehabilitation, 67*, 68.

Yunus, M. B., Holt, G. S., Masi, A. T., & Aldag, J. C. (1988). Fibromyalgia syndrome among the elderly: Comparison with younger patients. *Journal of American Geriatrics Society, 36*, 987–995.

Zeman, J., & Garber, J. (1996). Display rules for anger, sadness, and pain: It depends on who is watching. *Child Development, 67*, 957–973.

Zheng, Z., Gibson, S. J., Khalil, Z., McMeeken, J. M., & Helme, R. D. (2000). Age-related differences in the time course of capsaicin-induced hyperalgesia. *Pain, 85*, 51–58.

Zuckerman, B., Stevenson, J., & Bailey, V. (1987). Stomachaches and headaches in a community sample of preschool children. *Pediatrics, 79*, 677–682.

CHAPTER

6

Ethnocultural Variations in the Experience of Pain

Gary B. Rollman
Department of Psychology,
University of Western Ontario

Pain is experienced by persons, not groups. Still, researchers go to great effort to study interindividual factors such as sex, age, and culture as they relate to pain. That is done for a number of reasons: an understanding of predispositions to pain, the features that maintain it, and suggestions for tailored treatments.

The literature on sex and gender differences, for example, is quite sizeable now. Investigators have made considerable progress in considering the role of biological sex or gender identity in influencing the prevalence of pain conditions, the response to treatment, and the mechanisms used to cope with challenging pain syndromes. Typically, the majority of pain patients for many disorders is female (Berkley, 1997; LeResche, 1997; Unruh, 1996). This includes such conditions as headache, rheumatoid arthritis, fibromyalgia, irritable bowel disorder, and temporomandibular disorder. The data on prevalence have been supplemented (Fillingim, 2000; Mogil, Chesler, Wilson, Juraska, & Sternberg, 2000; Riley, Robinson, Wise, Myers, & Fillingim, 1998; Rollman & Lautenbacher, 2001) by research on biological, psychological, and sociocultural factors with the goal of understanding the underlying mechanisms, reducing the incidence of the problems, and improving the treatment of acute and chronic pain. We know, for example, that certain opioid drugs are more potent in males than in females (Craft & Bernal, 2001), that women have a moderate to large increase in sensitivity to experimentally-induced pain compared to men (Riley et al., 1998), that women are more likely than men to suffer from many forms of clinical pain

(Unruh, 1996), particularly those involving the musculoskeletal system (Rollman & Lautenbacher, 2001), and that both biological sex and psychological gender role are significant predictors of pain threshold, tolerance, and ratings of unpleasantness (Wise, Price, Myers, Heft, & Robinson, 2002).

In many respects, the rationale for studying ethnocultural differences in pain is identical, but culture is probably the most difficult and controversial of the biopsychosocial factors. This chapter critically examines the literature that suggests the individual's culture makes a critical difference in pain behavior and management.

Research on culture and pain has undergone three important stages. In the first, samples were small and poorly obtained and science often took a back seat to stereotypes. The second stage was marked by greater interest in both theory and methodology, but the validity of the findings was still often questionable. The third stage, which has recently emerged, is characterized by greater sophistication, larger sample sizes and population distributions, and closer attention to psychosocial factors which may mediate the results.

For reasons of convenience, most early studies of pain and culture took place in the laboratory. Typically, small numbers of persons from one cultural group were compared to small numbers of persons from one or two other groups, and sweeping generalizations were made. Wolff (1985) summarized a typical conclusion:

> Scandinavians are tough and stoic with a high tolerance to pain; the British are more sensitive but, in view of their ingrained "stiff, upper lip," do not complain when in pain; Italians and other Mediterranean people are emotional and overreact to pain; and Jews both overreact to pain and are preoccupied with pain and suffering as well as physical health. (p. 23)

Similarly, Sternbach and Tursky (1965) observed, "Old Americans have a phlegmatic, matter-of-fact, doctor-helping orientation; Jews express a concern for the implication of pain, and they distrust palliatives; Italians express a desire for pain relief, and the Irish inhibit expression of suffering and concern for the implications of the pain" (p. 241). To draw that conclusion, they asked questions about attitudes to pain and tested pain reactivity in American-born women from four different ethnic groups: Yankee (Protestants of British descent whose parents and grandparents were born in the United States), Irish, Italian, and Jewish (the last three born of parents who emigrated to the United States from Europe). There were sizeable differences in pain tolerance (the level at which participants indicated that the pain had reached the maximum level they wished to experience). The Yankee and Jewish subjects withstood significantly higher values than the Italians, with the Irish at an intermediate level.

These conclusions about the pain reactions of Old Americans, Jews, Italians, and Irish are interesting but unwarranted. Religion, ethnicity, and national origin are mixed. More importantly, 15 Massachusetts homemakers per sample hardly allow one to draw generalizations about either the attitudes or the pain responses of an ethnic or cultural group. Individuals vary enormously in their response to experimentally induced pain, and the differences between groups, even in large studies, is generally quite modest in comparison to the intergroup variability.

The same caveat applies to many clinical studies. Zborowski's book *People in Pain*, published in 1969, is often cited because of its early examination of how culture might shape the pain response. His conclusions—Old Americans are stoic, Italians loudly demand pain relief, and Jews seek relief but worry about the future implications of their disorder—all came from staff reports at a single New York Veterans Administration hospital. Likewise, Zola's (1966) study of interethnic differences in pain reporting and attitudes was based on interviews with patients at various outpatient clinics at the Massachusetts General Hospital. He focused on 63 Italians and 81 Irish new admissions of comparable age, education, and social class.

The study found that the Irish were markedly more inclined to locate their problem in the eye, ear, nose, or throat but were also more likely to say that the problem was not painful ("It was more a throbbing than a pain. It feels more like sand in my eye"). Moreover, the Irish described a specific problem. In contrast, the Italians tended to report diffuse discomfort, presented more symptoms, had complaints in more bodily locations, and indicated that they had more kinds of dysfunctions.

Zola speculated that "Italian and Irish ways of communicating illness may reflect major values and preferred ways of handling problems within the culture itself" and could be understood in terms of generalized expressiveness. So, for the Italians, the complaints may relate to "their expansiveness so often [seen] in sociological, historical, and fictional writing"—a "well seasoned, dramatic emphasis to their lives."

The Irish view of life, in Zola's view, is drab ("long periods of routine followed by episodes of wild adventure"). It was as if "life was black and long-suffering and the less said the better." Consequently, a patient when asked about her reactions to the pain of her illness stated, "I ignore it like I do most things." This sort of literary analysis is not uninteresting, but it is based on a Freudian perspective. Science is largely absent.

Lipton and Marbach (1984) presented a scholarly review of the literature on ethnicity and pain that had been collected until the early 1980s, noting its many inadequacies. Sometimes, responses from patients were examined in individual ethnic groups (e.g., American, British, Scandinavian, and Italian); at other times, these were simply combined into a single "White" group. Some studies focused deliberately on pain, whereas others included a few pain-related questions as part of a broader study of health beliefs and practices. Some used a short questionnaire, whereas others relied on interviews or caretaker impressions.

Lipton and Marbach proposed a model based upon three major areas of the pain experience. First was the physical experience—its intensity, quality, duration, and location—and the way in which the patient describes these sensations to others. Second was the patient's behavior in response to his or her pain. They introduced three subcategories here: cognitive interpretation (the interpretation and evaluation of the perceived pain), emotional responses (fear, anxiety, or depression and whether it is expressed openly or covertly), and function (how the pain affects social interaction and daily activities). The third area was medical intervention, dealing with the individual's action in response to pain and role as a pain patient (compliant and trusting or challenging and uncooperative).

Lipton and Marbach then applied this model to 476 consecutive patients of varied ethnic makeup seen at a facial pain clinic in a large hospital, concentrating on 50 patients in each of five groups: African American, Irish, Italian, Jewish, and Puerto Rican. There were some ethnic differences in pain description, a tendency for Italian and African American patients to attribute their pain to something they had done, the finding that African Americans and Puerto Ricans were less likely to hide their pain from family and friends, and relatively few ethnic differences in interference with daily functioning. The Irish, Italian, and Jewish patients were more likely to have consulted "quite a few doctors" before attending the clinic. Still, the similarities were considerably greater than the differences between the groups. The authors noted that the patients were all in one city, were often third-generation Americans (both their parents and themselves born in the United States), and generally saw their ethnic identity as American rather than foreign. As such, they were more likely to have adopted or become acculturated to at least some "American" norms for pain behaviors and attitudes. The Puerto Rican patients, who were most likely to have been immigrants, were also most likely to differ from the other groups, showing a high level of distress, strong friendship solidarity, dependency on members of their own ethnic group when sick, an emotionally expressive pain response, and great disruption in daily activities attributable to pain.

Although the earlier literature on medical care had suggested "ethnic group membership influences how one perceives, labels, responds to and communicates various symptoms, as well as from whom one selects to obtain care, when it is sought, and the types of treatment received," Lipton and Marbach showed that it is critically important to deconstruct the sociocultural determinants of pain behavior and attitudes. The social factor influences how families or local groups affect behavior and the practitioner–patient relationship, whereas the cultural factor influences an earlier stage, how symptoms are interpreted. Both are critical in understanding how individuals report or express their discomfort. Both are likely to change over time, particularly in a multicultural environment.

A related analysis of the cultural context of pain behaviors came from Calvillo and Flaskerud (1991). They presented the view that, "Cross-cultural studies have demonstrated that White Americans of Northern European origin react to pain stoically and as calmly as possible. This response to pain has become the cultural model or norm in the United States. It is the behavior expected and valued by health caregivers" (p. 16). In order to better understand such cultural norms, Carvillo and Flaskerud examined Mexican American pain expression, concluding:

> Many Mexican-American patients, especially women, moan when uncomfortable. Consequently, they are often identified by the nursing staff as complainers who cannot tolerate pain. In the Mexican culture, crying out with pain is an acceptable expression and not synonymous with an inability to tolerate pain. Crying out with pain does not necessarily indicate that the pain experience is severe or that . . . the patient expects the nurse to intervene. (p. 20)

Calvillo and Flaskerud suggested that crying and moaning may help the Mexican patient to relieve the pain rather than function as a request for intervention. Health practitioners, operating from the dominant culture model of response to pain, may, improperly, interpret crying and moaning as an indication that the patients are dramatic, emotional complainers with an inability to manage pain. Accordingly, there is an important need to understand culturally determined attitudes and pain reactions.

TREATMENT DISPARITIES

Recent studies have taken an epidemiological turn, studying the composition of patients seen in various medical clinics and, more importantly, whether treatment depends on ethnicity. For example, Todd, Samaroo, and Hoffman (1993) reviewed the charts at a major Los Angeles trauma center where it had been suggested that Hispanic patients were more likely than non-Hispanic White patients to receive no analgesia at all for arm or leg fractures. The evidence supported this impression, leading them to undertake a retrospective cohort study over a 2-year period. Of the 31 Hispanics who met the study criteria, 55% received no analgesic medication, compared to 26% of the non-Hispanic Whites. Analyses that controlled for sex, language, and insurance status, as well as severity of injury and physician characteristics, did not substantially change the evidence. Even where analgesics were offered, Hispanics tended to receive lower doses and fewer narcotics. Although they noted, "we cannot be sure that the injuries in each of the patient groups were equally painful," the authors suggested that physicians and other staff members may fail to adequately "recognize the presence of pain in patients who are culturally different from themselves" (p. 1539).

Ng, Dimsdale, Shragg, and Deutsch (1996) noted the uneven nature of studies on the relationship between ethnicity and pain, even in the 1990s. Most of the reports were based on anecdotal evidence, were based on small groups, and did not use well-validated assessment tools. Few studies controlled for acculturation. Ng et al. (1996) decided to extend the Todd et al. (1993) emergency room study on Hispanic and White patients, focusing on a much larger and more ethnically diverse sample of similar social class who were admitted to a San Diego clinic because of limb fracture and required an open reduction and internal fixation. Given the nature of the surgery and the hospitalization that followed, all were offered analgesic medications. Still, Whites received the highest dose of analgesics and a greater number of narcotics, followed by Blacks and Hispanics. They offered various theories regarding this outcome (the nurse's perception of the patient's pain, differences in the way patients demand pain control or expect pain to be eliminated, and, unlikely, pharmacokinetic differences across the ethnic groups), but concluded, "whether this difference reflects ethnic differences in analgesic requirements or reflects cultural biases in treatment remains to be determined" (p. 128).

One way to further explore this question is to look for ethnic group differences in the use of analgesics where the attitudes and expectations of the caregiver are not a factor. Patient-controlled analgesia (PCA), where the individual administers a drug such as morphine to himself or herself by pressing a hand switch attached to an infusion pump, provides such an opportunity. Ng, Dimsdale, Rollnik, and Shapiro (1996) examined the records for nearly 500 patients who were treated with PCA for postoperative pain and discovered that amounts of self-administered narcotics were not significantly different between Whites, Blacks, Hispanics, and Asians. What did vary was the initial PCA prescription ordered by the physician, so that a higher dose was ordered for Whites and Blacks than Hispanics. They interpreted their data to indicate that physicians predict Whites will have more pain, and prescribe accordingly, or that cultural factors influence communication (or lack thereof) between physician and patient, profoundly affecting the doctor's treatment plan.

Cleeland et al. (1994) also noted the discriminatory nature of patient care. They studied 1,300 consecutive outpatients who had been diagnosed with recurrent or metastatic cancer, asking both them and their physician to rate their level of pain and its interference with activity and sleep. Forty-two percent of the total group of patients received inadequate analgesia, but those seen at centers treating primarily patients representing minority groups were much more likely to have poorly controlled pain. The data do not provide encouragement about the management of cancer pain in this sample, but are also an indictment of the treatment of minority patients. A number of letters to the editor followed publication of this provocative article. One (Karnad, 1994) is short enough to print in its entirety: "I do not think the problem of pain control will be solved until we face the fact that much of it stems from our puritanical culture. In the recesses of our collective identity, we still embrace the notion that pleasure is bad and suffering is redemptive (no pain, no gain)" (p. 199).

Bonham (2001) carefully examined disparities in health care in the United States, indicating that "racial and ethnic minority groups often receive different and less optimal management of their health care than White Americans" (p. 52). He considered a number of possible reasons for this including stereotypes, language barriers, ineffective communication, a failure to understand the patient's expressions of pain and distress, and socioeconomic factors, concluding that adequate pain assessment is the most important step in reducing inadequate patient care.

Rathore et al. (2000) recruited 164 medical students to view one of two case presentations of angina, one involving a 55-year-old Black female patient actor and the other a 55-year-old White male. The scripts were identical, the clinical symptoms were sufficient for a diagnosis of definite angina, and the actors were in identical gowns and filmed in the same room. Students were less willing to provide a diagnosis of definite angina for the Black female (46%) than for the White male (72%), yet rated her quality of life as lower. The design did not allow a determination of whether this apparent bias in diagnosis and health status rating is based on race or sex or a combination of the two, but the data indicated that training in cultural awareness should be a required part of training for medical and other health care personnel.

Insensitivity to the needs of Central American residents of the Boston area is highlighted by three simple case studies presented by Flores, Abreu, Schwartz, and Hill (2000). A 3-year-old girl, who was later found to have a perforated appendix and peritonitis, was repeatedly sent home from a hospital emergency department because no interpreter was available and the staff lacked kindness, friendliness, and respect; a 2-year-old girl with shoulder pain was placed in the custody of the Department of Social Services because the resident thought that the caregiver's comment, "she was struck," meant she had suffered abuse, rather than the intended "she had fallen off her tricycle and struck her shoulder"; and the parents of a neonate with severe impairments were not informed of the poor prognosis and mistakenly believed the baby would soon recover and be released. In all cases, "failure to address language and cultural issues resulted in inferior quality of care, adverse outcomes, increased health care costs, and parental dissatisfaction" (p. 846).

It is important to test for disparities in health care or undertreatment of some ethnic groups in other societies. Sheiner, Sheiner, Shoham-Vardi, Mazor, and Katz (1999), in an investigation of the childbirth experience of Jewish and Bedouin women living in the Negev section of southern Israel, almost all of whom deliver at a major regional hospital, obtained ratings of pain (from the patient, physician, and midwife) at the initial active phase of labor. There were substantial demographic differences (the Bedouin women were younger, more likely to describe themselves as religious, less likely to be accompanied at labor by their husband, had less formal education, and did not attend childbirth education classes). Epidural analgesia was offered nearly twice as often to Jewish women as to the Bedouin (who preferred parenteral pethidine, a synthetic opioid analgesic).

The most interesting finding came from the concurrent visual analog scores of the mothers and the care providers. The self-assessments of the Jewish and Bedouin women were nearly identical (8.5 on a 10 point scale), but the ratings of the medical staff (almost all of whom were Jewish) indicated that they perceived the Bedouin women to experience less pain (6.9) than the Jewish ones (8.5). These data are different from some of those reported earlier, in that they do not show undertreatment of an ethnic group. Both groups of women had equal (albeit high) levels of pain at the time of assessment; what differed was the pain level judged by the delivery staff from the exhibited behavior. It is uncertain whether this difference was due to the behavior of the two groups, a bias on the part of the medical personnel, or their inability to recognize signs of pain in patients of a different culture.

Pain Expression

Diagnosis and treatment of pain are largely dependent on what the patient is willing to tell the health care provider or, for that matter, thinks is sufficiently important to report. The ethnocultural background of the practitioner is also likely to interact with that of the patient; a good physician or psychologist should examine his or her own attitudes and expectations about pain behavior. Davitz, Sameshima, and Davitz (1976), for example, asked over 500 nurses in the United States, Japan, Taiwan, Thailand, Korea, and Puerto Rico to read descriptions of patients and to judge their pain and psychological distress. The descriptions were brief and, in their own language, covered five disease categories, both sexes, three age levels, and two degrees of severity. The study found that Japanese and Korean nurses believed that their patients suffered a high degree of pain, while American and Puerto Rican nurses rated their patients' pain fairly low. These data run counter to the stereotype of Asian stoicism. Davitz et al. suggest that the Asian nurses distinguished between overt and covert expression of pain, so that they inferred far more pain than was observable through verbal or bodily expressions, whereas the U.S. nurses were more likely to assume congruence between pain experience and pain behavior. Consequently, Asian patients treated in North American hospitals might receive less treatment than their pain level would warrant. Interestingly, other stereotypes, which could be quite dangerous to the patient, were shared by the nurses in all six cultures. For one, males were seen as in less pain than females for similar degrees of emotional distress. For another, the nurses believed that children suffer far less psychological distress than adults for comparable levels of pain.

A cross-cultural study of both pain attitudes and reactivity to experimentally induced discomfort was conducted by Nayak, Shiflett, Eshun, and Levine (2000). They explored differences in beliefs about appropriate or normative pain behavior, extending the research of Kodiath and Kodiath (1992), who found that patients in India reported less suffering and anger about lack of pain relief than individuals in the United States with similar levels of pain. Nayak et al. had slightly over 100 undergraduates at universities in the United States and India complete a questionnaire about sex-appropriate public pain responses (grimacing, crying, talking about the pain, etc.) and tested pain tolerance and ratings in the cold pressor task (immersing the arm in a container of circulating ice water). Both males and females in India believed that overt expression of pain is less appropriate than did the U.S. undergraduates. Moreover, the Indian volunteers of both sexes kept their hand in the ice water longer than their American counterparts. The authors suggested:

> The greater willingness to express pain in American society could be due to the belief that pain is bad, need not be endured, and should be quickly eliminated. In addition, in American society today, the medical profession has taken on the primary role of pain relief, which, combined with the widespread availability and use of analgesics, provides a powerful reinforcement for pain expression. (p. 146)

Further studies with clinical rather than experimental pain and with a wider range of ages and socioeconomic conditions would be very helpful.

A relatively small sample of dentists and patients from three ethnic groups (Anglo-American, Chinese, and Scandinavian), all living in the greater Seattle area, were interviewed about their ways of coping with pain (Moore, 1990). Anglo-American patients sought pills and injections, denial of pain, and reassuring clinical contacts. Anglo-American dentists preferred to use drugs. In contrast, the Chinese patients preferred salves, oils, creams, and compresses and nontraditional medicine, although Chinese dentists (and the Scandinavian ones) shared the American preference for using pharmaceutical treatments. Interestingly, although Scandinavian patients did not want to be treated with local anesthetics, many volunteered that they accepted this treatment for their dentist's peace of mind.

Anthropological Studies. It is rare for anthropologists to go into the field in order to study pain behavior within an isolated cultural group. One exception is Sargent's (1984) study, conducted in the mid-1970s, of the Bariba, a major group of about 400,000 persons living in Benin and Nigeria who are "notable for consistently demonstrating an 'absence of manifest behavior' when confronted with apparently painful stimuli such as childbirth, wounds, or initiation ordeals" (p. 1299). Sargent interviewed 120 women of reproductive age in a small village regarding their behavioral ideals and actual behavior during delivery, spoke to numerous indigenous midwives and village leaders, and attended a number of deliveries. Tellingly, one local physician explained that the Bariba equate pain with cowardice, a source of enormous shame. They pride themselves on the courage of their men in war and their women in childbirth and disparage the behavior of other groups that express pain openly through complaints or behavioral expressions. Not surprisingly, the Bariba have few words with which to describe pain, although they do distinguish between pain sensation and suffering. Social modeling (Craig, 1986), from childhood, appears to shape the behavior of tribal members. Stoicism is not limited to pain; Bariba are expected to suppress grief and other negative emotions.

Honeyman and Jacobs (1996) went into the Australian outback to study pain behavior and beliefs among the members of a small aboriginal community. They observed that aboriginal children show few signs of distress and that adults minimize any overt pain behaviors. When questioned individually, community members acknowledged pain, including long-term low back pain, but none showed public pain or illness behaviors of the sort seen in Western society. Also, it was extremely rare for any of them to seek medical attention for pain problems. Honeyman and Jacobs proposed that:

> the concept of illness as a social process, separate from a biological malfunction termed disease, allows us to see these people as acting appropriately to their cultural setting. In this society there are strong community expectations about tolerating and not expressing or displaying pain. This was evidenced by the few public back pain reactions we saw and the reluctance to talk about pain in front of others. (p. 842)

Although back pain was quite common in the community, the inhabitants did not actively complain about it and it rarely appeared in health records.

The findings emphasize the need for sensitive questioning of patients about their symptoms, particularly when they may come from a group where emotional expression of symptoms is discouraged.

Pediatric Pain. Given the psychosocial perspective on cultural differences in pain, it would be interesting to look for evidence concerning ethnocultural variation in children's pain. The task is not easy because of problems in assessing pain in young children. Recent years have seen numerous advances in developing physiological measures, behavioral observations, and self-report measures (McGrath, 1995; McGrath et al., 2000; McGrath, Rosmus, Canfield, Campbell, & Hennigar, 1998) including analysis of facial expressions, scales involving faces and colors, and examination of drawings.

Little attention has been paid to the need to validate these scales in different cultural settings. Villarruel and Denyes (1991) developed alternative versions of the "Oucher" scale for Hispanic and African American children. The Oucher comprises a series of six photographs of a 4-year-old White boy showing facial expressions indicating various levels of pain. A pediatric patient is asked to point to the picture that best reflects his or her own level of hurt. Using photographs of Hispanic and African American children, taken when they were or were not experiencing pain, the authors established an ordering of six photographs that other children could agree represented a progression of pain expression. It remains to be established whether this particular measure will reveal any cross-cultural differences in children's pain levels, whether scales tailored to ethnic origin or race, although culturally sensitive, aid in either pain assessment or in strengthening communication between medical practitioners and children of different cultural groups, and whether culture-free measures (such as a series of face drawings; Chambers & Craig, 1998; Chambers, Giesbrecht, Craig, Bennett, & Huntsman, 1999) can achieve both validity and universality in pain assessment.

Abu-Saad (1984) interviewed Arab American, Asian American, and Latin American school children, asking what caused pain for them, what words they used to describe pain ("like a hurt" was the most common descriptor in each group), how they felt when they are in pain, and how they coped with pain. Given that all lived in the same urban environment, the finding that the similarities among the subjects are considerably greater than the differences is not surprising. Studies of this sort need to be conducted with large numbers of children, of varying age and in a range of countries, in order to help us to better understand at what age cross-cultural differences, if any, become apparent and what changes take place during infancy, childhood, and adolescence. They will also advance our understanding of the speed of cultural diffusion or adaptation. Pfefferbaum, Adams, and Aceves (1990) studied pain and anxiety in 37 Hispanic and 35 Anglo children with cancer at a hospital in Texas. The children were very similar in their behavioral responses. It was the parents who differed, with the Hispanic parents reporting significantly higher levels of anxiety than the Anglo ones.

Canadian-born Chinese and non-Chinese infants, receiving routine immunization at the age of 2 months, were compared for facial expressions and pain cries (Rosmus, Johnston, Chan-Yip, & Yang, 2000). This study is interesting because it provides an early examination of possible cultural differences in socialization. The authors, noting a literature on cross-cultural differences in infant development and the role of infant-care practices, assessed demographic information, degree of acculturation, the infant's feeding and crying patterns, and video recordings focused on the face during immunization. All babies exhibited facial and cry expressions, but the Chinese infants exhibited significantly greater brow bulges, duration of crying, and number of cry bursts. Anecdotal evidence indicated that the Chinese mothers were more interactive during the waiting period, possibly increasing the infants' arousal. The study is admittedly preliminary, but it opens the possibility that mothering patterns may either affect pain reactivity directly or influence the overall arousal response.

International Studies. An interesting cross-cultural study was recently reported by Litcher et al. (2001). The used the Children's Somatization Inventory, which assesses the frequency and severity of a comprehensive set of physical complaints, to compare children in Nashville with a large group of 10- to 12-year-olds in Kyiv, Ukraine, including many who had been evacuated from Chernobyl after the nuclear power plant accident there. The mothers of the children were given a similar questionnaire. Remarkably, the Ukrainian children reported fewer physical symptoms than the American ones of the same age, but their mothers reported nearly three times as many symptoms in their own children than those in Nashville. It is uncertain, of course, whether this reflects a generalized difference in awareness of bodily symptoms between American and Ukrainian women, developing at a later stage in life, or whether the Chernobyl incident fostered a more vigilant pattern in the latter group.

Another recent cross-cultural study (Levenstein et al., 2001) of symptom reporting compared the concerns of inflammatory bowel disease (IBD) patients in eight countries. Overall concern scores ranged from a high of 51 in Portugal to a low of 19 in Sweden, but the nature of the concerns also showed large inter-nation variability. Israeli patients were particularly concerned about pain and suffering whereas the Portuguese subjects worried about social stigma. Given the many behavioral consequences of chronic pain (McCracken, Zayfert, & Gross, 1992; Turk, Okifuji, Sinclair, & Starz, 1996), it is imperative to fully explore the sensory, affective, and cognitive reactions of pain patients, irrespective of ethnic background.

International studies of pain, particularly ones that focus on supposed ethnic or cultural differences, are influenced by differences in litigation or compensation systems in different countries. Hadjistavropoulos (1999), in a broad review of litigation and compensation, included a number of cross-cultural studies. Carron, DeGood, and Tait (1985), for example, found that back pain patients in the United States used more medication, experienced more disphoric mood states, and were more hampered in social-sexual, recreational, and vocational functioning than ones in New Zealand. At the onset of treatment, 49% of the U.S. sample was receiving pain-related financial compensation, in contrast to and only 17% of the New Zealand patients. Individuals in both countries who were receiving pretreatment compensation were less likely to report a return to full activity, although the relationship appeared more pronounced among those in the United States.

Other studies that demonstrate that certain expensive interventions are more likely to reduce acute pain (e.g., Macario, Scibetta, Navarro, & Riley, 2000) or that costly early interventions may reduce long-term disability (Borghouts, Koes, Vondeling, & Bouter, 1999; Hutubessy, van Tulder, Vondeling, & Bouter, 1999) suggest that national health care policies and budgets may influence both the nature and prevalence of pain syndromes.

Single-Society Studies. Many of the published studies of ethnocultural factors and pain have made broad generalizations based upon exceedingly small sample sizes. Thomas and Rose (1991) asked 28 African Caribbean males and females, 28 Anglo-Saxons, and 28 Asians in London, England, who were having an ear pierced with a piercing gun, to complete the McGill Pain Questionnaire. Asian subject scores were nearly twice those of the African Caribbeans, with Anglo-Saxon scores nearly as high, leading them to conclude, "the present results provide clear evidence that there are ethnic differences in pain experience in this test situation" (pp. 1064–1065).

Sanders et al. (1992) claimed that "American low back pain subjects had significantly higher pain intensity ratings than other cultures did" (p. 319) and that American, New Zealand, and Italian patients reported higher levels of psychosocial impairment than individuals living Japan, Mexico, or Colombia. Their subject pool consisted of 10 or 11 chronic low back pain patients from each of the six countries. Likewise, Brena, Sanders, and Motoyama (1990), evaluating 11 back pain patients from Tokyo and a like number of patients from Atlanta, reported, "Japanese low back pain patients were less psychosocially, vocationally, and avocationally impaired than similar American patients" (p. 122).

Sheffield, Kirby, Biles, and Sheps (1999) evaluated 124 Caucasians and 18 African Americans who had taken an exercise treadmill test which showed certain electrocardiographic abnormalities. Because 9 of the latter but only 34 of the former had angina during testing, they concluded, "African Americans reported anginal pain at twice the rate of Caucasians" (p. 107). A subsequent study of pain perception (Sheffield, Biles, Orom, Maixner, & Sheps, 2000) using a contact thermode to deliver noxious levels of heat to 27 Whites and 24 African Americans, showed that the latter group gave higher ratings than the former to each of 5 temperatures, leading them to indicate that "these data suggest that different pain mechanisms underlie race differences in pain perception" (p. 521) and to call for studies of acculturation and twin studies to better understand the specific factors.

Edwards and Fillingim (1999), testing 30 Whites and 18 African Americans, also found that the Whites had a greater thermal pain tolerance and gave lower unpleasantness ratings at the lower two of four temperatures in a scaling study, with no group differences in intensity ratings. There were also no group differences in questionnaire measures of pain reactivity or in pain complaints over the preceding month, although African Americans reported greater average pain severity and two pain sites rather than the Whites' number of 1.4. The two unpleasantness rating differences led to the proposal that there are racial differences in the affective-motivational dimension of pain. A significant correlation between pain tolerance and pain symptoms brought the suggestion that ethnic variation in affective-motivational judgments may account for the severity and number of pain sites. The authors presented the admittedly speculative suggestion that African Americans may require quantitatively greater degrees of pain treatment than Whites.

In a subsequent study of 68 African Americans and 269 Whites attending an interdisciplinary pain clinic, the African Americans reported significantly greater pain severity and pain-related disability than Whites (Edwards, Doleys, Fillingim, & Lowery, 2001), although no differences in the McGill Pain Questionnaire or measures of pain interference or affective distress. As well, the African Americans had shorter ischemic pain tolerance times for a tourniquet test (about 5 minutes vs. 9 for the White patients). The large difference in the latter, compared to a much smaller difference in clinical pain, led to the suggestion that coping styles, attitudes toward pain measurement, or differences in central pain modulating systems may distinguish the two groups. The inclusion of such diverse putative mechanisms underscores the risk of labeling any of the differences reported in this section as "racial" rather than "cultural." To the extent that the first term implies a genetic causation (a matter, as noted below, of considerable contention) and the second an environmental one, a confound of racial variation and socialization factors arises. This problem is exacerbated by the fact that members of a particular group may differ in both their culturally determined practices and in the manner in which they are treated by members of other groups in their society.

Some recent papers have started to correct the problem of small sample size. Ho and Ong (2001) used Singapore, a large multiethnic society, to examine the influence of group membership (Chinese, Malay, Indian, and other) on headache morbidity. No significant ethnic differences were found for lifetime or current headache prevalence within a sample of over 2,000 individuals, although there were some group differences in average headache intensity and frequency, with the Chinese lowest. Non-Chinese were also more likely to seek medical attention for their headaches and to have taken medical leave during the preceding year. The data do not allow one to determine whether genetic factors may have influenced the outcome of this study.

Allison et al. (2002) assessed musculoskeletal pain within a community sample of over 2,100 adults from the Indian, Pakistani, Bangladeshi, and African Caribbean communities in the area around Manchester, England, and compared the results to those obtained from a recent study of White residents using the same methodology. For the age range 45–64 years, musculoskeletal pain prevalence was higher in all ethnic groups (about 70 to 90%) than in White subjects, with the latter being about 53% for both males and females. When asked whether they had pain in "most joints," about 6 to 8% of Whites agreed compared to about 30 to 45% in the ethnic minority groups. There were no group differences, however, in disability scores. The authors cautioned that comparable studies need to be done in other geographical locations, because the data do not permit one to readily distinguish between differences in pain sensitivity or expression, the effects of change of culture and migration, and mental health issues. With respect to the last point, a study (Nelson, Novy, Averill, & Berry, 1996) with a relatively small sample of Black, White, and Hispanic patients in a southern U.S. community revealed different Minnesota Multiphasic Personality Inventory (MMPI) profiles, but the data also suggested that education level rather than ethnic group membership may be the more relevant characteristic.

McCracken, Matthews, Tang, and Cuba (2001), in one of the few studies of ethnic or racial group differences in the experience of chronic pain, asked 207 White and 57 African American patients seeking treatment at a pain management center about their physical symptoms, depression, disability, health care use, and pain-related anxiety. The two groups did not differ in age, education, or chronicity of their pain complaint. African Americans rated their pain higher and reported more avoidance of pain and activity, more fearful thinking about pain, and more pain-related anxiety. As well, they were higher on physical symptom complaints and on physical, psychosocial, and overall disability. The authors noted that many factors may explain these findings, including less social support, differences in social circumstances, beliefs about pain, and self-management strategies, and the possibility that African Americans may not seek or be referred for treatment unless they are suffering from high levels of distress.

A study by Jordan, Lumley, and Leisen (1998) compared pain control beliefs, use of cognitive coping strategies, and status of pain, activity level, and emotion among 48 African American and 52 White women with rheumatoid arthritis, controlling for the potentially confounding influence of income, marital status, and education. There were no group differences in pain, but the African American patients were less physically active and more likely to cope with pain by praying and hoping and diverting attention, whereas Whites were more likely to make coping statements and ignore the pain. Bill-Harvey, Rippey, Abeles, and Pfeiffer (1989) had earlier noted that 92% of low-income, urban African American arthritis patients used prayer to relieve their pain and discomfort. Cognitive behavior therapy and other treatments that encourage the use of increased coping attempts and decreased negative thinking can aid African Americans to manage experimentally induced pain (Gil et al., 1996) and are likely to be of clinical benefit.

Waza, Graham, Zyzanski, and Inoue (1999) found that Japanese patients who had been newly diagnosed with depression reported more total symptoms, particularly physical ones, than patients in the United States. Twenty seven percent of the Japanese patients reported only physical symptoms, whereas only 9% of the patients in the United States presented in this manner. A large proportion of the Japanese had pain complaints (generally abdominal pain, headache, and neck pain); comparable figures for the American patients were about 60 to 80% less. The authors propose that pain at specific body areas may arise because of cultural influences, possibly to avoid the stigma in Japan associated with emotional disorders. For example, many Japanese expressions use the term *hara* (abdomen) to verbalize emotion, and digestive-system complaints are the primary reason for outpatient medical visits in that country. Likewise, *katakori* (a pain in the neck) is a major medical complaint. Waza et al. suggested that the physical presentation of symptoms by Japanese patients may mean that many cases of depression are misdiagnosed.

Njobvu, Hunt, Pope, and Macfarlane (1999), in a review of pain among individuals from South Asian ethnic minority groups who live in the United Kingdom, observed that they more frequently attend medical clinics and report greater musculoskeletal pain. This leads to the question of whether South Asians also suffer greatly from pain in their countries of origin. Hameed and Gibson (1997) provided relevant data in a study of pain complaints among Pakistanis living in England and in Pakistan. Those living in England reported more arthritic symptoms and more nonspecific musculoskeletal pain, particularly among females. There are numerous possible explanations including the colder British climate, adjustment to life in a new society, and a greater willingness to report pain among the better educated Pakistanis living in Great Britain.

Sabbioni and Eugster (2001) also looked at immigrants, namely, Spanish and Italians living in Switzerland. Earlier studies had found that foreign patients in that country had worse medical outcomes after back injury than Swiss ones, but the migrants often worked in low-paying jobs with increased health hazards. There was no difference between groups in pain intensity or appraisal, but those immigrants with a high "degree of inclusion" (DI), as measured by type of work permit, age at immigration, and language fluency, were similar to Swiss citizens, and better than immigrants with low DI, with respect to general well-being, functional capacity, and mood.

A population-based study of low back pain (LBP) among about 4,000 Belgian adults (Skovron, Szpalski, Nordin, Melot, & Cukier, 1994) found that French Belgians (living in the southern region of Wallonia) had a greater likelihood than Flemish Belgians of ever having had LBP. The authors wondered whether the data are attributable to "a greater willingness among French speakers to share difficulties with the group in contrast with the more individualistic tendencies of the Flemish population," but they noted that it is also in this region where there are greater economic uncertainties, more heavy industry, and larger companies.

REFLECTIONS

The many studies reviewed here, and the many included in other reviews (Edwards, Fillingim, & Keefe, 2001; Lasch, 2000; Moore & Brodsgaard, 1999; Rollman, 1998), provide a fascinating view of ethnocultural variations in the experience of pain. The scholarly perspectives, nature of pain, research settings, variables investigated, and measures employed vary tremendously. Much has been learned, but much is still confusing. The results sometimes go in opposite directions. The samples are often small and based on convenience rather than sound epidemiological principles. Some studies investigated laboratory-induced pain whereas others examined acute or chronic clinical pain conditions. Some studies found differences that were statistically significant but likely to be clinically unimportant (such as a pain score of 55.7 for one group and 53.4 for the comparison one), yet they presented their data as confirming the presence of ethnic differences. On a subject as potentially contentious as ethnic or racial differences, it seems best to err on the side of caution.

Only one investigation compared both experimental and endogenous pain in the same individuals, ischemic pain tolerance in African American and White pain clinic patients (Edwards, Doleys, Fillingim, & Lowery, 2001). It is essential to go beyond pain threshold and tolerance measures and look into other measures of pain reactivity and inhibition (Gracely, Petzke, Wolf, & Clauw, 2002; Lautenbacher & Rollman, 1997; Lautenbacher, Rollman, & McCain, 1994; McDermid, Rollman, & McCain, 1996; Staud, Vierck, Cannon, Mauderli, & Price, 2001; Yang, Clark, & Janal, 1991) across ethnic groups.

Many factors, such as the subjects' education, psychological status, and assignment to ethnic categories, varied considerably, as did the training of the interviewers and quality of the assessment tools. The McGill Pain Questionnaire has been carefully validated in numerous languages (e.g., De Benedittis, Massei, Nobili, & Pieri, 1988; Hasegawa et al., 2001; Lazaro et al., 2001; Strand & Ljunggren, 1997), and there have been some interesting uses of the Brief Pain Inventory in various countries (Cleeland et al., 1996), but most other pain and coping measures have not been translated and validated.

Much remains to be learned about the process of acculturation or cultural diffusion and how it affects cognitions and behaviors. Bates's (Bates & Edwards, 1992) Ethnicity and Pain Questionnaire, which assesses an individual's ties to his or her ethnic group, indicates that later generations of families that came to the United States from abroad are likely to have acculturated to the culture of the majority group. In her New England sample, Central American, Italian, and Polish groups had the greatest heritage consistency, whereas Irish, French Canadians, and, especially, Anglo-Americans were more assimilated. Bates also assessed the psychological characteristics of her sample. Over 80% of the Central American participants reported an external locus of control, in contrast to the Polish group, where only 10% did so. Other studies have also suggested that there may be important cultural differences in responsibility, blame, and other attributional styles which moderate pain expression and suffering (Bachiocco, Credico, & Tiengo, 2002; Eccleston, Williams, & Rogers, 1997).

We assume that pain and emotion mean the same thing in all cultures, but we do not well understand the interaction between semantics and culture. We cannot answer the question, "Even if an Anglo-American has a headache, is the meaning the same as when a Chinese person says he or she has a headache?" (Moore & Brodsgaard, 1999). We are not good at judging facial expressions in other societies. Shiori, Someya, Helmeste, and Tang (1999) found that Japanese subjects experienced difficulties in recognizing some emotional facial expressions and misunderstood others. Russell (1991) provided a detailed review of the literature that indicates both similarities and differences in how emotions are categorized in different languages and cultures.

We should not assume that stoicism is good and expressiveness is bad, although that impression is often taken away from many of the studies reviewed here. One can easily argue the opposite and note that whatever cultural differences exist are not limited to pain or negative affect and that societies that openly express pain also seem to openly express joy or happiness.

We have not clarified the definitions of race and ethnicity, often using them interchangeably. Many scholars challenge the concept of "race-as-biology," arguing that it is, in fact, a social construct (Goodman, 2000). No genetic signature identifies individuals as members of a particular race, and even the term *ethnicity* leads to confusions (Dimsdale, 2000; Morris, 2001). A twin study of laboratory pain sensitivity (MacGregor, Griffiths, Baker, & Spector, 1997) found equally high correlations between both monozygotic and dizygotic twins, leading to the conclusion that "there is no significant genetic contribution to the strong correlation in pressure pain threshold that is observed in twin pairs. These findings reinforce the view that learned patterns of behavior within families are an important determinant of perceived sensitivity to pain" (p. 253).

A recent investigation by Raber and Devor (2002) showed that in rats the characteristics of a cagemate can largely override genetic predispositions to pain behavior, possibly through the influence of stress. They concluded:

Can the presence of social partners affect pain behavior without actually altering felt pain? In animals, we have no direct access to information of pain experience except as reflected in behavior. These questions, however, apply equally to humans, including oneself. Could genotype or social convention (including the presence of specific others) change outward pain behavior without actually affecting the "raw feel" of the pain? In humans, the answer is clearly yes, although intuitively one imagines that rodents are less bound by social context (innate or learned), and that pain behavior should therefore more faithfully reflect actual pain sensation. This caveat, however, cannot be ruled out. (p. 149)

Blacks from Africa, the Caribbean, and the United States have markedly different cultural experiences, even within their geographic region. Black, and White, and Asian groups within a single society such as the United States may have enormous differences in child-rearing practices, modeling, and behavioral reinforcement, in addition to whatever genetic factors might distinguish them.

One cannot legitimately lump together individuals from China, Japan, Thailand, the Philippines, Singapore, Korea, Indonesia, and so on and pretend that they share a single cultural identity that can be labeled "Asian." Moreover, in our increasingly multicultural societies, we have no easy way to classify the ethnicity of an individual whose parents come from different backgrounds, who has moved from one continent to another, or who has spent critical years being educated abroad.

This is not to say that there are no differences between racial or ethnic groups. Rather, it is to encourage extreme caution in statements based on small numbers in a single community. African Americans living in a major metropolitan area or a university town are not representative of all African Americans and are certainly not representative of all Blacks. We cannot have it both ways with regard to White participants: to proclaim the supposed differences between Irish, Italians, Poles, and Scandinavians, and then to randomly lump a cluster of them together as "Whites" or "Caucasians" when we need a group to contrast with Blacks or Asians.

It is misleading and potentially detrimental to generalize to all members of one group based on a handful of subjects, often obtained nonrandomly, and who differ from other members of their group in myriad respects. The NIH Guidelines for Inclusion of Women and Minorities as Subjects in Clinical Research (http://grants1.nih.gov/grants/funding/women_min/guidelines_amended_10_2001.htm) have the laudable goal of ensuring that there is broad inclusion of subjects and "no significant differences of clinical or public health importance in intervention effect based on sex/gender, racial/ethnic and/or relevant subpopulation comparisons." This does not mean that a group of researchers conducting a pain study that ends up with 43 White subjects, 9 African Americans, 7 Hispanics, and 5 Asians should present the findings as a study of ethnocultural variations.

To the extent that such research shows that there are ethnocultural differences in pain or the effects of analgesics or the degree of negative affect or the effects of psychosocial interventions, we have a responsibility to identify the evidence and take appropriate action to modify clinical practice guidelines. At the moment, it seems we are best able to say that all patients should be carefully evaluated and treated with respect. Irrespective of their ethnocultural status, their pain reports must be accepted and all efforts must be undertaken to reduce their pain and distress.

ACKNOWLEDGMENTS

Partial support for the preparation of this chapter came from a research grant from the Natural Sciences and Engineering Research Council of Canada. I wish to thank Heather Whitehead for her assistance in obtaining copies of the many papers on the topic of this review.

REFERENCES

Abu-Saad, H. (1984). Cultural group indicators of pain in children. *Maternal-Child Nursing Journal, 13*, 187–196.

Allison, T. R., Symmons, D. P., Brammah, T., Haynes, P., Rogers, A., Roxby, M., & Urwin, M. (2002). Musculoskeletal pain is more generalised among people from ethnic minorities than among white people in Greater Manchester. *Annals of the Rheumatic Diseases, 61*, 151–156.

Bachiocco, V., Credico, C., & Tiengo, M. (2002). The pain locus of control orientation in a healthy sample of the Italian population: Sociodemographic modulating factors. *Journal of Cultural Diversity, 9,* 55–62.

Bates, M. S., & Edwards, W. T. (1992). Ethnic variations in the chronic pain experience. *Ethnicity and Disease, 2,* 63–83.

Berkley, K. J. (1997). Sex differences in pain. *Behavioral and Brain Sciences, 20,* 371–380.

Bill-Harvey, D., Rippey, R. M., Abeles, M., & Pfeiffer, C. A. (1989). Methods used by urban, low-income minorities to care for their arthritis. *Arthritis Care and Research, 2,* 60–64.

Bonham, V. L. (2001). Race, ethnicity, and pain treatment: Striving to understand the causes and solutions to the disparities in pain treatment. *Journal of Law, Medicine and Ethics, 29,* 52–68.

Borghouts, J. A., Koes, B. W., Vondeling, H., & Bouter, L. M. (1999). Cost-of-illness of neck pain in The Netherlands in 1996. *Pain, 80,* 629–636.

Brena, S. F., Sanders, S. H., & Motoyama, H. (1990). American and Japanese chronic low back pain patients: Cross-cultural similarities and differences. *Clinical Journal of Pain, 6,* 118–124.

Calvillo, E. R., & Flaskerud, J. H. (1991). Review of literature on culture and pain of adults with focus on Mexican-Americans. *Journal of Transcultural Nursing, 2,* 16–23.

Carron, H., DeGood, D. E., & Tait, R. (1985). A comparison of low back pain patients in the United States and New Zealand: Psychosocial and economic factors affecting severity of disability. *Pain, 21,* 77–89.

Chambers, C. T., & Craig, K. D. (1998). An intrusive impact of anchors in children's faces pain scales. *Pain, 78,* 27–37.

Chambers, C. T., Giesbrecht, K., Craig, K. D., Bennett, S. M., & Huntsman, E. (1999). A comparison of faces scales for the measurement of pediatric pain: Children's and parents' ratings. *Pain, 83,* 25–35.

Cleeland, C. S., Gonin, R., Hatfield, A. K., Edmonson, J. H., Blum, R. H., Stewart, J. A., & Pandya, K. J. (1994). Pain and its treatment in outpatients with metastatic cancer. *New England Journal of Medicine, 330,* 592–596.

Cleeland, C. S., Nakamura, Y., Mendoza, T. R., Edwards, K. R., Douglas, J., & Serlin, R. C. (1996). Dimensions of the impact of cancer pain in a four country sample: New information from multidimensional scaling. *Pain, 67,* 267–273.

Craft, R. M., & Bernal, S. A. (2001). Sex differences in opioid antinociception: Kappa and "mixed action" agonists. *Drug and Alcohol Dependence, 63,* 215–228.

Craig, K. D. (1986). Social modeling influences: Pain in context. In R. A. Sternbach (Ed.), *The psychology of pain* (2nd ed., pp. 67–95). New York: Raven Press.

Davitz, L. J., Sameshima, Y., & Davitz, J. (1976). Suffering as viewed in six different cultures. *American Journal of Nursing, 76,* 1296–1297.

De Benedittis, G., Massei, R., Nobili, R., & Pieri, A. (1988). The Italian Pain Questionnaire. *Pain, 33,* 53–62.

Dimsdale, J. E. (2000). Stalked by the past: The influence of ethnicity on health. *Psychosomatic Medicine, 62,* 161–170.

Eccleston, C., Williams, A. C., & Rogers, W. S. (1997). Patients' and professionals' understandings of the causes of chronic pain: Blame, responsibility and identity protection. *Social Science and Medicine, 45,* 699–709.

Edwards, C. L., Fillingim, R. B., & Keefe, F. (2001). Race, ethnicity and pain. *Pain, 94,* 133–137.

Edwards, R. R., Doleys, D. M., Fillingim, R. B., & Lowery, D. (2001). Ethnic differences in pain tolerance: Clinical implications in a chronic pain population. *Psychosomatic Medicine, 63,* 316–323.

Edwards, R. R., & Fillingim, R. B. (1999). Ethnic differences in thermal pain responses. *Psychosomatic Medicine, 61,* 346–354.

Fillingim, R. B. (2000). Sex, gender, and pain: Women and men really are different. *Current Reviews of Pain, 4,* 24–30.

Flores, G., Abreu, M., Schwartz, I., & Hill, M. (2000). The importance of language and culture in pediatric care: Case studies from the Latino community. *Journal of Pediatrics, 137,* 842–848.

Gil, K. M., Wilson, J. J., Edens, J. L., Webster, D. A., Abrams, M. A., Orringer, E., Grant, M., Clark, W. C., & Janal, M. N. (1996). Effects of cognitive coping skills training on coping strategies and experimental pain sensitivity in African American adults with sickle cell disease. *Health Psychology, 15,* 3–10.

Goodman, A. H. (2000). Why genes don't count (for racial differences in health). *American Journal of Public Health, 90,* 1699–1702.

Gracely, R. H., Petzke, F., Wolf, J. M., & Clauw, D. J. (2002). Functional magnetic resonance imaging evidence of augmented pain processing in fibromyalgia. *Arthritis and Rheumatism, 46,* 1333–1343.

Hadjistavropoulos, T. (1999). Chronic pain on trial: The influence of litigation and compensation on chronic pain syndromes. In A. R. Block, E. F. Kremer, & E. Fernandez (Eds.), *Handbook of pain syndromes* (pp. 59–76). Mahwah, NJ: Lawrence Erlbaum Associates.

Hameed, K., & Gibson, T. (1997). A comparison of the prevalence of rheumatoid arthritis and other rheumatic diseases amongst Pakistanis living in England and Pakistan. *British Journal of Rheumatology, 36,* 781–785.

Hasegawa, M., Hattori, S., Mishima, M., Matsumoto, I., Kimura, T., Baba, Y., Takano, O., Sasaki, T., Kanemura, K., Senami, K., & Shibata, T. (2001). The McGill Pain Questionnaire, Japanese version, reconsidered: Confirming the theoretical structure. *Pain Research and Management, 6,* 173–180.

Ho, K. H., & Ong, B. K. (2001). Headache characteristics and race in Singapore: Results of a randomized national survey. *Headache, 41,* 279–284.

Honeyman, P. T., & Jacobs, E. A. (1996). Effects of culture on back pain in Australian aboriginals. *Spine, 21,* 841–843.

Hutubessy, R. C., van Tulder, M. W., Vondeling, H., & Bouter, L. M. (1999). Indirect costs of back pain in the Netherlands: A comparison of the human capital method with the friction cost method. *Pain, 80,* 201–207.

Jordan, M. S., Lumley, M. A., & Leisen, J. C. (1998). The relationships of cognitive coping and pain control beliefs to pain and adjustment among African-American and Caucasian women with rheumatoid arthritis. *Arthritis Care and Research, 11,* 80–88.

Karnad, A. B. (1994). Treating cancer pain. *New England Journal of Medicine, 331,* 199.

Kodiath, M. F., & Kodiath, A. (1992). A comparative study of patients with chronic pain in India and the United States. *Clinical Nursing Research, 1,* 278–291.

Lasch, K. E. (2000). Culture, pain, and culturally sensitive pain care. *Pain Management Nursing, 1,* 16–22.

Lautenbacher, S., & Rollman, G. B. (1997). Possible deficiencies of pain modulation in fibromyalgia. *Clinical Journal of Pain, 13,* 189–196.

Lautenbacher, S., Rollman, G. B., & McCain, G. A. (1994). Multi-method assessment of experimental and clinical pain in patients with fibromyalgia. *Pain, 59,* 45–53.

Lazaro, C., Caseras, X., Whizar-Lugo, V. M., Wenk, R., Baldioceda, F., Bernal, R., Ovalle, A., Torrubia, R., & Banos, J. E. (2001). Psychometric properties of a Spanish version of the McGill Pain Questionnaire in several Spanish-speaking countries. *Clinical Journal of Pain, 17,* 365–374.

LeResche, L. (1997). Epidemiology of temporomandibular disorders: Implications for the investigation of etiologic factors. *Critical Reviews in Oral Biology and Medicine, 8,* 291–305.

Levenstein, S., Li, Z., Almer, S., Barbosa, A., Marquis, P., Moser, G., Sperber, A., Toner, B., & Drossman, D. A. (2001). Cross-cultural variation in disease-related concerns among patients with inflammatory bowel disease. *American Journal of Gastroenterology, 96,* 1822–1830.

Lipton, J. A., & Marbach, J. J. (1984). Ethnicity and the pain experience. *Social Science and Medicine, 19,* 1279–1298.

Litcher, L., Bromet, E., Carlson, G., Gilbert, T., Panina, N., Golovakha, E., Goldgaber, D., Gluzman, S., & Garber, J. (2001). Ukrainian application of the Children's Somatization Inventory: Psychometric properties and associations with internalizing symptoms. *Journal of Abnormal Child Psychology, 29,* 165–175.

Macario, A., Scibetta, W. C., Navarro, J., & Riley, E. (2000). Analgesia for labor pain: A cost model. *Anesthesiology, 92,* 841–850.

MacGregor, A. J., Griffiths, G. O., Baker, J., & Spector, T. D. (1997). Determinants of pressure pain threshold in adult twins: Evidence that shared environmental influences predominate. *Pain, 73,* 253–257.

McCracken, L. M., Matthews, A. K., Tang, T. S., & Cuba, S. L. (2001). A comparison of blacks and whites seeking treatment for chronic pain. *Clinical Journal of Pain, 17,* 249–255.

McCracken, L. M., Zayfert, C., & Gross, R. T. (1992). The Pain Anxiety Symptoms Scale: Development and validation of a scale to measure fear of pain. *Pain, 50,* 67–73.

McDermid, A. J., Rollman, G. B., & McCain, G. A. (1996). Generalized hypervigilance in fibromyalgia: Evidence of perceptual amplification. *Pain, 66,* 133–144.

McGrath, P. A. (1995). Pain in the pediatric patient: Practical aspects of assessment. *Pediatric Annals, 24,* 126–128.

McGrath, P. A., Speechley, K. N., Seifert, C. E., Biehn, J. T., Cairney, A. E., Gorodzinsky, F. P., Dickie, G. L., McCusker, P. J., & Morrissy, J. R. (2000). A survey of children's acute, recurrent, and chronic pain: Validation of the pain experience interview. *Pain, 87,* 59–73.

McGrath, P. J., Rosmus, C., Camfield, C., Campbell, M. A., & Hennigar, A. (1998). Behaviours caregivers use to determine pain in non-verbal, cognitively impaired individuals. *Developmental Medicine and Child Neurology, 40,* 340–343.

Mogil, J. S., Chesler, E. J., Wilson, S. G., Juraska, J. M., & Sternberg, W. F. (2000). Sex differences in thermal nociception and morphine antinociception in rodents depend on genotype. *Neuroscience and Biobehavioral Reviews, 24,* 375–389.

Moore, R. (1990). Ethnographic assessment of pain coping perceptions. *Psychosomatic Medicine, 52,* 171–181.

Moore, R., & Brodsgaard, I. (1999). Cross-cultural investigations of pain. In I. K. Crombie, P. R. Croft, S. J. Linton, L. LeResche, & M. Von Korff (Eds.), *Epidemiology of pain* (pp. 53–80). Seattle, WA: IASP Press.

Morris, D. B. (2001). Ethnicity and pain. *Pain: Clinical Updates, 9,* 1–4.

Nayak, S., Shiflett, S. C., Eshun, S., & Levine, F. M. (2000). Culture and gender effects in pain beliefs and the prediction of pain tolerance. *Cross-Cultural Research, 34,* 135–151.

Nelson, D. V., Novy, D. M., Averill, P. M., & Berry, L. A. (1996). Ethnic comparability of the MMPI in pain patients. *Journal of Clinical Psychology, 52,* 485–497.

Ng, B., Dimsdale, J. E., Rollnik, J. D., & Shapiro, H. (1996). The effect of ethnicity on prescriptions for patient-controlled analgesia for post-operative pain. *Pain, 66,* 9–12.

Ng, B., Dimsdale, J. E., Shragg, G. P., & Deutsch, R. (1996). Ethnic differences in analgesic consumption for postoperative pain. *Psychosomatic Medicine, 58,* 125–129.

Njobvu, P., Hunt, I., Pope, D., & Macfarlane, G. (1999). Pain amongst ethnic minority groups of South Asian origin in the United Kingdom: A review. *Rheumatology (Oxford), 38,* 1184–1187.

Pfefferbaum, B., Adams, J., & Aceves, J. (1990). The influence of culture on pain in Anglo and Hispanic children with cancer. *Journal of the American Academy of Child and Adolescent Psychiatry, 29,* 642–647.

Raber, P., & Devor, M. (2002). Social variables affect phenotype in the neuroma model of neuropathic pain. *Pain, 97,* 139–150.

Rathore, S. S., Lenert, L. A., Weinfurt, K. P., Tinoco, A., Taleghani, C. K., Harless, W., & Schulman, K. A. (2000). The effects of patient sex and race on medical students' ratings of quality of life. *American Journal of Medicine, 108,* 561–566.

Riley, J. L. III, Robinson, M. E., Wise, E. A., Myers, C. D., & Fillingim, R. B. (1998). Sex differences in the perception of noxious experimental stimuli: A meta-analysis. *Pain, 74,* 181–187.

Rollman, G. B. (1998). Culture and pain. In S. S. Kazarian & D. R. Evans (Eds.), *Cultural clinical psychology: Theory, research, and practice* (pp. 267–286). New York: Oxford University Press.

Rollman, G. B., & Lautenbacher, S. (2001). Sex differences in musculoskeletal pain. *Clinical Journal of Pain, 17*, 20–24.

Rosmus, C., Johnston, C. C., Chan-Yip, A., & Yang, F. (2000). Pain response in Chinese and non-Chinese Canadian infants: Is there a difference? *Social Science and Medicine, 51*, 175–184.

Russell, J. A. (1991). Culture and the categorization of emotions. *Psychological Bulletin, 110*, 426–450.

Sabbioni, M. E., & Eugster, S. (2001). Interactions of a history of migration with the course of pain disorder. *Journal of Psychosomatic Research, 50*, 267–269.

Sanders, S. H., Brena, S. F., Spier, C. J., Beltrutti, D., McConnell, H., & Quintero, O. (1992). Chronic low back pain patients around the world: Cross-cultural similarities and differences. *Clinical Journal of Pain, 8*, 317–323.

Sargent, C. (1984). Between death and shame: Dimensions of pain in Bariba culture. *Social Science and Medicine, 19*, 1299–1304.

Sheffield, D., Biles, P. L., Orom, H., Maixner, W., & Sheps, D. S. (2000). Race and sex differences in cutaneous pain perception. *Psychosomatic Medicine, 62*, 517–523.

Sheffield, D., Kirby, D. S., Biles, P. L., & Sheps, D. S. (1999). Comparison of perception of angina pectoris during exercise testing in African-Americans versus Caucasians. *American Journal of Cardiology, 83*, 106–108, A8.

Sheiner, E. K., Sheiner, E., Shoham-Vardi, I., Mazor, M., & Katz, M. (1999). Ethnic differences influence care giver's estimates of pain during labour. *Pain, 81*, 299–305.

Shioiri, T., Someya, T., Helmeste, D., & Tang, S. W. (1999). Misinterpretation of facial expression: A cross-cultural study. *Psychiatry and Clinical Neurosciences, 53*, 45–50.

Skovron, M. L., Szpalski, M., Nordin, M., Melot, C., & Cukier, D. (1994). Sociocultural factors and back pain. A population-based study in Belgian adults. *Spine, 19*, 129–137.

Staud, R., Vierck, C. J., Cannon, R. L., Mauderli, A. P., & Price, D. D. (2001). Abnormal sensitization and temporal summation of second pain (wind-up) in patients with fibromyalgia syndrome. *Pain, 91*, 165–175.

Sternbach, R. A., & Tursky, B. (1965). Ethnic differences among housewives in psychophysical and skin potential responses to electric shock. *Psychophysiology, 1*, 241–246.

Strand, L. I., & Ljunggren, A. E. (1997). Different approximations of the McGill Pain Questionnaire in the Norwegian language: A discussion of content validity. *Journal of Advanced Nursing, 26*, 772–779.

Thomas, V. J., & Rose, F. D. (1991). Ethnic differences in the experience of pain. *Social Science and Medicine, 32*, 1063–1066.

Todd, K. H., Samaroo, N., & Hoffman, J. R. (1993). Ethnicity as a risk factor for inadequate emergency department analgesia. *Journal of the American Medical Association, 269*, 1537–1539.

Turk, D. C., Okifuji, A., Sinclair, J. D., & Starz, T. W. (1996). Pain, disability, and physical functioning in subgroups of patients with fibromyalgia. *Journal of Rheumatology, 23*, 1255–1262.

Unruh, A. M. (1996). Gender variations in clinical pain experience. *Pain, 65*, 123–167.

Villarruel, A. M., & Denyes, M. J. (1991). Pain assessment in children: Theoretical and empirical validity. ANS. *Advances in Nursing Science, 14*, 32–41.

Waza, K., Graham, A. V., Zyzanski, S. J., & Inoue, K. (1999). Comparison of symptoms in Japanese and American depressed primary care patients. *Family Practice, 16*, 528–533.

Wise, E. A., Price, D. D., Myers, C. D., Heft, M. W., & Robinson, M. E. (2002). Gender role expectations of pain: Relationship to experimental pain perception. *Pain, 96*, 335–342.

Wolff, B. B. (1985). Ethnocultural factors influencing pain and illness behavior. *Clinical Journal of Pain, 1*, 23–30.

Yang, J. C., Clark, W. C., & Janal, M. N. (1991). Sensory decision theory and visual analogue scale indices predict status of chronic pain patients six months later. *Journal of Pain and Symptom Management, 6*, 58–64.

Zborowski, M. (1969). *People in pain*. San Francisco: Jossey-Bass.

Zola, I. K. (1966). Culture and symptoms—An analysis of patients' presenting complaints. *American Sociological Review, 31*, 615–630.

Social Influences on Individual Differences in Responding to Pain

Suzanne M. Skevington
Victoria L. Mason
Department of Psychology,
University of Bath

This chapter explores how individuals respond to pain in the context of the wider social and cultural environment. Individual differences are discussed within the framework of a model of the psychological and social factors implicated in the generation and maintenance of a chronically painful illness (Skevington, 1995). This model is described and elaborated in the light of emerging empirical evidence in the field of pain to address the question of what determines how people respond to pain.

The medical model of disease is directed at understanding underlying pathology to obtain a diagnosis. The explanatory power of the medical model is limited when considering the response to tissue damage, which is complex and multifaceted. Fordyce (1976) argued that this model is inappropriate and ineffective when dealing with chronically painful diseases. Evidence to support this view comes from work showing that magnetic resonance imaging (MRI) scans show little statistical association with subjective reports of low back pain (Deyo, 1994). Although the case is equivocal, as recent research using fMRI imaging of the brain has shown that it is possible to isolate the brain activity associated with the pain response (e.g., Porro, Cettolo, Francescato, & Baraldi, 1998). Despite these new developments, the work of Deyo supports the notion that pain cannot be understood within the limits of the medical model that has tended to ignore the social, psychological, and cognitive variables that affect the way that individual's respond to pain.

Two areas have dominated the debate about the role of individual differences in understanding and managing pain until quite recently (Skevington, 1995). The first would be personality psychology, where the search for personality dispositions toward pain lasted several decades. Here the approach tended to use standardized questionnaires, like the Minnesota Multiphasic Personality Inventory (MMPI; Hathaway & McKinley, 1943) and its successor, the MMPI-2, to investigate stable dispositions, for example, the pain-prone personality, and to look at relationships between chronic pain and neurosis, and other types of psychopathology. The weakness of this approach was that it provided little information about how best to develop suitable treatments where other approaches, discussed later in this chapter, have succeeded. The personality approach also assumes that people have robust and enduring characteristics, which are not readily amenable to therapeutic interventions that require changes in behavior and lifestyle. The success of psychologically based interventions indicates that this assumption was unwarranted. Furthermore, it is clear from research and practice that relatively few pain sufferers fit these categories, and that for the majority, a psychiatric approach is quite inappropriate and can even be an impediment to rehabilitation. For example, the MMPI fails to predict self-reported outcomes of chronic lower back pain patients attending a pain management program (Chapman & Pemberton, 1994). Other approaches have had more success; for example, Main (1984) reported that levels of disability, current stress, and illness behavior are better predictors of outcome than either personality traits or pain intensity ratings. Furthermore, the persistent hunt for a personality disposition toward pain—for example, the rheumatoid personality—has hampered the creative process in searching for other lines of suitable psychological therapy (Skevington, 1995).

During the time span in which this search for stable personality features was undertaken, the area of individual differences was radically reconceptualized. Following the work of Mischel (1973, 1977), the orientation of personality theory changed from an exclusive and focused view of the person (or for ecological psychologists, the situation alone), to a much more holistic consideration of the person within their situation. Mischel proposed an interactionist model, whereby personality is influenced and moderated by a variety of external, environmental influences. He rejected the earlier idea of global personality traits, in favor of the role of person variables in predicting behavior. Indeed, Mischel argued that it was not the existence of individual differences per se that were important but their nature, causes, consequences, and utility (Mischel, 1968), mirroring the need to understand the person within the situation. This interactionist perspective of individual differences is utilized in this chapter, and sees the individual not as a slave to the dictates of the personality or simply a product of environmental forces but in a more active and dynamic role, integrating diverse information from these two sources.

The second area of investigation arises from behaviorism, out of which social learning theory was developed. Unlike studies of personality, behavioral approaches are process oriented, taking a fleeting glance at people's histories but focusing essentially on the environment in which they live and how their experiences and learning, in particular, shape their behavior as pain sufferers. Principles of reinforcement and punishment initially articulated by Fordyce (1976) have been successfully applied and extended in cognitive behavior therapy programs to help those with chronic pain deal with their disability. As family and health professionals are involved in providing reinforcement and punishment for pain behavior, the approach is necessarily "social" in orientation. However, positive reinforcements and punishments form only a small portion of the many events that encompass our social relationships with family, friends, colleagues, and so on. Although a neo-behaviorist approach has adopted a rationalist, cognitive style in adapting Fordyce's work, only relatively recently has the model explicitly incorporated and addressed important emotional factors that directly affect the experience, reporting, and management of pain. Likewise, the acknowledgment of social influences on pain behavior is present, but as yet, this is only selectively elaborated within the model, and hence in the model's clinical application.

Critical developments in understanding and managing pain in acute and chronic settings have also arisen from the application of the gate control theory (GCT) of pain (Melzack & Wall, 1965, 1982) and the subsequent demonstration of the plasticity of the nervous system. These advances in clarifying mechanisms and opening new avenues for pain relief are addressed extensively elsewhere (see chap. 1, this volume), but here we view them as representing important historical developments in understanding the biological basis of how and why individuals respond to pain, and in explaining the attenuation and persistence of pain. This perspective provides a foundation for understanding the role of the biopsychosocial model in the study of pain and pain treatments (see chap. 2, this volume). This systems theory approach (Engelbart & Vranken, 1984) has been used by health psychologists to develop comprehension and, from this perspective, psychological interventions suited to many different health problems and diseases. A social model of pain based on research evidence can be developed within this framework, by organizing social elements that affect and are affected by pain and then using the model to direct how treatment is conducted. Once the model is established, it can be reused to provide guidance on how therapeutic elements can be systematically changed and tested, with the aim of improving outcomes. In short, there is nothing as practical as a good theory, as GCT illustrates.

In this systems theory approach, all levels of organization are linked to each other hierarchically, so changes at one level will effect changes at others. This way, micro-level processes, for example, changes in heart rate, are nested in those at a macro level—for example, stereotypic professional views about people with chronic back pain. Consequently, changes at a micro level can have macro-level effects, and vice versa. Because biological processes connected with pain are commonly at the micro level, and psychological and social processes are more likely to be macro-level phenomena, it requires commitment to multidisciplinary thinking to be able to select and use this diverse multivariate information appropriately and effectively in problem solving. Work to date on biopsychosocial models already points to the urgent need to understand and address all three components in these models, if we are to create successful treatments (Taylor, 1999).

We argue here that pain researchers have been very successful with the application of biological approaches to pain relief (McQuay & Moore, 1998), and to some extent with psychological approaches, such as cognitive behavior therapy. But the contribution of social factors to the study of pain is poorly defined, weakly elaborated, and infrequently conducted, compared to other types of research on pain. It will be necessary to show which social factors directly and significantly affect and exacerbate pain if this approach is to gain acceptance as an important, independent, and equal contributor to the biopsychosocial triad. Important social factors will need to be properly evaluated for their potential to generate new types of treatment or styles of management. On the basis of existing evidence about the effectiveness of the model, it is increasingly clear that an integration of sociocultural factors is essential to achieving positive outcomes, relieving suffering, and diffusing action from the narrow medicalization of pain, in ongoing programs of care.

A MODEL OF THE PSYCHOSOCIAL FACTORS IMPLICATED IN THE ETIOLOGY AND MAINTENANCE OF CHRONICALLY PAINFUL ILLNESS

Although health professionals who work in pain research and practice have become pioneers in the design and running of smoothly functioning multidisciplinary teams, it is arguable that when examining the key social influences that affect pain and pain behavior, we have been slow to draw on contributions from the wider range of social science disciplines available, and to extend and apply them to improve our understanding of the pain response and its management. The model we present pays more attention to the social factors that affect pain, illness, and treatments, with the aim of il-luminating the inherently complex interaction between a pain sufferer and their psychosocial environment. Furthermore, it is not possible to do this properly without taking a multidisciplinary approach but within the per-spective of a different but overlapping set of disciplines.

The model developed by Skevington (1995) proposes four levels of un-derstanding that provide a framework within which the social aspects of chronic pain may be better appreciated, and this is shown in Fig. 7.1. Level 1 defines the individual processes affected by social influences, such as per-ceived bodily sensations. In contrast, Level 2 characterizes salient interper-sonal behaviors, in particular, that person's relationship with significant others. Level 3 defines group and intergroup behaviors such as group be-liefs, experience, and influences, whereas Level 4 encompasses some of the higher order factors that affect sociopsychological processing, such as health ideology and health politics. Although reductionist, this model aims to understand the processes within each level and the relationships be-tween levels, rather than assuming that each level can be better explained by looking at the level below. The model broadens our conceptualization of chronic pain by removing the individual from his or her social and cultural "black box." For the detailed empirical support for each element of this model, see Skevington (1995). The aim here is to extend the model and elab-orate it through a discussion of individual differences.

Level I: Individual Behaviors Affected by Social Processes

Individual behaviors affected by social processes include a multitude of subjective factors including perceived bodily sensations, the perceived se-verity of symptoms, lifetime personal and social schema, social and per-sonal emotions, individual representations, and personal motivation. This level of analysis is probably most familiar to those who work on chronic pain, and with pain patients where internal biological and psychological fac-tors have been investigated at a micro level. Although sensations superfi-cially appear to be physiologically determined, there is now extensive cross-cultural evidence to show that pain thresholds and pain tolerance lev-els are influenced by a wide variety of different social and cultural factors (Bates, 1987; McCracken, Matthews, Tang, & Cuba, 2001; Nayak, Shiflett, Eshun, & Levine, 2000; Zborowski, 1969; also see chap. 6, this volume). For instance, in the Hispanic culture, stoicism is highly prized (Juarez, Ferrell, & Bornemann, 1998), whereas in other cultures describing the pain in a vivid and extended detail is much more the norm (Zborowski, 1969). Reporting symptoms is known to be unreliable (Pennebaker, 1982), even when allow-ing for familial and social biasing influences that further explain the cross-

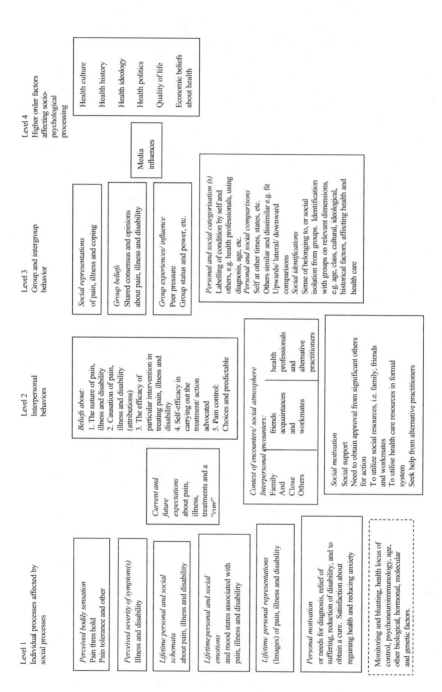

FIG. 7.1. Model of the psychosocial processes and social factors implicated in the generation and maintenance of a chronically painful illness. From Skevington (1995). *Psychology of Pain.* Chichester: John Wiley and Sons. Copyright © 1995. Adapted with permission.

184

cultural differences observed. Mechanic (1986) underscored this view when he suggested that sociocultural and sociopsychological factors affect the reporting of pain and illness. Indeed, according to Mechanic, cultural differences cannot be explained by learning and personality alone, but also require an appreciation of the sector of society to which people belong. Mechanic's observation raises interesting questions about how those working in pain might better explore social identity with their patients, and at the same time provides a link to a higher level of analysis in this model.

Pain severity also affects decisions about whether, when, and from whom to seek health care, and consequently has economic as well as social implications for mechanisms of health care delivery (Foster & Mallik, 1998). However, contrary to popular belief, people do not always seek help for their health when they are "sickest," but are more likely to do this when the symptoms interfere with their lives (Zola, 1973). Indeed, the point at which somebody obtains professional help may in some cases be a factor contributing to the transition from mild to severe pain, if the delay is considerable. Conceptually, it is worth considering the relationship between acute anxiety and depression, and the perceived severity of symptoms, as this combination is known to be a springboard to seeking help from others, whether this is self-referral to health professionals (Ingham & Miller, 1979), the utilization of lay networks, or help from alternative, spiritual, and other sources.

The way that individual pain patients behave is guided by how they see themselves, the way they organize knowledge about their bodies, the nature of the pain, the availability and accessibility of care, and information that determines whether treatments prescribed are acceptable. Abstract concepts, or schemata, are theories that pain patients hold about pain and treatment that influence the ways in which they selectively absorb new knowledge, remember it, and make use of it, to make sense of their painful experience and to inform decision making. Reality is structured and simplified, and these schemata mix and interpret past and present experience. Investigating and systematically recording the nature of these key concepts, and how those about the painful experience are stored and organized in the memory, allows us to better understand how patients think and therefore more readily anticipate what they may or may not do as a consequence. This is particularly important when trying to maximize concordance with medical advice or in outlining pain management strategies. By doing this, the twin goals of increasing self-efficacy and improving outcomes may be better achieved (Jensen, Turner, & Romano, 1991).

Emotions and mood states like depression are influenced by our social surroundings. Social support research shows how complex this process may be (e.g., Jensen et al., 2002). Moods are worth studying not only because they relate to the affective qualities of pain that are more commonly expressed by those in chronic pain (Skevington, 1995) but also because they are firmly grounded in coping behaviors, or shortage of them. In a study of humor related to pain and disability, Skevington and White (1998) found that patients with chronic arthritis (n = 100) reported they could readily change their own mood and that of others by using humor and jokes to deflect the social unease caused by visible evidence of their pain and disability. Linking into levels 2 and 3, the use of humor sets others more at their ease in this socially uncomfortable situation. Such studies reveal the potential for people to affect their social environment by adopting particular strategies. These studies could have important implications for managing social relationships while simultaneously managing pain.

Given the large body of literature illustrating the clear link between pain and depression (e.g., Ericsson et al., 2002; Maxwell, Gatchel, & Mayer, 1998; Rudy, Kerns, & Turk, 1988; Turk & Okifuji, 1994), this must also be seen as a key factor in the understanding of individual differences in pain. In a recent systematic review and meta-analysis, Dickens and colleagues looked at the strength of the relationship between rheumatoid arthritis (RA) and depression (Dickens et al., 2002). Examining 12 independent studies comparing depression in RA patients and healthy controls, they found that depression was more common in RA patients and could be attributed to the level of pain.

Other important psychological concepts include anxiety and fear avoidance (e.g., Fritz, George, & Delitto, 2001; George, Fritz, & Erhard, 2001; Vlaeyen & Linton, 2000), hypervigilance (e.g., Lorenz, 1998; Peters, Vlaeyen, & Kunnen, 2002), catastrophizing (e.g., Vlaeyen, deJong, Geilen, Heuts, & van Breukelen, 2001), worry (e.g., Eccleston, Crombez, Aldrich, & Stannard, 2001), and the emotional response to pain that is increasingly being employed (see chap. 2, this volume) to explain observations in the clinic. The fear–avoidance model has received considerable empirical attention recently, particularly in the development and maintenance of chronic musculoskeletal pain. Vlaeyen and Linton (2000) extensively reviewed the literature on fear–avoidance, the concept of fear of pain and methods of assessing pain-related fear. They concluded that the bulk of evidence pointed toward the importance of pain-related fear in explaining the differences observed in physical performance and self-reports of disability. Related to this concept is catastrophizing, where pain is interpreted as threatening. The perception of threat may be a precursor to fearing pain, and the consequent hypervigilance to bodily sensations (Vlaeyen & Linton, 2000). In a recent study, Sinclair (2001) examined the predictors of catastrophizing in a study of 90 female RA patients. Dispositional pessimism, passive pain coping, venting, and arthritis helplessness were found to predict catastrophizing (Sinclair, 2001). Sullivan and colleagues theoretically examined the concept of catastrophizing and suggested that social factors were implicated in the development and subsequent maintenance of catastrophizing

(Sullivan et al., 2001). Understanding these predictors underscores the susceptibility of different individuals to respond to pain in particular styles. The images or representations that patients hold about illness and disability are very important in their interpretation of pain sensations. Representations are a form of mental picture and several versions have been identified. Spatial representations for instance, provide images about how the body is organized in space. Looking at representations held by phantom limb patients, Katz and Melzack (1990) found them to be very elaborate. For example, amputated fingers felt as though they still had their rings on, many months later. People also have linear representations of events such as a sequential pattern of knowledge about their pain treatment or the history of their family's reaction to their pain, all of which impact on an individual's understanding of their current pain state. Furthermore, DeVellis and colleagues have shown that people with arthritis hold illness schemas that are relevant and meaningful not only for patients themselves, but also for health professionals (DeVellis, Patterson, Blalock, Renner, & DeVellis, 1997). These shared representations form part of the language used to express painful experience and facilitate communication between patients, health professionals, and significant others.

Among personal processes subject to social influence, there is the individual motivation to seek relief from suffering, obtain a clear diagnosis, reduce disability, and find a cure. Pain is a "powerful motivator" (Melzack & Dennis, 1978) and is a common reason for seeking medical help. Patients also prioritize their needs; for example, is the need to have a family holiday right now greater than the need to receive an epidural injection for low back pain, perhaps? Motivation to do something about the pain, however much such actions may lack an evidence base, is still a good predictor of treatment outcome (Grahn, Ekdahl, & Borgquist, 2000). Conceptually, motivation is also important in looking at self-efficacy, which explains the confidence that individuals have that they will be able to carry out a particular action such as seeking pain relief, or maintaining self-management strategies. Self-efficacy is explored in Level 2 of the model.

Although it would be impossible to be comprehensive in this very large and broad-ranging field, there are several other key biopsychosocial factors that we may consider in any analysis of individual differences at Level 1. The identification of characteristics such as the monitoring or blunting of attention, and health locus of control (HLC), have shown promise in understanding the individual's response to pain. During monitoring, there is a tendency to be highly attentive to threatening information, where the person selects salient information and focuses narrowly on bodily sensations. Blunting, in contrast, is used to ignore intruding sensations and to find distraction from them. Miller developed the Monitoring and Blunting Style Scale (Miller, 1987), originally to measure what appeared to be a personality trait but is now better conceptualized as a cognitive style that is situationally based. Concepts of monitoring and blunting have been used extensively to understand and explain different responses to pain. Miller, Brody, and Summerton (1988) found that those who were both high monitors and low blunters were highly likely to see their doctors faster, had mild problems, and did not improve much, but had the same level of distress, discomfort, and dysfunction as other people. So studies of cognitive style provide a somewhat different but equally informative set of explanations for individual reporting behavior than the more usual research on emotions.

Health locus of control (HLC) concerns the extent to which an individual sees health events as controllable by themselves or others (Wallston & Wallston, 1982). Measures of pain locus of control—for example, the Beliefs in Pain Control Questionnaire (Skevington, 1990)—have been standardized to assess under what circumstances a person in pain tends to adopt an internal or external locus of control. Conant has found an association between internal health locus of control and decreased pain perceptions in patients with spinal cord injury (Conant, 1998). HLC has also been used to explain patterns of analgesic use (Reynaert, Janne, & Delire, 1995). More generally, perceptions of control and control of pain are central to the experience of pain and understanding the response to pain. For example, Affleck and his colleagues (Affleck, Tennen, Pfeiffer, & Fifield, 1987) in a study of rheumatoid arthritis patients found that those who perceived that their illness was predictable believed that they were in control of their symptoms and the course of their disease. Furthermore, beliefs about control over specific symptoms were more important than control over the course of the disease, and positive moods were associated with those who felt that they had more control over their symptoms than their physicians. More recently, a study of patients undergoing abdominal hysterectomy, by Thomas, Heath, Rose, and Flory (1995), compared those receiving patient-controlled analgesia (PCA) with those receiving intramuscular injections (IMI). PCA gave significantly greater pain control, particularly among those with high levels of state anxiety. Furthermore, there were some direct cost implications, as PCA patients also required less analgesia and were discharged earlier than IMI patients. This study highlights both the importance of psychological variables associated with pain control and the advantages of allowing patients to take control of their analgesic use.

The field of psychoneuroimmunology (PNI) has been invaluable in cementing together the biopsychosocial model. In particular, it has shed new light on the relationship between emotions and the immune response, crossing the previous gap in the dualistic tradition of the separateness of mind and body. Evidence is emerging for the immunosuppressive effects of pain (Cheever, 1999; Kremer, 1999) that has important implications for the health of individuals with pain and highlights the complex interplay of factors that mediate the painful experience. Kiecolt-Glaser and colleagues recently reviewed considerable evidence and confirmed that stress delays wound healing (Kiecolt-Glaser, Page, Marucha, MacCullum, & Glaser, 1998). As pain is a prominent stressor, this has implications for the induction and perpetuation of chronic pain at physiological and neurological levels. Other research has shown that interpersonal stress is associated with an increase in disease activity in rheumatoid arthritis patients (Zautra et al., 1997), which points to the role of social factors in the inflammatory process. Taken together, this research highlights that the response to pain and its consequences can be influenced by factors external to the individual, and that this complex relationship has only just begun to be unraveled.

Aging and pain have also received empirical attention in recent years. Li and colleagues looked at whether pain perception differed between older and younger adults (Li, Greenwald, Gennis, Bijur, & Gallagher, 2001). Patients requiring a painful procedure—in this case, the insertion of an intravenous catheter during attendance at an emergency department—were asked to rate their pain on a visual analogue scale. The results showed that adults over 65 years reported significantly less pain than younger people, and this result was not influenced by gender. However, this study is unable to demonstrate whether such differences could be explained by a decline in sensitivity to pain or a reduced willingness to complain of pain, which may have implications for treatment. Having identified differences in the response to pain by people of different age groups, it follows that this is an important area of inquiry and should be considered when approaching the management of pain.

Other influences on the response to pain derive from the complex interplay of biological, hormonal, molecular, and genetic determinants, which are important at Level 1 of this model for understanding pain (see chap. 1 and chap. 3, this volume). Recently there has been an explosion of interest in the genetic mechanisms underlying pain, although this area of research is beyond the scope and direction of this chapter. Research examining these features of pain is well documented elsewhere; for example, for genetic variation see Hakim, Cherkas, Zayat et al. (2002), Mogil and Adhikari (1999), and Kest, Wilson, and Mogil (1999), and on the congenital insensitivity to pain, Indo (2002). Furthermore, these types of research are beginning to indicate that individuals respond differently to analgesics, and there has been some work to elucidate the possible mechanisms involved (Amanzio, Pollo, Maggi, & Benedetti, 2001).

Level 2: Interpersonal Behavior

Current and future expectations about pain, illness, treatments, and a "cure," link Level 1 to Level 2 of the model. Level 2 is characterized by beliefs about pain and treatment, the context of encounters, and social atmosphere and motivation. Beliefs about pain and treatment are socially shared, and include the nature of pain, illness, and disability, attributions about their causation, the efficacy of particular interventions, self-efficacy in implementing treatment, and aspects of pain control, such as choice and predictability. The social context of interpersonal encounters encompasses the social relationships with family, significant others, friends, acquaintances, workmates, colleagues, health professionals, and alternative practitioners. Social motivation incorporates social support, the need for approval of actions to utilize social resources such as family and friends and formal health care resources, and seeking help from alternative therapists.

Numerous beliefs, probably in the hundreds, need to be systematically documented and organized taxonomically to understand which are the most important predictors of the response to pain, illness, and treatment outcomes. Patients' beliefs tend to mirror the general and current views held by the society that they live in, being grounded in that culture. These interpersonal beliefs provides a backdrop for shared group and intergroup understandings at Level 3, and connect with higher order factors such as health culture at Level 4. Beliefs have considerable practical value in understanding how patients present their condition, and in predicting their response to advice and compliance with treatment, with erroneous beliefs being particularly prone to perpetuating persistent pain. Identifying several clusters of relevant beliefs, Jensen, Karoly, and Huger (1987) found that pain patients commonly believe that physicians will rid them of pain, that they themselves are not in control of the pain, that others are responsible for helping people in pain, that those in pain are permanently disabled, and that medication is the best form of treatment for pain. These beliefs are conceptualized as reflecting dependency, external health locus of control, absence of positive thoughts about rehabilitation, or catastrophizing, and medicalization, respectively. More recently, Jensen and Karoly (1992) found that among patients reporting low and medium levels of pain, a belief that they were disabled was related to lower activity levels, use of health care services, and poorer psychological functioning. They also found that where patients believed in a medical cure for their pain, this was related to more frequent use of health care services. These results highlight the importance of beliefs in adjustment to chronic pain (Jensen & Karoly, 1992), and it is these types of erroneous beliefs that need to be confronted in psychosocial interventions, such as self-management courses and cognitive behavior therapy, to enable patients to make gains and achieve a sense of control.

Much work has been carried out on the concept of self-efficacy in recent years, and numerous findings support the importance of self-efficacy beliefs in response to pain. For example, Jensen et al. (1991) found that self-efficacy beliefs were strongly related to coping efforts reported in a study of 114 chronic pain patients. Arnstein, Caudill, Mandle, Norris, and Beasley (1999) also found that pain intensity and self-efficacy contributed to the development of disability and depression in patients with chronic pain (n = 126). In line with this finding, they suggested that enhancing self-efficacy beliefs is an important therapeutic goal. Lin (1998), studying chronic cancer and low back pain patients, found that for both patient groups, perceived self-efficacy correlated negatively with pain intensity and interference with everyday life. Enhancing perceptions of self-efficacy has yielded significant and clinically meaningful results (Jensen et al., 1991). We return to self-efficacy in discussion of Level 3, where an application of this concept through the use of group processes is addressed.

Social learning theory and early behavior therapy contained a germ of an idea that spouses and "significant others" were playing a role in the maintenance of pain behaviors. It followed that they needed to be included in pain treatment programs, trained to help diminish damaging pain behaviors and to support the progress of the program at home. In many pain management programs running today, the inclusion of significant others as part of the program has disappeared, usually for reasons of cost, so the spotlight has again refocused on the individual, leaving a regrettable gap in attention to social factors. Fordyce (1976) gave tacit acknowledgment to the principle that health professionals needed to be trained in behaviorist techniques to provide the necessary environment for the program to work—that is, to "extinguish" pain behavior and "reinforce" or "reward" positive or health behavior. These social components are still an integral part of cognitive behavior therapy programs.

The focus now has shifted from the spouse or significant other to the response of the family and therefore to family therapy (see Carr, 2000, for review). This represents a much better understanding of the response of carers to the pain of a sick spouse. For example, the therapeutic progress of female rheumatoid arthritis patients was found to be substantially impaired when hostility was the predominant response of their husbands to their condition (Manne & Zautra, 1990). Of particular interest here are family adjustment and adaptation models (Kerns & Weiss, 1994). These emphasize the family as the primary unit of analysis, and the social context as the salient environment in which adaptation or maladaptation occurs. They examine the ways families approach and evaluate the stress of living with someone in a painful condition, and the family's capacity to deal with these challenges. When considering the individual's response to pain, it is impossible to ignore the impact of these influences.

This work links into an extensive social support literature (e.g., Newman, Fitzpatrick, Revenson, Skevington, & Williams, 1996). There is conflicting evidence about the impact of chronic pain on families; sometimes it is positive or neutral, but it is not always negative (Kerns & Payne, 1996). Sodergren and Hyland (2000) recently developed a Silver Lining scale, which could assess how people rise to the challenge of difficult painful situations. Although there are a number of studies about marital and sexual dysfunction, psychophysiological disorders and raised emotional distress, especially depression (Ahern, Adams, & Follock, 1985), these are often poorly controlled. Revenson and Majerovitz (1991) concluded on the basis of the available evidence that it is not clear whether chronic pain sufferers really do have higher levels of distress compared to others. However, Kerns and Turk (1984) found that support from a spouse is capable of reducing depression among chronic pain patients.

Level 3: Group and Intergroup Behavior

In Level 3 we look at how people in pain as a group, with a common social or cultural heritage, view their pain and how group processes, in turn, can change the way people manage it. This level includes examining social representations of pain, illness, and coping; group beliefs such as shared opinions and consensus about pain, illness and disability, and group experience; and influence including peer pressure, group status, and power. Level 3 also encompasses personal and social categorizations, such as the process of labeling the condition by self and others. Other aspects of this are personal and social comparisons with self at other times and with similar and dissimilar others. To do this, upward, downward, and lateral comparisons can be used to compare with those who are better off, worse, or the same as self. Social identification or a "sense of belonging" to a particular group also appears to be influential at the points in time where people recognize themselves as disabled, a "loser," and so on, in identification with similar others.

Shared views and consensus about experiences and beliefs emerge from an examination of groups. Self-management courses designed by Lorig and colleagues during the last 15 years successfully utilize group dynamics, group beliefs, and group experience to help those with chronic illness to help themselves. A major strength of this new intervention arises from a reorientation in thinking, whereby those with chronic illness are seen as "expert" in their own condition. As such, they must be active decision makers in their own care (not passive recipients), so that they become self-confident and less dependent. The psychological components of this group approach include cognitive symptom management, problem solving, resource utilization, communications with professionals, and the formation of a partnership, as well as making lifestyle changes to improve exercise, nutrition, and so on. The program is explicitly orientated toward building self-efficacy in every activity that is undertaken, and it is this psychological process that is of paramount importance; the content is of lesser interest (e.g., Lorig, Gonzalez, Laurent, Morgan, & Laris, 1998).

In evaluating this intervention, Lorig, Mazonson, and Holman (1993) followed up patients from their self-management programs for 4 years. Even after 4 years, they found that pain was still 20% less than at baseline, physician visits were 40% less frequent, and that the physical disability of this chronic arthritis group had only increased by 9% over the same period. Based on physician fees, they calculated that had the program been implemented nationwide, savings of $648 could be made for each participating rheumatoid arthritis patient, and $189 in a case of osteoarthritis, amounting to savings of millions of dollars to the U.S. health care budget. These economic costs were additional to those from wages lost due to work absenteeism and the incalculable human costs of pain, disability, despair, anger, bitterness, and more. Self-management programs are currently being implemented nationally in Britain and the United States.

From many diverse sources of health research, there is now clear evidence that giving people information or education about their disease and treatment alone is really not sufficient to make them change their lifestyle to improve their health. Looking laterally, there are, in fact, many commonalities to the problems and concerns faced by those with nonmalignant painful chronic conditions such as arthritis, heart disease, and back pain, as well as those that are more normally pain free, such as diabetes and epilepsy, as they have to deal not only with their illness but also with the effects that it has on their lives, particularly their emotions (Lorig et al., 1998; von Korff et al., 1998).

Lorig's self-management groups are lead by lay people with chronic illnesses themselves who are properly trained and equipped, and it is known that they can be as effective in leading self-management groups as health professionals. Because the program is user led, leaders from different cultures (and subcultures) can reach disadvantaged groups in the community in a culture-sensitive way, so this program provides a unique opportunity to tackle demonstrable inequalities in health and health care. Although the empowerment of patients is central to the success of this endeavor, at the same time, the success of these groups requires changes to health professional attitudes, so that the newly self-confident patient is not seen as a threat (Lorig et al., 1998).

Group members categorize beliefs in meaningful ways—for example, by shared images, beliefs, and labels of those who are disabled. These group processes also impact on the treatment of groups by society as a whole. Some people with painful illness refuse to concede that they are ill; for example, in a study of rheumatoid arthritis patients, Donovan and colleagues (Donovan, Blake, & Fleming, 1989) found that most arthritis patients who visited a general practitioner said their arthritis was inconvenient, but less than half refused to use the label of being ill. These labels are socially shared with others, and a diagnosis is a good example of a label that patients share with their physicians. Elder (1973) found that the majority of rheumatoid arthritis patients said they learned the label from their physicians and the rest learned it from lay people, from the television, or said that they just know it. These studies provide examples and evidence of social categorization. However, patients do not always share the same label as their physicians; for example, in painful conditions where there is not a definitive diagnosis, patients and doctors may hold different views about the etiology and the label given. This may generate conflict and frustration, and place a strain on the doctor–patient relationship. Certain groups of patients may also be stigmatized due to the presence of diffuse and unverifiable symptoms, for example, with fibromyalgia (Asbring & Narvanen, 2002).

Bendelow and Williams (1996) used qualitative techniques to examine lay beliefs about "pain clinics," in the United Kingdom. They found that the term *pain clinic* represented the "end of the road" for many participants, that is, the last possible hope of obtaining relief from pain. The authors suggested that there was a feeling among participants that medicine had failed them. Studies such as this one highlight the power of beliefs around treatment underscored by the medical model, and the power of the medical system in representing the only possible route to relief. When this medical model fails, there is a strongly held belief that there is no viable alternative. It also fuses a connection between previous comments on patient beliefs at Level 2 and higher order factors from Level 4.

Work has also been carried out using alternative models of understanding the beliefs people hold about their medical conditions. Bodily changes pose a threat to the integrity of the self and identity, and Leventhal and colleagues developed a model outlining several components that underpin lay beliefs about illness and symptoms. There are five clusters of beliefs: First is the identity of the disease or condition that is formulated from the symptoms and the illness label. Then perceived causes such as germs, accidents, and genetic mutations are considered and derived. Third, the timeline of the disease is of some concern, and is deduced from onset, duration, and recovery time. Fourth, for consequences, people consider death, disability, pain, and social and economic loss. Finally, under the heading of controllability, people consider the intractability of their condition versus their susceptibility to self-treatment, medicine, or surgery (Leventhal, Meyer, & Nerenz, 1980). The content and organization of these attributes vary among individuals, and within individuals as time passes, such as in the transition from an acute to a chronically painful disease (Leventhal, Idler, & Leventhal, 1999). Leventhal's framework has been applied to numerous medical conditions and helps us to understand the way that people struggle to make sense of an unfolding, and sometimes unpredictable, milieu of symptoms. Pain and illness may stimulate various coping procedures such as self-treatment, social comparisons (see below) and seeking medical care, but not all symptoms activate self-evaluation procedures. The Leventhal et al. (1999) work implies that the presence of pain creates pressure to reformulate the self, in response to disabling illness. Where this occurs and can be identified, we suggest that it provides a "window" of opportunity for clinicians to make progress with treatment.

Social comparison theory has been an enduring and useful model within which to view people with conditions characterized by pain. Blalock and DeVellis found that making comparisons with others who share similar or dissimilar health affects self-esteem and progress of rehabilitation (Blalock et al., 1988; Blalock, DeVellis, & DeVellis, 1989). Comparisons can be intrapersonal, so that you compare yourself now with other memorable times, perhaps when healthy, young, and so on. There can be interpersonal comparisons, such as with others who have better (upward comparisons) or worse health (downward) than you, or the same (lateral). Those who were ill applied the use of social comparisons strategically, to enhance their own mood if they could, and particularly to boost their self-esteem (Blalock et al., 1988, 1989). Sick people also employed higher order social comparisons based on what more abstract groups like "society," their own sociocultural groups, and the medical profession (as represented by their doctors), expected from someone of their age, sex, stage of illness, and so on (Skevington, 1994).

Together, categorization and comparisons lead to identification with a group or isolation from it. Pain has often been associated with feelings of isolation (Rose, 1994) and alienation. Addressing the identities of those in pain at a group level could be a more appropriate and cost effective method than individual consultations. This could be brought about through the use of newsletters, meetings, support groups, and trained lay leaders in self-management groups. In a study looking at how sense is made of the causes of chronic pain, Eccleston and colleagues found that pain challenges the identities of patients and health professionals when responsibility and blame are taken away from the sufferer and healer. These findings clearly have interactive implications for the way that patients and health professionals respond to each other (Eccleston, Williams, & Rogers, 1997).

The media plays a pivotal role in presenting, reflecting, and reinforcing society's message about those in pain. A hard-wired model of how migraine is relieved, presented in a well-known analgesic advertisement in Britain, propagates the erroneous image of a pain mechanism that predates the advances made by the gate control theory of pain and makes it harder to manage the beliefs of those who seek treatment. It perpetuates the view that medication is the only solution to pain, ignoring other important strategies and influences. The reverse side of media influence has been recently illustrated in an Australian study (Buchbinder, Jolley, & Wyatt, 2001), where a population based multimedia campaign intervention was designed to alter beliefs about back pain. Buchbinder et al. found that positive messages improved beliefs among the population, and in health professionals about pain, and positively influenced the better management of pain. Studies such as this highlight the power of the media in influencing beliefs about pain and people's response to it.

Level 4: Higher Order Factors

Level 4 represents the higher order factors affecting social and psychological processing that influence the response to pain, such as health culture, history, ideology and politics, quality of life, and economic beliefs about health. For health culture we must ask how particular cultural beliefs foster sickness and wellness in the community. There was a Western cultural tradition of prescribing extended bed rest for all low back pain sufferers until the results of Deyo's seminal study (Deyo, Diehl, & Rosenthal, 1986) showed how this recommendation was contraindicated for those without malignancy or herniated disc and indeed, could be iatrogenic.

In a wider sense of the word, this issue is also about whether culture encourages or discourages people from, for example, taking up and maintaining exercise that would prevent or retard the onset of a painful condition, or enable people to better cope with it when present. In a recent community study conducted in a town in northern England noted for its high immigrant population, a health promotion scheme was set up to enable Bangladeshi women to cultivate vegetables in publicly owned plots. At the end of the project these formerly housebound women had improved physical, psychological, and social health and quality of life: in particular, a boost to their confidence relating to self-efficacy, and less depression. This was as a result of regular contact with other Bangladeshi women, participating in culturally acceptable forms of physical exercise through gardening, and improving their family's diet by cultivating fresh vegetables suited to Asian dishes, to take home (NHS Health Development Agency, UK, 2001). By providing a rationale for exercise, distraction, and social support, such community pilot projects have the potential to retard the onset of pain, and where pain and disability are present, to maintain mobility, and other aspects of quality of life including good mental health.

Health history encompasses the sociocultural history of seeking medical care for pain and other problems, and the reactions of health professionals and significant others on each event, not simply the traditional record of previous illnesses. These higher order factors also relate to the apparent legitimacy of a person's complaint and help-seeking behavior, that is, whether or not a person's symptoms are deemed severe enough to justify seeking professional help, particularly when dealing with a phenomenon that other people cannot see.

Health ideology and politics at an individual differences level have rarely been studied in detail in pain research but are necessarily reflected by the predominant premises adopted by the very different health services delivery systems that have been implemented around the world. Those who believe in a socialist medical system, such as the National Health Service in Britain, may wait uncomplainingly on a waiting list for a physiotherapy appointment or scan, despite having trouble sleeping, walking, and working, because they believe that health care should be free at the point of use— that in the current politico-economic context of limited resources and with the assumption of a fair system, they must necessarily wait their turn. In countries where health care is provided through fee for service or health insurance, those without financial resources or health insurance often suffer without professional care. An individual assessment of health economics, within the ideology of a patient-centered system, might include an evaluation of how people in pain believe the resource should be shared out. There is likely to be a continuum from those who hold highly individualistic views, to those who believe that the resources should be used to benefit the greatest number of those in pain. Here, government policy and funding are pertinent issues and are likely to impact indirectly on how people respond to symptoms, like pain. Policies to withdraw formerly available treatments on the grounds of inconclusive findings of evidence-based medicine may, in the psychological terms of reactance theory (Brehm, 1966; Brehm & Brehm, 1981), make the treatment all the more attractive, and the pain worse as a result of the treatment's newly inaccessible status. Indeed, recent research has shown a link between patient noncompliance and reactance (Fogarty, 1997; Fogarty & Youngs, 2000). Thus, people are inclined to react adversely when told they must do something.

Global inequities in pain relief arising from different governmental policies, have been extensively documented by Stjernsward (1993). This is particularly evident in the field of palliative care concerning the use or withholding of morphine. Recently McQuay argued that politics, prejudice, and ignorance prevent the most appropriate use of opioid analgesics (McQuay, 1999). Fears of addiction have hindered the effective use of strong pharmaceuticals for pain relief. This has some resonance with the question of individual response to pain, not only at a physiological or biochemical level, but also psychologically, as dominant attitudes toward the prescription of strong analgesics can influence the beliefs, attitudes, and behavior of people with acute and chronic pain.

We must also include a consideration of the variable impact of pain on quality of life in health. Without knowing how satisfying or problematic the pain and disability can be, and how much it affects many different aspects of life, we can barely begin to evaluate individual problems. Too often researchers and clinicians have erroneously subscribed to a deficit theory, in the erroneous assumption that the greater the pain intensity, the poorer is the quality of life. There is now substantial empirical data for the quality-of-life literature to show that many of the patients who are in intense pain do not necessarily also have very poor quality of life. Similarly, relatively low pain intensity can be extremely troublesome. This is because the meaning of pain is very different for different people; for some, pain is very threatening and debilitating, whereas for others with the same level of intensity, it plays a less significant role and does not appear to greatly impair their well-being or lifestyle. We need to invest in understanding the variables that mediate this and other important factors and elucidate the impact that living with pain has on a person's quality of life. Ultimately, quality of life is about people's "goals expectations, standards and concerns" (WHOQOL Group, 1995) and how far these are satisfied. A person's quality of life and well-being may impact on his or her response to pain, and vice versa (Skevington, 1998; Skevington, Carse, & Williams, 2001). In addition, beliefs about quality of life may be mediated by these concepts that are heavily culturally determined (WHOQOL Group, 1995), and all the processes identified in the model impact on decision making regarding quality of life.

Before summing up, two additional sections have been added to satisfy different purposes. In the first, we outline an example of a pertinent sociocultural issue that reflects and is reflected by individual differences, and seek to show how key issues may be addressed in different ways, cutting across all levels of the model. Although no claim is made for the comprehensiveness of the model's components, such examples illustrate that there is some semblance of gestalt, with the whole being more than the sum of the parts. Gender was chosen as the example because it represents an important issue that has widespread influence on individual differences in terms of pain experience and report. The second section provides some limited observations on methods in this area.

GENDER: AN EXAMPLE OF FEATURES THAT MAY BE ADDRESSED AT ALL LEVELS OF THE MODEL

Central to the debate around gender and pain is epidemiological evidence of more frequent symptom reporting and/or help seeking by women than men (Berkley, 1997; Unruh, 1996), and the greater prevalence of certain conditions, like fibromyalgia, in women (Yunus, 2002). Individual differences explained by gender are conceptually important at all levels of the proposed model, although there has been a tendency to focus on a limited number of gender differences at the expense of what are seen as less interesting but more frequently occurring similarities. Gender is biologically determined at Level 1. However, as we move through Levels 1 to 4, we see the increasing importance of socialized gender patterns and sociocultural expectations of pain reporting and help seeking, which shape the behavior of men and women. At Levels 2 and 3, women are seen as highly social in the ways they seek out social information for decision making and actions relating to pain. In interaction with health professionals, women communicate in different styles and receive different treatments for the same conditions (Verbrugge, 1989; Verbrugge & Steiner, 1984, 1985). Differential perceptions of various aspects of quality of life (WHOQOL Group, 1995), and gendered ideologies, histories, and cultures connected with health and health care, as well as lower income, are indicated as relevant factors at Level 4.

Factors addressing features from all these levels seem to be evident in Bendelow's (1993) in-depth qualitative study, which explored women and men's experience of and beliefs about causes of pain. Both gender groups believed that women were better able to cope with pain, and provided sophisticated biological and sociocultural explanations for this. Bendelow also found that pain was seen as "normal" for women because of painful experiences associated with the reproductive process, particularly childbirth. In contrast, men were not only discouraged from expressing pain but at the same time were encouraged to deny pain and be stoic. More recently, experimental research with the cold-pressor task has shown differences in the perception of and response to coping with pain among men and women. This was particularly evident where sensory- or emotion-focused coping instructions were given (Keogh & Herdenfeldt, 2002). Other evidence points to the role of catastrophizing (Keefe et al., 2000; Sullivan, Tripp, & Santor, 2000) and negative emotions (Keogh & Mansoor, 2001) in explaining apparent gender differences in the response to pain. In general, it appears that women are more vulnerable to pain than men but they have a larger repertoire of ways to deal with it (Berkley & Holdcroft, 1999). The importance of understanding gender issues around pain hinges on the ability of therapists to maximize therapies or interventions designed to relieve or improve the management of pain, including a greater understanding of differential patterns of expressing pain. For more on gender and pain, see Berkley and Holdcroft (1999).

MEASURING THE RESPONSE TO PAIN AT ALL LEVELS

The literature on measurement of pain (see chap. 8, this volume) and its correlates has burgeoned in recent years, and this has led to a "pick and mix" of measures and instruments, with a claim to assess or quantify some aspect of pain or pain treatment, so it is not possible to provide an extensive review here. Increasingly, attention is being paid to the reliability of instruments purporting to measure pain and, in particular, to the challenging issue of pain measurement in pediatrics.

The social context of pain measurement has also been studied; for example, Kelleher and colleagues provided preliminary evidence that pain scores are influenced by the social context in which they are obtained (Kelleher, Rennell, & Kidd, 1998). This provides additional support for the model outlined in this chapter and the importance of including, accounting for, and exploring the social factors that mediate the response to pain.

Countless instruments and indexes are used in the clinic and for research into the complex, multifactorial response to pain. For example, based on a cognitive affective model of pain where pain interrupts and demands attention (Eccleston & Crombez, 1999), the Pain Vigilance and Awareness Questionnaire (McCracken, 1997) was developed, and this was recently adapted this for use with a subclinical sample, including diagnoses other than low back pain (McWilliams & Asmundson, 2001). In this small cluster of studies we can see how a biopsychosocial theory generated by health psychologists has been applied in the development of a theoretically based measure, and the theory itself is then available to provide guidance and a reference point should the scale require adjustment, and in subsequent adaptations. In this way the articulation of an initial theoretical direction adds value to the practical endeavor of relieving suffering.

Thus, measuring the response to pain is often driven by the need to test a particular theory or set of variables that are hypothesized to impact on, or predict, how individuals and groups will react to perceived pain, with the goal of explaining the largest proportion of variance. Reliable and valid measures for those in pain are important given the unreliability of proxy assessment, as, for example, displayed by the discordance between patient and physician ratings of pain (Mantyselka, Kumpusalo, Ahonen, & Takala, 2001). Existing and new measures can be utilized to assess many of the psychosocial processes and social factors outlined in this model of the response to pain: from the relatively straightforward visual analogue scale appropriate to pain intensity or severity in Level 1, to more complex multidimensional assessments of quality of life in Level 4. When integrated, these results could provide a holistic outcome assessment that is long overdue.

CONCLUSIONS

The model presented here is a working model that is incomplete. It includes elements representing a body of research that has already been published (see Skevington, 1995, for a resumé) but there may be other important factors that have not yet been identified, or if identified they may not as yet, be assessed properly. As we move across the levels from 1 to 4, there is less confidence in the robustness of the evidence about exactly how some of these social factors influence the experience and expression of pain and outcomes of treatment. Level 1 of the model represents the first conceptual level that must be examined to appreciate the individual's unique response to pain. Although grounded in the biological and psycho-logical aspects of the pain experience, it reveals how these factors can be influenced by social processes, as shown by PNI, for instance, and should not be seen in isolation from the other levels. Level 2 represents the complex interplay between a person and immediate and salient aspects of their social environment, such as significant others and health care professionals. Level 3 shows how the individual is deeply embedded in their particular culture, and highlights the importance of aspects of group and intergroup relations for the understanding of responding to a highly individualized and private experience such as pain. The effect of higher order processes outlined in Level 4 may be quite insidious, and not immediately apparent to the person experiencing pain or the health care professional who is caring for them. However, these aspects are deeply rooted in cultural beliefs, norms, and experience, and reflect and are reflected by a long history of being a patient within a particular culture. It seems likely that research into these higher order factors will clarify the emerging picture about the response to pain and help to further understand and explain the existence of sociocultural differences.

We have presented just some of the important social issues that have been raised in the literatures on pain, health and social factors in recent years. Some are well researched by those working in pain research, whereas others have been largely ignored, or "lip service" has been paid to their value. Nevertheless, these factors affect people's response to chronic pain, including the variety of ways in which they respond to treatments and consultations, particularly given the largely interpersonal context of health care interactions. Although a few salient examples have been used to demonstrate key issues, empirical evidence can be found in many other sources (e.g., Skevington, 1995). The model shows how each level can mediate individual differences. Understanding the individual's response to pain has considerable theoretical value, but perhaps more importantly can facilitate recovery from pain and promote the rehabilitation process. Indeed, a further elucidation of key individual differences is essential if we are to improve the way treatments are delivered to ensure that treatment outcomes are maximized through the inclusion of patient preferences and a consideration of cultural differences. Increased and more extended multidisciplinary working will bring about cross-fertilization of ideas to give a more holistic picture of the experience and treatment of pain to ensure better targeted interventions to account for patient variability, and the development of more comprehensive treatment programs, in addition to an understanding of patterns of concordance and adherence with treatment regimens. Enthusiasm for empirical work in relatively new avenues of inquiry such as psychoneuroimmunology will add to the understanding of pain and facilitate the development of more comprehensive theory.

We need to take a more holistic view of the patient in his or her social and environmental context, and this requires several actions; in particular, it requires multidisciplinary teamwork. We should be harnessing the energy and ideas of health economists, policymakers, medical sociologists, and anthropologists into pain research in order to better understand individual well-being, or lack of it. This is already happening in studies of health more generally (e.g., Blaxter, 1990; Bowling, 1993, 1995) and needs to be applied in the study of pain. There is also a need to create gender- and culture-sensitive psychosocial therapies that could take account of individual differences, and that are better tailored to meet the particular needs of the social groups who participate. In addition, we need to account for the variability and complexity of individual differences through developing ways of systematically investigating and assessing all possibilities, to ensure that important factors are not being overlooked.

The structure of the model outlined in this chapter could also be used as an interview framework for a semistructured interview to generate an overall assessment in a systematic social assessment. Not all elements of the model have yet been properly operationalized; some may need multidimensional scales to be developed, rather than answers to single items. Once this is done, we can evaluate the elements of the model collectively, to look at how each factor contributes to overall patient well-being and to a greater understanding of how the individual responds to pain. When this information is available, we shall be in a better position to say more precisely which factors best predict outcomes for chronic pain patients. The relative importance of these elements may well point to the value of social interventions that could be applied simultaneously alongside biological interventions, like medication, epidural anesthetic, and psychological interventions, like self-management regimes or cognitive behavior therapy.

ACKNOWLEDGMENTS

Professor Skevington thanks the Irish Pain Society for the opportunity to present an early draft of this chapter at their Inaugural Scientific meeting in Dublin, 2001.

REFERENCES

Affleck, G., Tennen, H., Pfeiffer, C., & Fifield, J. (1987). Appraisals of control and predictability in adapting to a chronic disease. *Journal of Personality and Social Psychology, 53*, 273–279.

Ahern, D., Adams, A., & Follock, M. (1985). Emotional and marital disturbance in spouses of chronic low back pain patients. *Clinical Journal of Pain, 1*, 69–74.

Amanzio, M., Pollo, A., Maggi, G., & Benedetti, F. (2001). Response variability to analgesics: A role for non-specific activation of endogenous opioids. *Pain, 90*, 205–215.

Arnstein, P., Caudill, M., Mandle, C. L., Norris, A., & Beasley, R. (1999). Self-efficacy as a mediator of the relationship between pain intensity, disability and depression in chronic pain patients. *Pain, 80*, 483–491.

Asbring, P., & Narvanen, A. L. (2002). Women's experience of stigma in relation to chronic fatigue syndrome and fibromyalgia. *Qualitative Health Research, 12*, 148–160.

Bates, M. S. (1987). Ethnicity and pain: A biocultural model. *Social Science & Medicine, 24*, 47–50.

Bendelow, G. (1993). Pain perceptions, emotions and gender. *Sociology of Health and Illness, 15*, 273–294.

Bendelow, G. A., & Williams, S. J. (1996). The end of the road? Lay views on a pain-relief clinic. *Social Science & Medicine, 43*, 1127–1136.

Berkley, K. J. (1997). Sex differences in pain. *Behavioral and Brain Sciences, 20*, 371–380.

Berkley, K. J., & Holdcroft, A. (1999). Sex and gender differences in pain. In P. D. Wall & R. Melzack (Eds.), *Textbook of pain* (4th ed., pp. 951–965). London: Churchill Livingstone.

Blalock, S. J., DeVellis, B. M., & DeVellis, R. F. (1989). Social comparisons among individuals with rheumatoid arthritis. *Journal of Applied Social Psychology, 19*, 665–680.

Blalock, S. J., DeVellis, B. M., DeVellis, R. F., & Sauter, S. H. (1988). Self-evaluation processes and adjustment to rheumatoid arthritis. *Arthritis & Rheumatism, 31*(10), 1245–1251.

Blaxter, M. (1990). *Health and lifestyles*. London: Tavistock.

Bowling, A. (1993). *Measuring health*. Buckingham: Open University Press.

Bowling, A. (1995). *Measuring disease*. Buckingham: Open University Press.

Brehm, J. W. (1966). *A theory of psychological reactance*. New York: Academic Press.

Brehm, S. S., & Brehm, J. W. (1981). *Psychological reactance: A theory of freedom and control*. New York: Academic Press.

Buchbinder, R., Jolley, D., & Wyatt, M. (2001). 2001 Volvo Award winner in clinical studies: Effects of a media campaign on back pain beliefs and its potential influence on management of low back pain in general practice. *Spine, 26*, 2523–2542.

Carr, A. (2000). Evidence-based practice in family therapy and systematic consultation II—Adult focused problems. *Journal of Family Therapy, 22*, 273–295.

Chapman, S. L., & Pemberton, J. S. (1994). Prediction of treatment outcome from clinically derived MMPI clusters in rehabilitation for chronic low-back-pain. *Clinical Journal of Pain, 10*, 267–276.

Cheever, K. H. (1999). Pain, analgesic use, and morbidity in appendectomy patients. *Clinical Nursing Research, 8*, 267–282.

Conant, L. L. (1998). Psychological variables associated with pain perceptions among individuals with chronic spinal cord injury pain. *Journal of Clinical Psychological Medicine, S5*, 71–90.

DeVellis, R. F., Patterson, C. C., Blalock, S. J., Renner, B. R., & DeVellis, B. M. (1997). Do people with rheumatoid arthritis develop illness-related schemas? *Arthritis Care and Research, 10*, 78–88.

Deyo, R. A. (1994). Magnetic-resonance-imaging of the lumbar spine. *New England Journal of Medicine, 331*, 1526.

Deyo, R. A., Diehl, A. K., & Rosenthal, M. (1986). How many days of bedrest for acute low back pain? A randomised clinical trial. *New England Journal of Medicine, 315*, 1064–1070.

Dickens, C., McGowan, L., Clark-Carter, D., & Creed, F. (2002). Depression in rheumatoid arthritis: A systematic review of the literature with meta-analysis. *Psychosomatic Medicine, 64*, 52–60.

Donovan, J. L., Blake, D. R., & Fleming, W. G. (1989). The patient is not a blank sheet: Lay beliefs and their relevance to patient education. *British Journal of Rheumatology, 28*, 58–61.

Eccleston, C., & Crombez, G. (1999). Pain demands attention: A cognitive-affective model of the interruptive function of pain. *Psychological Bulletin, 125*, 356–366.

Eccleston, C., Crombez, G., Aldrich, S., & Stannard, C. (2001). Worry and chronic pain patients: A description and analysis of individual differences. *European Journal of Pain, 5*, 309–318.

Eccleston, C., Williams, A. C. D., & Rogers, W. S. (1997). Patients' and professionals' understandings of the causes of chronic pain: Blame, responsibility and identity protection. *Social Science & Medicine, 45*, 699–709.

Elder, R. G. (1973). Social class and lay expectations of the etiology of arthritis. *Journal of Personality and Social Psychology, 14*, 28–38.

Engelbart, H. J., & Vrancken, M. A. (1984). Chronic pain from the perspective of health: A view based on systems theory. *Social Science & Medicine, 19*, 1383–1392.

Ericsson, M., Poston, W. S., Linder, J., Taylor, J. E., Haddock, C. K., & Foreyt, J. P. (2002). Depression predicts disability in long-term chronic pain patients. *Disability and Rehabilitation, 24*, 334–340.

Fogarty, J. S. (1997). Reactance theory and patient noncompliance. *Social Science & Medicine, 45*, 1277–1288.

Fogarty, J. S., & Youngs, G. A. (2000). Psychological reactance as a factor in patient noncompliance with medication taking: A field experiment. *Journal of Applied Social Psychology, 30*, 2365–2391.

Fordyce, W. E. (1976). *Behavioral methods for chronic pain and illness.* St. Louis, MO: Mosby.

Foster, S., & Mallik, M. (1998). A comparative study of differences in the referral behaviour patterns of men and women who have experienced cardiac-related chest pain. *Intensive Critical Care Nursing, 14*, 192–202.

Fritz, J. M., George, S. Z., & Delitto, A. (2001). The role of fear-avoidance beliefs in acute low back pain: Relationships with current and future disability and work status. *Pain, 94*, 7–15.

George, S. Z., Fritz, J. M., & Erhard, R. E. (2001). A comparison of fear-avoidance beliefs in patients with lumbar spine pain and cervical spine pain. *Spine, 26*, 2139–2145.

Grahn, B., Ekdahl, C., & Borgquist, L. (2000). Motivation as a predictor of changes in quality of life and working ability in multidisciplinary rehabilitation. A two year follow-up of a prospective controlled study in patients with prolonged musculoskeletal disorders. *Disability and Rehabilitation, 22*, 639–654.

Hakim, A. J., Cherkas, L., El Zayat, S., MacGregor, A. J., & Spector, T. D. (2002). The genetic contribution to carpal tunnel syndrome in women: A twin study. *Arthritis and Rheumatism, 47*, 275–279.

Hathaway, S. R., & McKinley, J. (1943). *Minnesota Mutliphasic Personality Inventory.* Minneapolis: University of Minnesota Press.

Indo, Y. (2002). Genetics of congenital insensitivity to pain with anhidrosis (CIPA) or hereditary sensory and autonomic neuropathy type IV. Clinical, biological and molecular aspects of mutations in TRKA (NTRK1) gene encoding the receptor tyrosine kinase for nerve growth factor. *Clinical Autonomic Research, 12*, 120–132.

Ingham, J. G., & Miller, P. M. (1979). Symptom prevalence and severity in a general practice population. *Journal of Epidemiology and Community Medicine, 33*, 191–198.

Jensen, M. P., Ehde, D. M., Hoffman, A. J., Patterson, D. R., Czerniecki, J. M., & Robinson, L. R. (2002). Cognitions, coping and social environment predict adjustment to phantom limb pain. *Pain, 95*, 133–142.

Jensen, M. P., & Karoly, P. (1992). Pain-specific beliefs, perceived symptom severity, and adjustment to chronic pain. *Clinical Journal of Pain, 8*, 123–130.

Jensen, M. P., Karoly, P., & Huger, R. (1987). The development and preliminary validation of an instrument to assess patients attitudes toward pain. *Journal of Psychosomatic Research, 31,* 393–400.

Jensen, M. P., Turner, J. A., & Romano, J. M. (1991). Self-efficacy and outcome expectancies: Relationship to chronic pain coping strategies and adjustment. *Pain, 44,* 263–269.

Juarez, G., Ferrell, B., & Borneman, T. (1998). Influence of culture on cancer pain management in Hispanic patients. *Cancer Practice, 6,* 262–269.

Katz, J., & Melzack, R. (1990). Pain 'memories' in phantom limbs: Review and clinical observations. *Pain, 43,* 319–336.

Keefe, F. J., Lefebvre, J. C., Egert, J. R., Affleck, G., Sullivan, M. J., & Caldwell, D. S. (2000). The relationship of gender to pain, pain behavior, and disability in osteoarthritis patients: The role of catastrophizing. *Pain, 87,* 325–334.

Kelleher, D. J. A., Rennell, B., & Kidd, B. L. (1998). The effect of social context on pain measurement. *Journal of Musculoskeletal Pain, 6,* 77–86.

Keogh, E., & Mansoor, L. (2001). Investigating the effects of anxiety sensitivity and coping strategy on the perception of cold pressor pain in healthy women. *European Journal of Pain, 5,* 11–25.

Keogh, E., & Herdenfeldt, M. (2002). Gender, coping and the perception of pain. *Pain, 97,* 195–201.

Kerns, R. D., & Payne, A. (1996). Treating families of chronic pain patients. In R. J. Gatchel & D. C. Turk (Eds.), *Psychological approaches to pain management: A practitioner's handbook* (pp. 283–304). New York: The Guilford Press.

Kerns, R. D., & Turk, D. C. (1984). Depression and chronic pain: The mediating role of the spouse. *Journal of Marriage and the Family, 46,* 845–852.

Kerns, R. D., & Weiss, L. H. (1994). Family influences on the course of chronic illness: A cognitive-behavioral transactional model. *Annals of Behavioral Medicine, 16,* 116–130.

Kest, B., Wilson, S. G., & Mogil, J. S. (1999). Sex differences in supraspinal morphine analgesia are dependent on genotype. *Journal of Pharmacology & Experimental Therapy, 289,* 1370–1375.

Kiecolt-Glaser, J. K., Page, G. G., Marucha, P. T., MacCullum, R. C., & Glaser, R. (1998). Psychological influences on surgical recovery—Perspectives from psychoneuroimmunology. *American Psychology, 53,* 1209–1218.

Kremer, M. J. (1999). Surgery, pain and immune function. *CRNA, 10,* 94–100.

Leventhal, H., Idler, E. L., & Leventhal, E. A. (1999). The impact of chronic illness on the self-system. In R. J. Contrada & R. D. Ashmoore (Eds.), *Self, social identity and physical health: Interdisciplinary explorations* (pp. 185–208). New York: Oxford University Press.

Leventhal, H., Meyer, D., & Nerenz, D. (1980). The common-sense representations of illness danger. In S.Rachman (Ed.), *Medical psychology* (pp. 7–30). New York: Guilford Press.

Li, S. F., Greenwald, P. W., Gennis, P., Bijur, P. E., & Gallagher, E. J. (2001). Effect of age on acute pain perception of a standardized stimulus in the emergency department. *Annals of Emergency Medicine, 38,* 644–647.

Lin, C. C. (1998). Comparison of the effects of perceived self-efficacy on coping with chronic cancer pain and coping with chronic low back pain. *Clinical Journal of Pain, 14,* 303–310.

Lorenz, J. (1998). Hyperalgesia or hypervigilance? An evoked potential approach to the study of fibromyalgia syndrome. *Zeitschrift fur Rheumatologie, 57,* 19–22.

Lorig, K., Gonzalez, V. M., Laurent, D. D., Morgan, L., & Laris, B. A. (1998). Arthritis self-management program variations: Three studies. *Arthritis Care Research, 11*(6), 448–454.

Lorig, K. R., Mazonson, P. D., & Holman, H. R. (1993). Evidence suggesting that health education for self-management in patients with chronic arthritis has sustained health benefits while reducing health care costs. *Arthritis & Rheumatism, 36*(4), 439–446.

Main, C. J. (1984). *Must we play the MMPI game? Or is the MMPI the only game in town?* Paper presented to the Annual Meeting of the British Pain Interest Group.

Manne, S. L., & Zautra, A. J. (1990). Couples coping with chronic illness: Women with rheumatoid arthritis and their healthy husbands. *Journal of Behavioural Medicine, 13,* 327–342.

Mantyselka, P., Kumpusalo, E., Ahonen, R., & Takala, J. (2001). Patients' versus general practitioners' assessments of pain intensity in primary care patients with non-cancer pain. *British Journal of General Practice, 51,* 995–997.

Maxwell, T. D., Gatchel, R. J., & Mayer, T. G. (1998). Cognitive predictors of depression in chronic low back pain: Toward an inclusive model. *Journal of Behavioural Medicine, 21,* 131–143.

McCracken, L. M. (1997). "Attention" to pain in persons with chronic pain: A behavioral approach. *Behaviour Therapy, 28,* 271–284.

McCracken, L. M., Matthews, A. K., Tang, T. S., & Cuba, S. L. (2001). A comparison of blacks and whites seeking treatment for chronic pain. *Clinical Journal of Pain, 17,* 249–255.

McQuay, H. (1999). Opioids in pain management. *Lancet, 353,* 2229–2232.

McQuay, H., & Moore, R. A. (1998). *An evidence-based resource for pain relief.* Oxford: Oxford University Press.

McWilliams, L. A., & Asmundson, G. J. G. (2001). Assessing individual differences in attention to pain: Psychometric properties of the Pain Vigilance and Awareness Questionnaire modified for a non-clinical pain sample. *Personality and Individual Differences, 31,* 239–246.

Mechanic, D. (1986). The concept of illness behaviour: Culture, situation and personal predisposition. *Psychological Medicine, 16,* 1–7.

Melzack, R., & Dennis, S. G. (1978). Neurophysiological foundations of pain. In R. A. Sternbach (Ed.), *The psychology of pain* (pp. 1–26). New York: Raven Press.

Melzack, R., & Wall, P. D. (1965). Pain mechanisms—A new theory. *Science, 150,* 971–979.

Melzack, R., & Wall, P. D. (1982). *The challenge of pain.* Harmondsworth: Penguin.

Miller, S. M. (1987). Monitoring and blunting—Validation of a questionnaire to assess styles of information seeking under threat. *Journal of Personality and Social Psychology, 52,* 345–353.

Miller, S. M., Brody, D. S., & Summerton, J. (1988). Styles of coping with threat: Implications for health. *Journal of Personality and Social Psychology, 54,* 142–148.

Mischel, W. (1968). *Personality and assessment.* New York: Wiley.

Mischel, W. (1973). Toward a cognitive social learning reconceptualization of personality. *Psychological Review, 80,* 252–283.

Mischel, W. (1977). The interaction of person and situation. In D. Magnusson & N. S. Endler (Eds.), *Personality at the crossroads: Current issues in interactional psychology.* Hillsdale, NJ: Lawrence Erlbaum Associates.

Mogil, J. S., & Adhikari, S. M. (1999). Hot and cold nociception are genetically correlated. *Journal of Neuroscience, 19,* RC25.

NHS Health Development Agency, UK. (2001, July). Great oaks from little acorns grow. *Health Development Today,* pp. 20–23.

Nayak, S., Shiflett, S. C., Eshun, S., & Levine, F. M. (2000). Culture and gender effects in pain beliefs and the prediction of pain tolerance. *Cross-cultural Research, 34,* 135–151.

Newman, S., Fitzpatrick, R., Revenson, T. A., Skevington, S., & Williams, G. (1996). Social support and family relationships. In *Understanding rheumatoid arthritis* (pp. 140–168). London: Routledge.

Pennebaker, J. W. (1982). *The psychology of physical symptoms.* New York: Springer-Verlag.

Peters, M. L., Vlaeyen, J. W., & Kunnen, A. M. (2002). Is pain-related fear a predictor of somaosensory hypervigilance in chronic low back pain patients? *Behaviour Research Therapy, 40,* 85–103.

Porro, C. A., Cettolo, V., Francescato, M. P., & Baraldi, P. (1998). Temporal and intensity coding of pain in human cortex. *Journal of Neurophysiology, 80,* 3312–3320.

Revenson, T. A., & Majerovitz, S. D. (1991). The effects of chronic illness on the spouse: Social resources as stress buffers. *Arthritis Care and Research, 4,* 63–72.

Reynaert, C., Janne, P., & Delire, V. (1995). To central or to be controlled—From health locus of control to morphine control during patient-controlled analgesia. *Psychotherapy and Psychosomatics, 64,* 74–81.

Rose, K. E. (1994). Patient isolation in chronic benign pain. *Nursing Standard, 8,* 25–27.

Rudy, T. E., Kerns, R. D., & Turk, D. C. (1988). Chronic pain and depression: Toward a cognitive-behavioral mediation model. *Pain, 35,* 129–140.

Sinclair, V. G. (2001). Predictors of pain catastrophizing in women with rheumatoid arthritis. *Archive of Psychiatric Nursing, 15,* 279–288.

Skevington, S. M. (1990). A standardized scale to measure beliefs about controlling pain (B.P.C.Q.): A preliminary study. *Psychology and Health, 4,* 221–232.

Skevington, S. M. (1994). Social comparisons in cross cultural research quality of life assessment. *International Journal of Mental Health, 23,* 29–47.

Skevington, S. M. (1995). *Psychology of pain.* Chichester: John Wiley & Sons.

Skevington, S. M. (1998). Investigating the relationship between pain and discomfort and quality of life, using the WHOQOL. *Pain, 76,* 395–406.

Skevington, S. M., Carse, M. S., & Williams, A. C. D. (2001). Validation of the WHOQOL-100: Pain management improves quality of life for chronic pain patients. *Clinical Journal of Pain, 17,* 264–275.

Skevington, S. M., & White, A. (1998). Is laughter the best medicine? *Psychology & Health, 13,* 157–169.

Sodergren, S. C., & Hyland, M. E. (2000). What are the consequences of illness? *Psychology & Health, 15,* 85–97.

Stjernsward, J. (1993). Palliative medicine—A global perspective. In D. Doyle, G. W. C. Hanks, & N. MacDonald (Eds.), *Oxford textbook of palliative medicine* (pp. 803–816). Oxford: Oxford University Press.

Sullivan, M. J., Thorn, B., Haythornthwaite, J. A., Keefe, F., Martin, M., Bradley, L. A., & Lefebvre, J. C. (2001). Theoretical perspectives on the relation between catastrophizing and pain. *Clinical Journal of Pain, 17,* 52–64.

Sullivan, M. J. L., Tripp, D. A., & Santor, D. (2000). Gender differences in pain and pain behavior: The role of catastrophising. *Cognitive Therapy Research, 24,* 121–134.

Taylor, S. E. (1999). *Health psychology* (4th ed.). Singapore: McGraw-Hill.

Thomas, V., Heath, M., Rose, M., & Flory, P. (1995). Psychological characteristics and the effectiveness of patient-controlled analgesia. *British Journal of Anaesthesia, 74,* 271–276.

Turk, D. C., & Okifuji, A. (1994). Detecting depression in chronic pain patients: Adequacy of self-reports. *Behaviour Research Therapy, 32,* 9–16.

Unrah, A. M. (1996). Gender variations in clinical pain experience. *Pain, 65,* 123–167.

Verbrugge, L. M. (1989). The twain meet: Empirical explanations of sex differences in health and mortality. *Journal of Health and Social Behaviour,* 36, 282–304.

Verbrugge, L. M., & Steiner, R. P. (1984). Another look at physician's treatment of men and women with common complaints. *Sex Roles,* II, 11–12.

Verbrugge L. M., & Steiner, R. P. (1985). Prescribing drugs to men and women. *Health Psychology, 4*(1), 79–98.

Vlaeyen, J. W., deJong, J., Geilen, M., Heuts, P. H., & van Breukelen, G. (2001). Graded exposure in vivo in the treatment of pain-related fear: A replicated single-case experimental design in four patients with chronic low back pain. *Behaviour Research Therapy, 39,* 151–166.

Vlaeyen, J. W., & Linton, S. J. (2000). Fear-avoidance and its consequences in chronic musculo-skeletal pain: A state of the art. *Pain, 85,* 317–332.

von Korff, M., Moore, J. E., Lorig, K., Cherkin, D. C., Saunders, K., Gonzalez, V. M., Laurent, D., Rutter, C., & Comite, F. (1998). A randomized trial of a lay person-led self-management group intervention for back pain patients in primary care. *Spine, 23,* 2608–2615.

Wallston, K. A., & Wallston, B. S. (1982). Who is responsible for your health? The construct of health locus of control. In G. S. Sanders & J. Suls (Eds.), *Social Psychology of health and illness* (pp. 65–95). Hillsdale, NJ: Lawrence Erlbaum Associates.

WHOQOL Group. (1995). The World Health Organisation Quality of Life Assessment (the WHOQOL): Position paper from the World Health Organisation. *Social Science & Medicine, 41,* 1403–1409.

Yunus, M. B. (2002). Gender differences in fibromyalgia and other related syndromes. *Journal of Gender Specific Medicine, 5,* 42–47.

Zautra, A. J., Hoffman, J., Potter, P., Matt, K. S., Yocum, D., & Castro, L. (1997). Examination of changes in interpersonal stress as a factor in disease exacerbations among women with rheumatoid arthritis. *Annals of Behavioural Medicine, 19,* 279–286.

Zborowski, M. (1969). *People in pain.* San Francisco, CA: Jossey-Bass.

Zola, I. K. (1973). Pathways to the doctor—From person to patient. *Social Science & Medicine, 7,* 677–689.

Assessment of Chronic
Pain Sufferers

Dennis C. Turk
Elena S. Monarch
Arthur D. Williams
Department of Anesthesiology
University of Washington

When patients suffering with pain are referred to a mental health professional, there are a number of specific questions that need to be addressed related to the purpose of the assessment. A primary care physician may simply conduct a mental status assessment to assist in routine treatment planning and to identify any significant emotional problems that need to be addressed. Referral questions might be initiated by a governmental agency related to disability determination or vocational issues. A specific referral question from a third-party payer may focus on the issue of malingering. The referral question might be related to decisions that will influence initiation of a particular treatment. For example, a surgeon might refer a patient for assessment in order to determine whether the patient is a good candidate for a particular surgery or neuroaugmentation procedure (i.e., implantation of a spinal cord stimulator or implantable drug delivery system). Alternatively, a physician may seek advice concerning whether there are any contraindications for initiating a course of chronic opioid therapy. Another referral question may concern the appropriateness of a patient for enrollment in a rehabilitation program that involves self-management.

Each of the referral questions and purposes pose some unique features that need to be covered. However, there is a core set of areas that need to be addressed for all chronic pain patients, regardless of the referral question. In addition to responding to referral questions, for patients who are being treated, there is a need for ongoing assessment to evaluate progress. Methods for process assessment are also included in our discussion.

209

In this chapter we describe a comprehensive approach to the assessment of the person with chronic pain. We also include discussion and recommendations for methods, procedures, and measures that address the more specific questions. We begin by presenting a general model of assessment based on a biopsychosocial perspective. Description of this perspective is essential as it serves as an outline for the composition of a comprehensive assessment. We highlight the set of psychosocial factors (i.e., cognitive, affective, and behavioral) that appear to contribute significantly to the experience of pain and suggest ways to include each of these factors in brief screenings and, when indicated, in comprehensive assessments. We include a specific guide, with procedures, methods, and instruments (and their limitations), for assessing chronic pain sufferers based on research findings. We note methods to address the different referral questions posed. An underlying theme of our approach is that we need to consider and assess the person, within his or her social context, who reports pain, and not just the pain and underlying physical pathology. Throughout our discussion, we describe how to use assessment data to generate recommendations and guide treatment planning. Finally, we discuss the importance of ongoing assessment for these patients and suggest ways to approach reassessment.

BIOPSYCHOSOCIAL MODEL OF PAIN ASSESSMENT

The biopsychosocial model (see also chap. 2, this volume) proposes that dynamic and reciprocal interactions between biological, psychological, and sociocultural variables shape the experience of pain (Turk, 1996a; Turk & Monarch, 2002). According to the biopsychosocial model, the pain experience usually begins when peripheral nociceptive stimulation produces physiological changes, although there may be central mechanisms involved in the initiation of pain, and the experience is thoroughly modulated by a person's unique genetic endowment, learning history, individual difference characteristics, affective state, and behavior.

Given the same nociceptive stimulations, two people may respond very differently. People's reports of pain severity and impact will vary depending on a range of contributions and will not be solely the result of physical pathology or perturbations within the nervous system. One person may ignore the pain and continue working, socializing, and engaging in previous levels of activity, whereas another may leave work, refrain from all activity, become emotionally distressed, and assume the "sick role." In both instances, the noxious input may be identical but the experience and response are colored by the unique characteristics of the each person. The biopsychosocial perspective forces an evaluator to consider not only the nature, cause, and characteristics of the noxious stimulation but the presence of the sensations reflected against a history that preceded symptom onset. These unique characteristics will determine the person's total experience.

The biopsychosocial model incorporates cognitive-behavioral concepts in understanding chronic pain. For example, proponents of this model suggest that both the person and the environment reciprocally determine behavior. People not only respond to their environment but elicit environmental responses by their behavior. In a very real sense, people create their environments. The person who becomes aware of a physical event (e.g., shooting pain in the neck) and decides the symptom requires attention from a health care provider initiates a set of circumstances different from the individual with the same symptom who chooses to self-manage symptoms. Another assumption of the cognitive-behavioral perspective is that people are active agents and capable of change. People with chronic pain, no matter how severe, despite their common beliefs to the contrary, are not helpless pawns of fate. The passive role many patients have in traditional physician–patient relationships often reinforces their beliefs that they have minimal ability to impact their own recovery. In the cognitive-behavioral perspective, people are active participants in learning and carrying out more effective modes of responding to their environment and their plight.

Chronic pain sufferers often develop negative expectations about their own ability to exert any control over their pain. From a biopsychosocial perspective, maladaptive appraisals about one's condition, situation, and personal efficacy in controlling the pain experience may lead to overreaction to nociceptive stimulation, reduced perseverance in the face of difficulty, and diminished activity. Negative expectations may also lead to psychological distress such as feelings of frustration and demoralization. Together, negative cognitions and emotional distress can lead pain sufferers to further maladaptive behaviors and adoption of passive coping strategies such as inactivity, medication use, or substance abuse. They also may absolve themselves of personal responsibility for managing their pain and, instead, rely on family and health care providers. Research studies show that these potentially controllable factors (e.g., passivity) contribute to the exacerbation, attenuation, and maintenance of pain, pain behaviors, affective distress, and dysfunctional adjustment to chronic pain (Jensen, Romano, Turner, Good, & Wald, 1999; Jensen, Turner, Romano, & Lawler, 1994). The specific thoughts and feelings that people experience prior to, during, or after an episode of pain, will greatly influence the experience of pain. Thus, each of these factors is considered in a biopsychosocial pain assessment.

From the biopsychosocial perspective, the physical factors that initiated the original report of pain play a diminishing role in disability over time; secondary problems associated with deconditioning may exacerbate and maintain the problem. We believe that inadequate assessment of biopsychosocial factors, particularly ones described in more detail later, can impede successful rehabilitation.

The Challenge of Assessing the Person
with Chronic Pain

When patients report pain, health care professionals have the important and challenging task of assessment. Seasoned clinicians, particularly those working in multidisciplinary settings, know that assessing a patient's pain is not solely a matter of attempting to uncover the physical etiology of the pain. Regardless of the etiology, converging threads of evidence suggest that numerous factors contribute to the experience of pain in addition to physical pathology. In fact, pain symptoms and experiences are not tightly linked to degree of physical pathology. This is why the biopsychosocial model has such heuristic appeal. A thorough evaluation of a patient involves assessing the myriad of psychosocial and behavioral factors that contribute to the experience and report of pain. The importance of evaluating the range of potentially important contributing factors cannot be overstated, as successful outcomes rest on how adequately these factors are addressed.

Inadequate assessment of pain problems may stem from the fact that patients and health care professionals alike often ignore the distinction between nociception and pain. Nociception is limited to a sensory event beginning with noxious peripheral chemical, thermal, or mechanical energy. Pain is a subjective perceptual experience. Although pain is likely to follow from nociception, nociception does not necessarily precede the subjective experience of pain. Cognitive and emotional processes moderate and modulate the experience of pain. The International Association for the Study of Pain (Merskey, 1986) recognized the distinction between nociception and pain by defining pain as "an unpleasant sensory *and* emotional experience associated with actual or potential tissue damage or described in terms of such damage" (emphasis added, p. S217).

In the majority of cases, biomedical factors lead to initial reports of pain. In chronic pain (i.e., extending over many months and years) other factors, particularly psychosocial and behavioral ones, are capable of maintaining and exacerbating pain, influencing adjustment, and contributing to excessive disability. Because research shows that these non-biomedical factors, including fear, anxiety, anger, beliefs, and contextual influences, can contribute to the experience of pain (e.g., Turk & Okifuji, 2002), they should be considered integral parts of the assessment of any patient reporting persistent pain and related symptoms.

In fact, psychosocial factors have been shown to be significant predictors of pain, distress, treatment seeking, disability, and response to any treatment (e.g., Boothby, Thorn, Staud, & Jensen, 1999; Pfingsten, Hildebrandt, Leibing, Carment, & Saur, 1997). For example, many chronic back pain sufferers view back surgery as a necessary treatment for back pain relief. One might believe that back surgery is a drastic step taken because it is the only road toward recovery. Unfortunately, however, some back-surgery patients do not improve. In one study, 39% of patients who underwent circumferential lumbar fusions because of chronic low back pain reported that, in retrospect (at least 2 years postsurgery), they would not go through it again for the same outcome, with half of those patients stating that they felt the same or worse than before their surgeries (Slosar et al., 2000). The reason patients may respond differently to treatments may be accounted for, in part, by pretreatment psychosocial differences.

By and large, researchers and clinicians are increasingly adopting the view that every individual who becomes a pain patient has a unique set of circumstances that will affect his or her prognosis. Thus, our assessments of pain patients need to encompass a wide range of areas and, at times, need to be tailored toward the individual patient. For example, Gatchel (2001) recommended taking a "stepwise approach" when conducting biopsychosocial assessments, noting that assessments can have greater impact when the order of the steps are arranged to meet the needs of each specific patient.

Although chronic pain is a major health care problem in the United States and has enormous individual, social, and economic consequences, there is currently no treatment that totally eliminates pain problems for the majority of chronic pain sufferers. As a consequence, people will likely continue to experience pain for years, even decades, despite the best efforts of health care providers. The longer pain persists, the more impact it will have on the pain sufferer's life and the more psychosocial variables will play a role.

PSYCHOLOGICAL ASSESSMENT OF CHRONIC PAIN SUFFERERS

Optimal treatment cannot begin without appropriate assessment, and appropriate assessment must attend to cognitive, affective, and behavioral factors. This assessment can be a brief psychological screening or a comprehensive psychological evaluation. The overall objectives of both types of assessment (described next) are to determine the extent to which cognitive, emotional, or behavioral factors are exacerbating the pain experience, interfering with functioning, or impeding rehabilitation.

Initial Screening

In some settings, such as hospitals, health professionals are asked to conduct bedside pain evaluations or provide pain consultation service for physicians treating patients with complicated symptoms or on rehabilitation units. Under these circumstances, a brief *psychological screening* may be all that is feasible. This screening should supplement the routine assessment of pain that has become a requirement of the Joint Commission on the Accreditation of Rehabilitation Facilities (JCAHO) in the United States and the U.S. Veterans Administration (VA). In those instances, patients are routinely queried as to pain severity, location, and characteristics. In addition, the VA recommends that, when feasible, patients should be asked about the impact of pain on their activities (e.g., socializing, eating, ambulating), current and past treatments for pain, and patients' expectations for pain relief. In addition, behavioral manifestations of pain should be observed (e.g., limping, protective body postures, moaning) and changes in these should be noted.

A first consideration is the purpose for the screening (e.g., "Is this patient significantly depressed?" "Why is the patient noncompliant?" "Why is the patient being so uncooperative?"). The evaluator must be responsive to the referral question; however, one of the main objectives of any psychological screening is to determine whether a comprehensive pain assessment is warranted. In many instances, initial screenings can be conducted by physicians, nurses, or other health professionals with the understanding that if particular concerns are detected, they should refer the patient to a pain psychologist for a comprehensive evaluation.

Under ideal circumstances, psychological screenings can take as little as 15 minutes, particularly if patients complete paper-and-pencil questionnaires ahead of time. We discuss the use of surveys, inventories, and questionnaires in a later section.

Physicians and other health care providers should conduct a brief screening with all chronic pain patients to determine whether they require a more comprehensive psychological evaluation. Table 8.1 includes areas that should be examined and some sample questions. When a patient demonstrates problems in response to 6 of the 16 areas included in the inquiry or shows a particularly worrisome response to any one of the questions included in Table 8.1, we recommend referral for a comprehensive psychological assessment. We next expand on several of the areas covered in Table 8.1 to provide additional clarification.

Inappropriate Medication Use/Substance Abuse

A significant percentage of people with chronic pain treated in primary care are prescribed one or more analgesic medications with a substantial percentage receiving prescriptions for opioid medication (Clark, 2002). Patients

TABLE 8.1

Screening Questions

If a combination of more than 6 "Yes" to the first 13 questions and "No" to the last 3 questions below or if general concerns in any one area, consider referral for psychological assessment.

1. Has the patient's pain persisted for three months or longer despite appropriate interventions and in the absence of progressive disease? [Yes]
2. Does the patient repeatedly and excessively use the health care system, persist in seeking invasive investigations or treatments after being informed these are inappropriate, or use opioid or sedative-hypnotic medications or alcohol in a pattern of concern to the patient's physician (e.g., escalating use)? [Yes]
3. Does the patient come in requesting specific opioid medication (e.g., dilaudid, oxycontin)? [Yes]
4. Does the patient have unrealistic expectations of the health care providers or the treatment offered ("Total elimination of pain and related symptoms")? [Yes]
5. Does the patient have a history of substance abuse or is he or she currently abusing mind altering substances? [Yes] Patients can be asked, "Have you ever found yourself taking more medication than was prescribed or have you used alcohol because your pain was so bad?" or "Is anyone in your family concerned about the amount of medication you take?"
6. Does the patient display a large number of pain behaviors that appear exaggerated (e.g., grimacing, rigid or guarded posture)? [Yes]
7. Does the patient have litigation pending? [Yes]
8. Is the patient seeking or receiving disability compensation? [Yes]
9. Does the patient have any other family members who had or currently suffer from chronic pain conditions? [Yes]
10. Does the patient demonstrate excessive depression or anxiety? [Yes]. Straightforward questions such as, "Have you been feeling down?" or "What effect has your pain had on your mood?" can clarify whether this area is in need of more detailed evaluation.
11. Can the patient identify a significant or several stressful life events prior to symptom onset or exacerbation? [Yes]
12. If married or living with a partner, does the patient indicate a high degree of interpersonal conflict? [Yes]
13. Has the patient given up many activities (recreational, social, familial, in addition to occupational and work activities) due to pain? [Yes]
14. Does the patient have any plans for renewed or increased activities if pain is reduced? [No]
15. Was the patient employed prior to pain onset? [No] If yes, does he or she wish to return to that job or any job? [No]
16. Does the patient believe that he or she will ever be able to resume normal life and normal functioning? [No]

---

seeking pain relief may inadvertently become psychologically dependent on prescription medications. Adherence to prescribed medications should be explored. In addition to asking about what analgesic medications have been prescribed, the evaluator should inquire about the frequency of medication use, whether the patient alters the recommended schedule of medication use, what the patient does when he or she has an exacerbation of pain, and what the patient does if he or she uses up the supply of available medication. When patients make frequent requests for increased or stron-

216   TURK, MONARCH, WILLIAMS

ger medications, rely solely on medications for relief, or when there are indications that the patient may be overmedicated (e.g., the patient can no
longer do his or her job because of being too sedated), urine screening and
a thorough psychological evaluation may be warranted.

Patients may also make use of alcohol and illicit drugs to palliate their
symptoms. A particular concern is that of substance abuse. Patients with
histories of substance abuse may be at particular risk for becoming psychologically dependent on and abusing pain medications. Reviewing the
chart and conducting a detailed history of previous and current prescription and substance use may help ascertain whether this area warrants further inquiry.

Excessive Physical, Work, Family, or Social Dysfunction

Patients who abandon their exercise routines, employment, family, and social activities are at greater risk for problems associated with persistent
pain. Lack of physical activity can lead to weakened and more vulnerable
muscles, which are more susceptible to exacerbation of pain. Physical deconditioning through further reduction in activity can lead to even greater
loss of muscle strength, flexibility, and endurance.

Disengagement from family, social activities, or employment can have a
number of repercussions, such as leading the patient to greater isolation
and diminished self-esteem, and ultimately greater disability. If pain patients demonstrate poor social and physical functioning, particularly in
light of their degree of objective physical pathology, a comprehensive evaluation may clarify their situation, and help to identify areas to be addressed in a comprehensive treatment plan. One way to assess patient
functioning is to inquire, "Are there things that you used to do that you no
longer do because of your pain?" The clinician should note whether the patient has modified activities in healthful ways (e.g., switching from a karate
class to a yoga class) or has completely abandoned them.

Involvement in Litigation/Disability Compensation

Financial compensation from litigation or disability payments can serve as
positive reinforcement for reports of pain. Financial compensation, especially when combined with other factors, such as those listed above, may
contribute to disability. In order to briefly address this area in a screening,
patients can be asked direct questions such as, "Have you hired an attorney
to assist you?" "What are your monthly disability payments?" "What percent of your previous salary is covered by disability payments?"

Beliefs About Current and Future Pain and Functioning

Finally, the way patients think about their pain can exacerbate their symptoms. When patients have catastrophic beliefs about their situation or express hopelessness about their future, they should be referred for a comprehensive evaluation. Clinicians can also ask patients questions about their beliefs, such as, "What do you believe is the cause of your pain?" and "Do you believe that your pain will improve?" Alternatively, they may administer self-report questionnaires such as the Survey of Pain Beliefs and Attitudes (Jensen, Karoly, & Huger, 1987) or the Pain Beliefs and Perceptions Inventory (Williams & Thorn, 1989).

In addition to gathering information through an interview, health care professionals can administer any of a number of standardized self-report measures in addition to the ones we mentioned. These instruments are efficient means for obtaining relevant detailed information. Some of these measures require psychological expertise for interpretation; however, a number of instruments require little training (see Turk & Melzack, 2001). Note that many of these instruments were not developed specifically for chronic pain patients. As a result, it is always best to corroborate information gathered from the instruments with other sources, such as interviews with the patient and significant others, and chart review. An important caveat: The results of such brief screening should not be used to diagnose but rather to determine whether a more comprehensive psychological evaluation is warranted.

PURPOSES OF A COMPREHENSIVE PSYCHOLOGICAL EVALUATION

When health care professionals suspect that cognitive, emotional, or behavioral factors play a role in patients' suffering (six or more items identified in Table 8.1 or a particularly concerning area identified during the initial screening), a comprehensive psychological evaluation is appropriate. Experienced health psychologists are best able to perform these evaluations. A thorough psychological evaluation will reveal aspects of the patient's history that are relevant to the current situation. For example, the psychologist will gather information about psychological disorders, substance abuse or dependence, vocational difficulties, and family role models for chronic illness. In terms of current status, topics covered include recent life stresses, vocational, social and physical functioning, sleep patterns, and emotional functioning. The purpose of the evaluation is to examine whether historical or current factors are influencing the way the patient perceives and copes with pain.

The psychological evaluation cannot provide definitive information about the cause(s) of pain and other symptoms. Moreover, if psychological factors are identified as contributing to pain and disability, this does not preclude the possibility of physical pathology, just as the presence of positive physical findings does not necessarily preclude the possibility that psychological factors are contributing to the patient's pain.

PREPARATION OF PATIENTS FOR PSYCHOLOGICAL EVALUATIONS

Many patients with persistent pain may not see the relevance of a psychological evaluation. They tend view their symptoms as physical and they are not accustomed to a biopsychosocial approach. Many believe that identification and treatment of the physical cause of their pain is the only road toward finding relief for their symptoms. When compensation or litigation issues are involved, patients may be particularly sensitive to the implications of a psychological evaluation. They may wonder, "Is this psychologist trying to figure out if I am exaggerating my symptoms?" Another concern they may have is that their health care providers believe they are "crazy" or that their pain is "all in their head."

When health care providers refer patients for a psychological evaluation, they can save the patient considerable grief and enhance patient cooperation by engaging in a brief discussion about why they were referred for such an evaluation. Specifically, the provider can inform the patient that an evaluation helps his or her providers ensure that factors in the person's life, such as stress, are not interfering with their treatment and not contributing to suffering. Patients can then be told that, used in conjunction with other treatments, patients with persistent pain have found that psychological techniques can reduce their symptoms and help them better manage their pain and their lives. Table 8.2 includes a transcript with some guidance for discussing a referral to a psychologist. Although it is not ideal, when referral agents do not prepare patients for psychological evaluations, pain psychologists can provide the rationale for the evaluation themselves. One way to establish rapport with these patients is to begin the evaluation with less "psychologically charged" questions. Instead, begin by asking patients to describe their pain and its onset. The transcript included in Table 8.2 can be modified for a psychologist to use during the introduction to the assessment.

COMPONENTS OF A PSYCHOLOGICAL EVALUATION

A comprehensive psychological evaluation covers the same information as screening but in much greater depth and breadth. Results of comprehensive psychological evaluations can be combined with physical and voca-

TABLE 8.2
Preparation for Referral for a Psychological Evaluation

- Acknowledge that you believe the patient's experience of pain is real.
- Inform them that they are being referred to a psychologist because when pain persists it begins to affect all aspects of life.
- Note that the purpose of the referral is to help formulate a comprehensive treatment plan that addresses both the physical factors involved with pain and the impact of pain on the patient's life.
- Inform them that information provided to a psychologist will be confidential and shared only with other health care professionals. If third-party payers are to obtain information the patient will be alerted to this. Limitations of confidentiality, as required by law, need to be stated.

The following is a transcript of an interaction where a health care provider is preparing a patient for a referral for a psychological evaluation.

"When people have persistent pain, fatigue, and other distressing symptoms and they have been referred for a psychological evaluation, they often think, 'Does my doctor think that my symptoms are all in my head (imaginary)?' 'Does he or she think I am exaggerating or, making everything up, faking?' 'Does my doctor think I am a hopeless case and is he or she trying to get rid of me?' Others may think, 'I'm not depressed, why do I need to see a psychologist?'

"There is no question that your pain and other symptoms are real. I'm referring you to a psychologist because I understand you have been having unremitting symptoms for a long time and I know that this can affect all areas of your life. Psychologists do not just deal with people who have severe emotional problems. They also work with patients who have to adapt to a disorder with distressing symptoms. As you know all too well, living with pain is difficult, can create many problems, and interfere with all aspects of your life—household activities, work, marital, family, and social relations, work, and more. There is no question that pain and associated symptoms cause a lot of stress. Do you agree? It is not surprising that people with pain become irritable, angry, frustrated, worried, and yes, depressed. To provide you with the best treatment, then, requires that we understand your situation and work with you as a whole person (not just a set of body parts that are broken) and provide you with a comprehensive treatment.

"Some of the things that a psychologist might ask you about include how chronic pain has affected your life and how you have been coping with the many symptoms. Based on the psychological evaluation, the psychologist may recommend ways to help you adjust your life style to reduce pain and disability, relaxation methods to help you control your body, a number of stress management skills and ways to help you cope with your physical symptoms and your distress, and methods to help you improve your marital, family, and social relations. I hope I have addressed some of your concerns about my recommending a psychological evaluation. Do you have any questions?"

Note. From "Psychological Evaluation of Patients with Fibromyalgia Syndrome: A Comprehensive Approach," by D. C. Turk, E. S. Monarch, & A. D. Williams, 2002, *Rheumatic Disease Clinics of North America, 28*, 219–233. Copyright 2002 by W. B. Saunders Company. Reprinted with permission.

tional evaluations conducted by physicians or physical therapists and vocational counselors, respectively, or can stand alone.

Interview

A central component of a psychological evaluation is the interview. A number of topics roughly fitting within 10 general areas are covered in the interviews.

Description of Symptoms. Pain psychologists are interested in how patients experience their pain, what types of things exacerbate or alleviate the symptoms, and what thoughts and feelings they have about their pain. For example, does the patient believe that they have no control over symptoms? Are they able to detect any patterns in their pain experience? Or do they notice that their behaviors influence their symptoms to some extent and that there are predictable patterns with respect to their pain?

It is also useful to ask patients to rate their pain on a 0–10 scale (e.g., 0 equals no pain at all and 10 equals the most intense pain possible). They might be asked to rate their pain "right now," "over the past weeks," "usual or average pain," "most severe pain," and how much their pain affects their regular activities. These ratings can be informative in generating hypotheses and might also be used to evaluate progress during treatment. A patient who assigns very low ratings but grimaces and limps while moving about the clinic may be underreporting his or her pain. On the other hand, a patient who assigns a 10 as the lowest pain experienced may be making a plea for help. The patients might also be asked about the location and changing (spreading) of pain, the characteristics of pain (e.g., burning, aching), the effect of pain on activities, and what they do when their pain is particularly severe, as well as how they typically control their pain. These questions can be presented orally or patients can be asked to complete a questionnaire addressing these topics. There is no simple way to assess a person's pain level, but *how* a patient describes his or her pain might be as useful as knowing the pain level itself.

Difficulties sleeping frequently accompany chronic pain and can create a vicious circle of suffering. Lack of sleep can contribute to pain, and experiencing pain can make it more difficult to sleep soundly. In a comprehensive evaluation, patients should be asked about their sleep—specifically, do they have any difficulty initiating or maintaining sleep? Do they feel rested when they awaken? If the patient endorses any of these difficulties, psychologists can probe further and help determine whether there are (often easy) changes that can be made. For example, does the patient discontinue caffeine consumption eight hours and alcohol four hours before bedtime?

What does the patient do when he or she wakes up in the middle of the sleep cycle?

Prior Treatments. Patients should be asked about what treatments they have tried in the past and are using presently. How effective were (are) these treatments? Also, are they or health care providers considering additional treatments in the future, such as surgery for their pain? If there is a pending treatment, what does the patient know about the procedure(s) being considered, what are the patient's expectations about the likely results, how confident are they in the potential of this treatment? How worried are they about the treatments being considered, what do their significant others think about the treatment(s) being contemplated? Answers to these questions are useful in evaluating whether patients have already assumed a self-management role or whether they see themselves as reliant on others for all their care.

Compensation and Litigation Status. When patients with persistent pain seek compensation for lost wages or are involved in litigation, these processes can add an additional layer of distress. Keeping up with paperwork, phone calls, visits to physicians and hospitals, and meetings with attorneys are often undesirable activities. They may have realistic concerns about the potential outcomes of the assessment. Moreover, patients involved in litigation are usually in the awkward position of having to "prove" how disabled they are as a result of an injury. The more they attend to their limitations, the less they attend to their improvements. Yet an important part of rehabilitation is taking note of capabilities and maximizing a "wellness" role. Psychologists should ask patients about these areas in order to assess whether compensation or litigation statuses might inadvertently be contributing to and maintaining the patients' symptoms. The psychologist needs to be vigilant for the potential of secondary gains coloring the patient's presentation.

A number of studies (e.g., Rohling, Binder, & Langhinrichen-Rohling, 1995) have demonstrated that litigation and compensation can influence reports of pain and response to treatment. This cannot, however, be taken as an indication that those involved with litigation and receiving disability compensation are dissimulating or exaggerating. There are a number of factors (e.g., the process of litigation, the nature of work of those seeking compensation) that may influence their responses. Moreover, although the studies suggest that litigation and compensation are predictors of disability these factors are only *relative* predictors. That is, not every patient who is involved with litigation or who is receiving compensation will ipso facto respond poorly to treatment or report higher levels of pain (Turk, 1997). The clinician must be cautious not to overemphasize the role of these factors in his or her evaluation of chronic pain sufferers and in treatment recommendations.

Patients' Responses to Their Symptoms and Responses From Significant Others. This part of the interview is particularly important. How has the patient changed his or her life as result of the pain? Has the patient ceased engaging in favorite activities? Has a significant other taken over household responsibilities? When the patient experiences an increase in pain, does he or she complain about it to significant others? How do significant others respond?

From a biopsychosocial perspective, antecedents and consequences of pain symptoms and associated behaviors can potentially shape future experiences and behaviors. Pain psychologists use this information to formulate hypotheses about what behavioral factors in a person's life may serve to maintain or exacerbate the pain experience. It is helpful to gather this information through interviews with patients and significant others together as well as separately. During conjoint interviews the psychologist should observe interactions between the significant others and responses by significant others to patients expressions of pain and suffering.

Coping Efforts. People who feel that they have a number of successful methods for coping with pain may suffer less than those who behave and feel helpless, hopeless, and demoralized. Thus, assessments should focus on identifying factors that exacerbate and ameliorate the pain experience. Does the patient continue to engage in enjoyable activities? Does he or she have a history of coping well with stressors? Is he or she so overwhelmed by pain and other stressors that he or she has little resources left to cope with his symptoms? Does emotional stress increase his or her perceived pain level? If so, he or she may meet the criteria for a pain disorder associated with both psychological factors and a general medical condition (if diagnosed by a physician) in the *Diagnostic and Statistical Manual* (American Psychiatric Association, 1994). Does the patient have problems with pacing activities, so that he or she does more when the patient feels better, which leads to increased pain and subsequent sedentary behavior? Do relaxation techniques reduce the pain level? Is reliance on pain medication the primary way pain is reduced?

The psychologist should not only focus on deficits and weakness in coping efforts and coping repertoire but also strengths. What has the patient tried and what has been helpful? How has the patient coped with other problems (illnesses, stress) in the past? How successful does the patient feel he or she was in coping with problems prior to pain onset? What is the extent of his or her coping repertoire?

Educational and Vocational History. Does the patient have a history of achievement, consistent work, and adequate income? Patients without these may be at a further disadvantage in terms of future successes (Dworkin, Richlin, Handlin, & Brand, 1986). What was (is) the nature of the patient's work? What are the physical demands required? Does the patient believe that he or she will be able to return to previous occupation? How did the patient get along with coworkers, supervisors, and employees? Did the patient like his or her job and does he or she wish to return to the same or a related job? What plans has the patient made regarding return to work or to resumption of usual activities? If psychologists learns that these factors may impede progress, they can include recommendations for referral to a vocational counselor.

Social History. Did anyone in the patient's family of origin live with chronic pain? If so, what did the patient learn from that? Does the patient currently have a supportive network of family or friends? Do significant others unwittingly reinforce pain behaviors? Is his or her marriage or home life chaotic? Has it changed since the onset of pain? A comprehensive evaluation and subsequent report can guide recommendations about these issues. Severe difficulties in these areas may warrant a referral to a psychotherapist or family counselor.

History and Current Alcohol and Substance Use. Has the patient coped with difficulties in the past by turning to alcohol? Is the patient self-medicating? Does his or her substance use interfere with his ability to manage symptoms? It is helpful to use an interview such as the Structured Clinical Interview for the *DSM–IV* (SCID; American Psychiatric Association, 1997) (described later) to determine if the patient meets the criteria for substance abuse or dependence. Patients who are reliant on substances will need additional services for proper treatment.

Psychological Dysfunction. It is important to assess whether patients have a prior history of psychiatric illness. Are they currently being treated for psychological problems? If yes, did treatment begin prior to pain onset, or is treatment related to current pain? How helpful does the patient feel psychological treatments have been (are)? Are there any additional factors from the patient's history that may impede rehabilitation? Is the patient so overwhelmed by his or her current situation that he or she has become suicidal? Patients with psychological dysfunction may benefit from additional support, therapy, or consultation with a psychiatrist for psychotropic medications. Information acquired during the SCID may help determine if the patient meets *DSM–IV* criteria for several diagnostic categories. The interview may also differentiate if depression is a primary factor or is secondary to chronic pain.

The SCID–I and SCID–II (1997) can be used to determine whether the patient suffers from any Axis I (primary psychiatric diagnosis) or Axis II (personality disorder) *DSM–IV* diagnoses (American Psychiatric Association, 1994). It is helpful to differentiate if depression or anxiety predated the onset of pain symptoms, is related to a primary psychiatric diagnosis, such as major depressive disorder, or is secondary to chronic pain. Significant depressive symptoms secondary to chronic pain may meet the criteria for depressive disorder not otherwise specified. It is also necessary to determine whether the patient's symptoms meet the *DSM–IV* criteria for a pain disorder associated with psychological factors (code 307.80) or a pain disorder associated with both psychological factors and a general medical condition (code 307.89) (which would need to be diagnosed by a medical doctor) (American Psychiatric Association, 1994). For example, the pain may be exacerbated by maladaptive responses to stress.

The SCID–I for Axis I disorders also includes a comprehensive set of questions regarding substance use. If a patient is abusing or is dependent on substances, this may adversely affect his or her ability to adaptively manage pain.

Concerns and Expectations for the Future and Treatments. Patients should be asked about their beliefs and expectations about the future of their pain problem. Are they convinced that they will not be cured unless they have a surgery? What would they do if their pain were eliminated? What would be the first sign that they were on the road to recovery? These questions are meant not only to assess the patient's thoughts (beliefs, expectations, attitudes) surrounding their pain problem but also to assess whether the patient has considered that rehabilitation is possible. To what extent have they internalized the disability role? Are they expecting to improve?

Table 8.3 describes each of these areas in some more detail and provides additional examples of helpful questions. It is important to note that the categories are listed as if they are independent. Actually they are interrelated and, ultimately, will allow the evaluators to identify specific areas for rehabilitation.

Observation. Observation of patients' behaviors (ambulation, body postures, facial expressions) can occur while they are being escorted to interview, during the interview, and when exiting interview (observation checklists are available to assist in assessing pain behaviors; Keefe, Williams, & Smith, 2001; Richards, Nepomuceno, Riles, & Suer, 1982). Observation of significant others' responses to patients can occur at the same time.

TABLE 8.3
Areas Covered in Comprehensive Interview

Experience of Pain and Related Symptoms
- Location and description of pain (e.g., "sharp", "burning")
- Onset and progression
- Perception of cause (e.g., trauma, virus, stress)
- What have they been told about their symptoms and condition? Do they believe that what they have been told is accurate?
- Exacerbating and relieving factors (e.g., exercise, relaxation, stress, massage). "What makes your pain worse?" "What makes your pain better?"
- Pattern of symptoms (e.g., symptoms worse certain times of day or following activity or stress)
- Sleep habits (e.g., difficulty falling to sleep or maintaining sleep, sleep hygiene)
- Thoughts, feelings, and behaviors that precede, accompany, and follow fluctuations in symptoms

Treatments Received and Currently Receiving
- Medication (prescribed and over-the-counter). How helpful have these been?
- Pattern of medication use (prn [as needed], time-contingent), changes in quantify or schedule
- Physical modalities (e.g., physical therapy). How helpful have these been?
- Exercise (e.g., Do they participate in a regular exercise routine? Is there evidence of deactivation and avoidance of activity due to fear of pain or exacerbation of injury?). Has the pattern changed (increased, decreased)?
- Complementary and alternative (e.g., chiropractic manipulation, relaxation training). How helpful have these been?
- Which treatments have they found the most helpful?
- Compliance/adherence with recommendations of health care providers
- Feelings about previous health care providers

Compensation/Litigation
- Current disability status (e.g., receiving or seeking disability, amount, percent of former job income, expected duration of support)
- Current or planned litigation (e.g., "Have you hired an attorney")

Responses by Patient and Significant Others
- Typical daily routine ("How much time do you spend sitting, standing, lying down?")
- Changes in activities and responsibilities (both positive and obligatory) due to symptoms ("What activities did you use to engage in prior to your symptoms?" "How has this changed since your symptoms began?")
- Changes in significant other's activities and responsibilities due to patient's symptoms
- Patient's behavior when pain increases or flares up ("What do you do when your pain is bothering you?" "Can others tell when your pain is bothering you?" "How do they know?")
- Significant others' responses to behavioral expressions of pain ("How can significant others tell when your pain is bad?" "What do your significant others do when they can tell your pain is bothering you?" "Are you satisfied with their responses?")
- What does the patient do when pain is not bothering him or her (uptime activities, well behaviors)?
- Significant other's response when patient is active ("How does your significant other respond to your engaging in activities?")
- Impact of symptoms on interpersonal, family, marital, and sexual relations (e.g., changes in desire, frequency, or enjoyment)
- Activities that patient avoids because of symptoms
- Activities continued despite symptoms
- Pattern of activity and pacing of activity (can use activity diaries that ask patients to record their pattern of daily activities [time spent sitting, standing, walking, and reclining] for several days or weeks)

(Continued)

TABLE 8.3

(Continued)

Coping

- How does the patient try to cope with his or her symptoms? (e.g., "What do you do when your pain worsens?" "How helpful are these efforts?"). Does patient view himself or herself as having any role in symptom management? "What role?"
- Current life stresses
- Pleasant activities ("What do you enjoy doing?")

Educational and Vocational History

- Level of education completed (any special training)
- Work history
- How long at most recent job?
- How satisfied with most recent job and supervisor?
- What do they like least about most recent job?
- Would they like to return to most recent job? If not what type of work would they like?
- Current work status (including homemaking activities)
- Vocational and avocational plans

Social History

- Relationships with family or origin
- History of pain or disability in family members
- History of substance abuse in family members
- History of, or current, physical, emotional, and sexual abuse. Was the patient a witness to abuse of someone else?
- Marital history and current status?
- Quality of current marital and family relations.

Alcohol and Substance Use

- History and current use of alcohol (quantity, frequency)
- History and current use of illicit psychoactive drugs
- History and current use of prescribed psychoactive medications
- Consider the CAGE questions as a quick screen for alcohol dependence (Mayfield, McLeod, & Hall, 1987). Depending on response consider other instruments for alcohol and substance abuse (Allen & Litten, 1998).

Psychological Dysfunction

- Current psychological symptoms/diagnosis (depression including suicidal ideation, anxiety disorders, somatization, posttraumatic stress disorder). Depending on responses, consider conducting formal SCID (American Psychiatric Association, 1997).
- Is the patient currently receiving treatment for psychological symptoms? If yes, what treatments (e.g., psychotherapy or psychiatric medications). How helpful?
- History of psychiatric disorders and treatment including family counseling
- Family history of psychiatric disorders

Concerns and Expectations

- Patient concerns/fears (e.g., Does the patient believe he/she has serious physical problems that have not been identified? Or that symptoms will become progressively worse and patient will become more disabled and more dependent? Does the patient worry that he or she will be told the symptoms are all psychological?)
- Explanatory models ("What have you been told is the cause of your symptoms?" "Does this explanation make sense?" "What do you think is the cause of your pain now?")
- Expectations regarding the future and regarding treatment (will get better, worse, never change)
- Attitude toward rehabilitation versus "cure."
- Treatment goals

Note. From "Psychological Evaluation of Patients with Fibromyalgia Syndrome: A Comprehensive Approach," by D. C. Turk, E. S. Monarch, & A. D. Williams, 2002, *Rheumatic Disease Clinics of North America, 28,* 219–233. Copyright 2002 by W. B. Saunders Company. Reprinted with permission.

SIGNIFICANT OTHER INTERVIEW

Because significant others may unwittingly contribute to pain expression and disability, whenever possible a chronic pain evaluation should include an interview with a significant other. It is best to interview the significant other (e.g., spouse, partner, family member, close friend) individually, because he or she might feel more comfortable discussing details of the patient's situation. The rationale offered to the patient is that by interviewing a significant other, the treatment team can learn more about the patient and ultimately can provide better treatment. It is also helpful to mention that significant others are frequently affected by the patient's persistent pain and appreciate the opportunity to express their feelings and concerns.

When possible, it is also helpful to interview the patient and significant other together. As mentioned previously, it is useful to observe patient and significant other interactions, noting any behaviors that might be related to the patient's disability. For example, are there indications that the significant other inadvertently reinforces pain behaviors? How does the significant other respond to the patient as he or she describes the pain and distress (e.g., reaches out to touch the patient, frowns, or contradicts)?

CASE EXAMPLE

A 34-year-old truck driver, Mr. C, injured his back while unloading boxes at work one year earlier. He experienced immediate lower back pain that he rated as a 9 on an 11-point scale (0–10, with 10 representing the worst pain possible). At present he reports that his pain is at level 7 most of the day and is worst in the morning.

Mr. C reports he has difficulty falling asleep due to discomfort and recurring worry about his future. He states that he goes to bed at 11:00 p.m. but does not fall asleep until around 2:00 a.m. Mr. C indicates that he wakes up three to four times per night every night due to pain. When he wakes up, he notes that he watches television or "surfs" the Internet. Mr. C reports that he awakens for the day at 5:30 a.m. feeling tired. He notes that he takes 2-hour naps in the afternoon most days. He acknowledges that he smokes one pack of cigarettes per day, the last one being immediately before going to bed. He then smokes one to two cigarettes when he awakens during the night. Mr. C reports that he consumes five cups of coffee per day, the last being about 2 hours before going to bed. He describes poor sleep hygiene and would benefit from interventions to help him fall asleep and maintain his sleep. He indicates that he has been depressed since his injury. Chronic sleep deprivation and a disrupted sleep cycle can lead to increased pain, increased stress, depressed or anxious mood, decreased concentration, and irritability.

Mr. C notes that he drinks four beers per day and this has been his pattern since he was 21. He has his last "night cap" close to bedtime. He may be using alcohol to reduce his perceived pain. He acknowledges that he had one arrest for driving while intoxicated when he was 20.

Mr. C displayed the following pain behaviors during the interview: holding his lower back, wincing periodically, moaning when sitting down and getting up out of the chair, and changing position frequently. His wife expresses sympathy verbally and helps him to get out of the chair. She reports that she feels sorry for him and gives him massages several times a week. Both Mr. C and his wife admit that he is irritable and that his wife has had to take over many of the household chores he used to do prior to his injury. Mrs. C acknowledges that she is getting frustrated with her husband as he "orders me around and does little to help me or himself."

Mr. C indicates that he has difficulty with most physical activities of daily living, such as lifting, bending, pushing, pulling, and carrying. Pain increases with these activities as well as emotional stress. He appears to have difficulty pacing his activities, tending to do more when he feels better. This leads to increased pain, which in turn leads to decreased activity.

The *DSM–IV* Axis I diagnoses would be: Pain disorder associated with both psychological factors (and a general medical condition [code 307.89], which would need to be diagnosed by a medical doctor), and depressive disorder not otherwise specified (code 311), because the depressive symptoms are secondary to the pain disorder.

STANDARDIZED SELF-REPORT INSTRUMENTS

A large number of psychological instruments have been used to assess domains relevant to patients with chronic pain. A word of caution about psychological measures is in order. Many of these instruments were not developed on patients with medical problems. For example, Piotrowski (1998) conducted a survey of psychologists who were engaged in the assessment of chronic pain patients and reported that the most frequently used measures in order of frequency of use included the Minnesota Multiphasic Personality Inventory (MMPI; Hathway & McKinley, 1967; Hathway, McKinley, & Butcher, 1989), Beck Depression Inventory (BDI; Beck, Ward, Mendelson, Mock, & Erbaugh, 1961), McGill Pain Questionnaire (MPQ, Melzack, 1975), and SCL–90R (Derogatis, 1983), and the Multidimensional Pain Inventory (MPI; Kerns, Turk, & Rudy, 1985). Only the MPQ and MPI were specifically developed for use with chronic pain sufferers.

Data gathered from measures not specifically developed or normed on a chronic pain sample should be interpreted with caution as the patient's medical condition may influence some of the responses. Items such as "I have few or no pains," "I am in just as good physical health as my friends," and "I am about as able to work as I ever was" (from the original MMPI) illustrate the concern (Pincus, Callahan, Bradley, Vaughn, & Wolfe, 1986). It is reasonable to assume that the sensitivity of these measures may be relatively low and there may be a tendency of "overpathologize" patients.

Cutoffs for depression on standard measures, such as the Beck Depression Inventory, do not apply to chronic pain patients (Novy, Nelson, Berry, & Averill, 1995). In addition, it is unclear how pain medications might affect the way patients respond to psychological instruments. As mentioned earlier, it is best to corroborate findings from psychological measures with other sources of information, such as the patient or significant other interview or medical records. In some cases, it will not be possible to corroborate information and interpretations should be made cautiously.

Decisions regarding which measures to select will depend, at least to some extent, on the information obtained during the interview and data derived from the initial psychological screening instruments. Still, standardized assessment instruments can provide an alternate source of information about areas that appear to be influencing patients' adaptation to their pain and their response to treatment. For example, if a high level of marital distress was identified during the interview, the psychologist may request that a patient and his or her spouse both complete a marital adjustment inventory (e.g., Spanier, 1976) to identify areas of conflict and congruence between the two partners. If a patient demonstrates a high degree of defensiveness and unusual personality characteristics during the interview, the examiner may request that he or she complete the MMPI/MMPI-2 to corroborate the clinical impression obtained during the interview.

It is beyond the scope of this chapter to review all of the assessment measures that have been developed to assess people with chronic pain (for a comprehensive review see Turk & Melzack, 2001). Mikail, DeBreuil, and D'Eon (1993) attempted to delineate a core assessment battery for use with chronic pain patients. They factor-analyzed nine self-report measures commonly used to assess chronic pain patients. Based on this analysis they concluded that a core assessment should evaluate general affective distress, social support, pain descriptions, and functional capacities. De Gagne, Mikail, and D'Eon (1995) followed up on the Mikail et al. (1993) study and suggested that a set of measures including the MPI, BDI, and MPQ would be adequate to cover the four domains and suggest this set should form the core assessment. Similarly, Bernstein, Jaremko, and Hinkley (1995) reported that scales of the MPI correlated highly with measures of psychosocial adjustment including the SCL-90R (Derogatis, 1983) and physical functioning, suggesting that there is no need to add an additional measure of psychological adjustment or a measure of functional activities to the MPI. Nevertheless, Burton and colleagues (1999) suggest that the

Basic Personality Inventory (Jackson, 1989) would be a useful complementary tool to the MPI.

We suggest supplementing the set recommended by De Gagne et al. (1995) with a functional activity scale such as the Oswestry Disability Index (Fairbank, Couper, Davies, & O'Brien, 1980), as it includes much more specific activities of daily living, whereas the MPI assess more general activities. This set of instruments should require less than 1 hour for a patient to complete. We consider adding a personality measure as a supplement to the core battery if there were some reason to believe that this information would be of value in addressing a specific referral question or if we identified concerns during the interview.

Cognitive Testing

Patients can be queried about their ability to complete tasks that require cognitive and motor skills, such as driving (e.g., "Are you able to drive?" "Have you been in any car accidents since your pain began?" "Are you able to follow recipes when cooking?"). After considering the information together (subjective report, brief cognitive tests, and queries about activities of daily living), if psychologists suspect cognitive impairments, they can refer patients for further neuropsychological testing. In addition, they can suggest that medical professionals ensure that the patient has understood treatment guides and instructions. In addition to questions included in the interview, there are a number of formal neuropsychological tests available. There are some data regarding the appropriateness and sensitivity of these measures for chronic pain patients (Hart, Martelli, & Zasler, 2000). We return to discuss some of these when we address specific referral questions regarding disability and impairments later in this chapter.

Ongoing Assessment and Reassessment

Once areas of concern are identified from the evaluation, it is important to develop a plan for how to assess progress. Because conducting repeat comprehensive evaluations will often not be feasible, one way to reassess patients is to use the psychological screening described earlier. The screening should be supplemented with questions about the particular areas of concern that were detected in the prior comprehensive evaluation. In general, however, psychologists should look for signs that the patients' psychosocial, physical, and behavioral functioning have improved or declined. Several brief measures have been developed that may be used during process ratings (Pain Disability Index [Tait, Chibnall, & Krause, 1990], 8 items; Short Form of the MPI [von Korff, 1992], 8 items; Brief Pain Inventory–Short Form, 15 items [Cleeland, 1989]).

Patients may also be asked to complete diaries in which they report (daily, several times a day) the activities they performed (e.g., number of hours sitting, standing, walking), their mood (e.g., fear, anxiety, depression), medication usage, thoughts, use of coping strategies, and sleep quality. Be advised that patients may not comply with the requested frequency. For example, instead of completing ratings three times a day, they may fill in all ratings at the end of the day or fill in the data that was supposed to be recorded daily at the end of the week.

There are additional reasons to be cautious, however, in the selection of measures. If too little time has elapsed since the original evaluation, results of the measures may not be valid. Also, some psychological measures, such as the MMPI, were not designed to assess state variables. Instead, most personality inventories are designed to measure traits and traits should not be expected to change over the course of pain treatment. Hence, they should not be used as indicators of progress. Finally, frequent recording may draw attention to pain and emotional distress when the treatment may be encouraging distraction from symptoms. Thus, the responses may be reactive. There are several solutions to these problems. For example, the patient may complete and mail individual pages each day. Hand-held computers with paging capability can prompt patient responses and lock out access to previous ratings (e.g., Stone, Briderick, Porter, & Kaell, 1997). There are strengths and weaknesses of each approach; however, it is incumbent on those who are treating patients to make efforts to evaluate progress during the course of the treatment.

PSYCHOLOGICAL ASSESSMENT PRIOR TO INVASIVE AND INITIATION OF LONG-TERM OPIOID TREATMENT

At this time, many surgeons and interventional anesthesiologists strongly advocate pretreatment psychological assessments (e.g., Carragee, 2001; Prager & Jacobs, 2001) prior to operations and implantation of spinal cord stimulators and drug delivery systems. Some suggest that a comprehensive psychological assessment should be performed before initiating long-term opioid therapy (Robinson et al., 2001). Treatment providers are noting the advantages of psychological pre-assessment as a way to improve their outcomes as there are sufficient studies demonstrating wide variability in response to ostensibly identical treatments (Turk, 2002). This is becoming more important with the emphasis on evidence-based medicine and the requirement to demonstrate clinical effectiveness and cost-effectiveness of any treatment in order to obtain reimbursement.

Psychosocial variables have been shown to be among the strongest predictors of spinal surgery outcome (Schade, Semmer, Main, Hora, & Boos,

1999). Psychologists are being asked to help physicians and surgeons predict which candidates are poor risks for controversial, invasive, and often costly treatments. The comprehensive assessment protocol we described earlier is appropriate for addressing this referral question. Psychologists should not provide a simple yes–no response, as the evidence is not adequate to warrant definite statements. Rather, psychologists should indicate whether there are any apparent impediments to initiating the treatment and also what might be done either prior to treatment or following treatment to improve the outcomes. For example, a psychologist might suggest that a patient be treated for substance abuse prior to implantation of a spinal cord stimulator. A patient might be scheduled to meet with a psychologist and physical therapist following surgery to help the patient with his fear of certain activities. The psychologist might recommend family counseling to coincide with initiation of chronic opioid therapy.

Despite our general cautionary tone, there do appear to be some relative indicators of poorer outcomes for the types of invasive treatments and long-term opioids. Some of these are intuitive and based on clinical experience (e.g., Nelson, Kennington, Novy, & Squitieri, 1996; and see Turk, 1996b, for a listing of guidelines for use of chronic opioid therapy). Table 8.4 contains the suggested exclusion criteria for patients being considered for implantation of spinal cord stimulators. This list is based on clinical experience and has not been validated.

Epker and Block (2001) suggest that three general areas have been shown to have an influence on lumbar surgery: personality-emotional, cognitive-behavioral, and environmental-historical. These areas may be equally relevant for implantation of spinal cord stimulators (Prager & Jacobs, 2001) and long-term opioid therapy (Robinson et al., 2001). Epker and Block (see also Robinson & Riley, 2001, for a review) recommended the use of the MMPI and particularly emphasize elevations of scales 1 (Hypochondriasis), 2 (Depression), 3 (Hysteria), 4 (Psychopathic Deviate), and 7 (Psychasthenia) as risk factors for the personality domain. In the coping domain

TABLE 8.4
Proposed Exclusion Criteria for Implantation
of a Spinal Cord Stimulator (Nelson et al., 1996)

- Active psychosis
- Active suicidality
- Active homicidality
- Untreated or poorly treated major mood disorders such as major depression
- An unusually high-level somatization or other somatoform disorders
- Substance abuse disorder
- Unresolved workers' compensation or litigation cases
- Lack of appropriate social support
- Cognitive defects that compromise adequate reasoning and memory

they note that the Coping Strategies Questionnaire (Rosensteil & Keefe, 1983) may be a useful predictor. They suggest that patients who engage in more active coping strategies are more likely to have better responses to surgery. In terms of environmental influences, they suggest that patients with significant others who reinforce pain behaviors may have poorer outcomes. Epker and Block also noted the role of litigation and compensation status as an indicator of treatment response. Based on the available literature they suggested that those patients with litigation pending or receiving compensation are poorer risks. In general they suggested that the presence of a psychiatric diagnosis predicts relatively poorer results. Marital relations and history of substance abuse round out the set of factors associated with poorer prognosis. Some combination of these factors should be used to contribute to the psychologist's recommendation regarding the likelihood of a successful outcome to surgery.

A history of childhood physical and sexual abuse has been reported to be prevalent in chronic pain patients (e.g., Linton, 1997). Schofferman, Anderson, Hines, Smith, and White (1992) tested for an association between childhood traumas in general and outcome following lumbar spine surgery. Patients who had three or more of a possible five serious childhood traumas (which included abuse) had an 85% likelihood of an unsuccessful surgical outcome compared to a 5% failure rate for those without a trauma history. Although a high percentage of patients with early trauma had unsuccessful surgical outcomes, not all patients with abuse histories have poor surgical outcomes. It may well be that no one factor by itself is sufficient but combinations of factors identified by Epker and Block (2001) may be implicated.

Although there is some evidence for the importance of the factors outlined by Epker and Block (2001) and a history of abuse, there are limited data to support the predictive validity. Moreover, we need to realize that these predictors are of *relatively* better or poorer outcome. Data reported are based on groups and there is no guarantee that all people with the poor prognostic factors will have an equally poor treatment outcome. Such actuarial data combined with other information may, at least, alert the referring surgeon to potential problems, some of which may be treatable and lead to improved outcomes.

IMPAIRMENT, DISABILITY, AND VOCATIONAL ASSESSMENT

Decisions regarding impairment and disability associated with pain are a difficult area, as pain is a subjective experience and there are no objective signs that can validate reports of pain. Thus, physicians and psychologists have to rely on base-rate information regarding functioning in response to particular physical impairments, in conjunction with history, physical examination (in the case of physicians), observations, collateral information, and importantly self-reports. Four areas of functioning are particularly relevant in deciding the impact of pain (disability), namely, activities of daily living; social functioning; concentration, persistence, and pace; and adaptability to stress. Activities of daily living include the following areas: self-care, physical activities (e.g., ability to sit, stand, walk, lift, have sex, bathe, write, dress, cook, clean), cognition (e.g., attention, memory, concentration), sensory functions (e.g., see, hear), sleep, and basic interpersonal and social activities.

In addition to the functional activities outlined, the abilities to understand, remember, and perform work procedures, follow instructions, and persist at tasks are central. The patient's ability to request assistance, respond to criticism; get along with coworkers; and maintain socially appropriate behavior and along with job satisfaction have been found to be related to return to work following work-related injuries (Turk, 1997). Psychologists can inquire about some of these areas during an interview. In addition, the clinician can make use of standardized measures and may request a functional capacity evaluation from a trained occupational therapist to supplement report.

In addition to some of the measures described, there are other instruments that can be used to assess functional activities. For example, recently an instrument labeled the Impairment Impact Inventory (I^3; Turk, Robinson, Cocchiarella, & Hunt, 2001) was developed for use in assessment pain-related impairment. This measure was designed for use with the fifth edition of American Medical Association's *Guides to the Evaluation of Permanent Impairment* (Cocchiarella & Andersson, 2001). Preliminary data on the reliability, validity, and ability to detect exaggerated responding suggest this may be a promising measure (Robinson, Turk, & Aulet, 2002; Turk, Robinson, & Aulet, 2002).

For vocational evaluations, it is helpful to know how the patient responds to changes at work and is aware of typical hazards. Many patients with chronic pain report having difficulties related to cognitive functioning. Review of the studies reveals that some chronic pain patients, who have not suffered from traumatic brain injuries or neurological disorders, display deficits in attentional capacity, processing speed, and psychomotor speed (Hart et al., 2000). A gross assessment of mental status can be obtained with very brief measures such as the Mini-Mental State Examination (Folstein, Folstein, & McHugh, 1975). When a pain patient performs below expected levels on cognitive tests, however, results need to be interpreted in light of their pain medication use, potentially disrupted sleep, emotional factors, and other symptoms.

Malingering

For some referral sources there are concerns about malingering. This is a contentious issue. Many third-party payers believe that in the absence of sufficient objective physical pathology, reports of pain are motivated by secondary gains, especially financial compensation. The actual base rate for malingering in chronic pain is believed to be quite low (e.g., Mendelson, 1986). Dramatic cases, however, are very salient and induce high levels of suspicion. Of course, the real incidence is unknown. As a consequence, the low base rate and unknown incidence make the task even more difficult for the clinician and only extreme circumstances can conclusions be drawn with any confidence.

When asked to address the question of malingering, the clinician will need to rely on multiple converging sources of information including archival data (previous history), collateral sources of information, knowledge of incentives, litigation status, responsiveness to previous treatments, evidence of physical pathology, performance of tasks of physical functioning, observable behavior in the interview and other unobtrusive situations (e.g., observation of patient in waiting room, as exiting the office), facial expressions, and self-report (i.e., content, quality, and clarity of information provided during the interview, responses to self-report questionnaires that can be compared to appropriate comparison groups or that include "validity scales"). Each of these sources of information and the consistency among them contribute to the clinician's determination of the credibility of the patient's report.

Given the psychometric limitations of tests of malingering and the inherent difficulty with finding appropriate criterion groups for research in this area, it is best to rely on behavioral decision rules. Williams (1998) suggested that psychologists should use three major areas in which discrepancies occur to construct a malingering index for traumatic brain injury. Some of these concepts are also relevant to chronic pain patients. The first is the relationship of injury severity to cognitive functioning. The severity of the injury is directly related to the severity of the expected impairment. The second area involved noting the interrelationship of the tests and subtests. Williams opined, "Inconsistencies are expressed as scores that are sufficiently disparate that they violate the known relationships between the tests" (p. 122). The third area involved the relationship between preinjury status and current test results and, by extension, current functioning. In a forensic report the psychologist may point out inconsistencies but leave the determination of veracity to the "trier of fact."

Conscious dissimulation is possible with any self-report measure. This dissimulation is often referred to as *response bias*. Response biases may also occur unwittingly as when the response is influenced by poor memory.

Conscious dissimulation is particularly a concern when there is an incentive such as disability compensation based on performance deficits. Highly contentious situations often surround assessment of pain-related impairment and disability such as worker compensation, social security disability, veterans' disability compensation, civil litigation related to accidental injuries (e.g., automobile accident, product liability), and access to controlled substances. The validity scales of instruments such as the MMPI and the Eysenck Personality Inventory (Eysenck & Eysenck, 1975) and the variable response scale for the MPI (Bruehl, Lofland, Sherman, & Carlsom, 1998) are at times use in an effort to detect possible biases in patients' responses. In a preliminary study, Lofland, Semenchuk, and Cassisi (1995) concluded the MPI "appears to be a good screening measure to detect patients who are exhibiting symptom exaggeration." It is important to reiterate, that the exaggeration detected may or may not be conscious.

There have been numerous attempts to identify specific psychological profiles of litigation and compensation patients. There is, however, no conclusive evidence that specific characteristics differentiate those who are litigating or who are receiving disability compensation from those who are not (Kolbison, Epstein, & Burgess, 1996).

Recently, Turk et al. (2002) conducted a preliminary study comparing three groups of people with chronic pain to determine whether a group being evaluated by physicians performing an independent medical examination (IME) who completed a self-report measure assessing pain, emotional distress, and functional limitations (I^3; Turk et al., 2001) responded differently than groups of chronic pain patients being treated in rehabilitation facilities (a group of fibromyalgia syndrome patients and a heterogeneous group of chronic pain patients attending an interdisciplinary pain clinic). The authors found no difference in the responses to any of the three sections of the instrument—pain severity, emotional distress, and functional activities. The authors concluded that clinicians should not assume that patients who potentially have something to gain by poor performance (disability seeking) will inevitably exaggerate the burden of their pain and the resultant disability.

Waddell and colleagues (Waddell, McCulloch, Kummel, & Venner, 1980) developed a system of behavioral signs designed to determine the validity of a psychological basis for a given patient's pain report. Presumably, those patients showing a higher number of nonanatomic (nonorganic) signs with their pain report have a high degree of psychological factors contributing to their pain report. Other investigators have examined facial expressions of pain: the ability of observers to distinguish exaggerated pain expressions from healthy subjects and pain sufferers' "real" expressions of pain (Craig, Hyde, & Patrick, 1991; Poole & Craig, 1992).

Physical tests to evaluate suboptimal performance have also been used to detect malingering (Robinson, O'Connor, Riley, Kvaal, & Shirley, 1994).

Some efforts are made to ask patients to repeat standard physical tasks and use discrepancy of performance ("index of congruence") as an indication of motivated performance. Reviewing efforts to detect deception led Craig, Hill, and McMurtry (1999) to the following conclusion: "Definitive, empirically validated procedures for distinguishing genuine and deceptive report are not available and current approaches to the detection of deception remain to some degree intuitive" (p. 41).

There is a growing body of information concerning the ability of neuropsychological tests to detect malingering (Inman & Berry, 2002). Additional research is needed, however, before strong conclusions should follow from performance on these measures. At best performance on neuropsychological test should be combined with other confirmatory information.

LINKING ASSESSMENT WITH TREATMENT

During any assessment, it is helpful to think about how the data gathered will be used in treatment and, ultimately, how a patient's assessment might be related to his or her outcome. Being mindful of treatment implications can assist the pain psychologist in asking better questions during the assessment. Additionally, psychologists need to ensure that their evaluations have addressed the referral question(s), that their reports are informative, and that they have made reasonable, appropriate, and helpful recommendations.

Patient Differences and Treatment Matching

There is a common assumption among many health care providers that patients who have the same medical diagnosis require identical treatment. Some have suggested that there should be a general diagnosis of "chronic pain syndrome." Clinicians are perplexed when the outcomes for patients with the same diagnosis vary widely. One explanation is that there are important variables beyond the common medical diagnosis that differentiate patients. To psychologists this may be intuitively obvious, as they are taught to be concerned about individual variation. However, even some psychologists tend to treat chronic pain patients with one or a few approaches from the number that are available. The selection of treatment is likely based more on training then attention to unique patient differences. Do all chronic pain patients with the same medical diagnosis require the same treatment? Recent research efforts are beginning to show that data gleaned from comprehensive assessments might be used to facilitate patient–treatment matching. It appears that particular treatment strategies are more effective for patients with particular characteristics (Turk, Okifuji, Sinclair, & Starz, 1998a).

There is some evidence that patients respond differentially to treatment based on their pretreatment assessment. Although psychological treatments appear to be effective, not all patients benefit equally. A number of studies have identified subgroups of patients based on psychosocial and behavioral characteristics (e.g., Mikail, Henderson, & Tasca, 1994; Turk & Rudy, 1988, 1990). Dahlstrom and colleagues (Dahlstrom, Widmark, & Carlsson, 1997) found that when patients were classified into different subgroups based on their psychosocial and behavioral responses during assessment, they responded differentially to treatments. Similarly, Turk, Okifuji, Sinclair, and Starz (1998b) noted differential responses to a common treatment for patients with distinctive psychological characteristics but identical physical diagnoses.

Chronic pain syndromes are made up of heterogeneous groups of people, even if they have the same medical diagnosis (Turk, 1990). Patients with diseases and syndromes as diverse as metastatic cancer, back pain, and headaches show similar adaptation patterns, whereas patients with the same diagnosis can show marked variability in their degrees of disability (Turk et al., 1998). Research studies looking only at group effects may mask important issues related to the characteristics of patients who successfully respond to a treatment.

Only a handful of studies have actually begun to demonstrate that matching treatments to patient characteristics, derived from assessments, is of any benefit (e.g., Turk, Rudy, Kubinski, Zaki, & Greco, 1996; Turk, Okifuji, Sinclair, & Starz, 1998b). More studies targeted toward matching interventions to specific patient characteristics are needed (Turk, 1990). Developing treatments that are matched to patients' characteristics should lead not only to improved outcomes but also to greater cost-effectiveness.

In order to advance the area of pain assessment, additional studies of how these assessments can inform and improve treatments are desirable. Moreover, as we learn more about patient–treatment matching, pain assessment procedures should reflect this progress.

CONCLUSION

Symptoms of chronic pain are extremely distressing and many times there is no cure or treatment capable of substantially reducing all symptoms. At the present time, rehabilitation, including improvement in emotional functioning, physical functioning, and quality of life, is the goal. Rehabilitation in spite of pain is a daunting task even for patients with ample coping skills.

The high levels of emotional distress, disability, and reduced quality of life noted in many chronic pain patients suggest that psychological screening is essential; in the majority of cases, a thorough psychological evaluation is called for. Biopsychosocial assessment allows health care professionals to tailor treatment to meet individual needs and preferences. A comprehensive assessment is a complex task, involving an exploration of broad range of areas, and should be administered by an experienced health psychologist. The importance of psychologists in the assessment and treatment of chronic pain has been accepted by a number of agencies and governmental bodies in the United States, Canada, and England (e.g., U.S. Veterans Administration; U.S. Social Security Administration, Ontario Workplace Safety and Insurance Board). In fact, the Commission on the Accreditation of Rehabilitation Facilities in the United States *requires* involvement of psychologists in treatment for multidisciplinary treatment programs to be certified.

In contrast to acute pain where the focus of assessment and treatment is on cure, in chronic pain the focus is often on self-management. However, self-management requires many skills. A thorough psychological assessment allows health care professionals to examine what factors in a patient's history and current situation, including emotional well-being, social support, and behavioral factors, might interfere with their functioning. Strengths identified during assessment may inform treatment planning. The information obtained should assist in treatment planning, specifically the matching of treatment components to the needs of individual patients. Once the whole person is evaluated, treatment can focus on an individual's unique needs and characteristics.

ACKNOWLEDGMENTS

Preparation of this chapter was supported in part by grants from the National Institute of Arthritis and Musculoskeletal and Skin Diseases (AR/AI44724, AR47298) and the National Institute of Child Health and Human Development/National Center for Medical Rehabilitation Research (HD33989) awarded to Dennis C. Turk.

REFERENCES

Allen, J. P., & Litten, R. Z. (1998). Screening instruments and biochemical screening. In A. W. Graham, T. K. Schultz, & B. B. Wilford (Eds.), *Principles of addiction medicine* (pp. 263–272). Chevy Chase, MD: American Society of Addiction Medicine.

American Psychiatric Association. (1994). *Diagnostic and statistical manual of mental disorders* (4th ed.). Washington, DC: American Psychiatric Association Press.

American Psychiatric Association. (1997). *User's guide for the Structured Clinical Interview for DSM–IV axis I disorders SCID–1: Clinician version.* Washington, DC: American Psychiatric Association.

Beck, A. T., Ward, C. H., Mendelson, M., Mock, J., & Erbaugh, J. (1961). An inventory for measuring depression. *Archives of General Psychiatry, 4*, 561–571.

Bernstein, I. H., Jaremko, M. E., & Hickley, B. S. (1995). On the utility of the West Haven–Yale Multidimensional Pain Inventory. *Spine, 20*, 956–963.

Boothby, J. L., Thorn, B. E., Stroud, M. W., & Jensen, M. P. (1999). Coping with pain. In R. J. Gatchel & D. C. Turk (Eds.), *Psychosocial factors in pain: Critical perspectives* (pp. 343–359). New York: Guilford Press.

Bruehl, S., Lofland, K. R., Sherman, J. J., & Carlson, C. R. (1998). The variable responding scale for detection of random responding on the Multidimensional Pain Inventory. *Psychological Assessment, 10*, 3–9.

Burton, H. J., Kline, S. A., Hargadon, R., Cooper, B. S., Shick, R. D., & Ong-Lam, M. C. (1999). Assessing patients with chronic pain using the basic personality inventory as a complement to the multidimensional pain inventory. *Pain Research and Management, 4*, 121–139.

Carragee, E. J. (2001). Psychological screening in the surgical treatment of lumbar disc herniation. *Clinical Journal of Pain, 17*, 215–219.

Clark, J. D. (2002). Chronic pain prevalence and analgesic prescribing in a general medical population. *Journal of Pain and Symptom Management, 23*, 131–137.

Cleeland, C. S. (1989). Measurement of pain by subjective report. In C. R. Chapman & J. D. Loeser (Eds.), *Issues in pain assessment* (pp. 391–403). New York: Raven Press.

Cocchiarella, L., & Andersson, G. B. J. (2001). *Guides to the evaluation of permanent impairment* (5th ed.). Chicago Illinois: American Medical Association.

Craig, K. D., Hill, M. L., & McMurtry, B. W. (1999). Detecting deception and malingering. In A. R. Block, E. F. Kremer, & E. Fernandez (Eds.), *Handbook of pain syndromes* (pp. 41–58). Mahwah, NJ: Lawrence Erlbaum Associates.

Craig, K. D., Hyde, S., & Patrick, C. J. (1991). Genuine, suppressed, and faked facial behavior during exacerbation of chronic low back pain. *Pain, 46*, 161–172.

Dahlstrom, L., Widmark, G., & Carlsson, S. G. (1997). Cognitive-behavioral profiles among different categories of orofacial pain patients: Diagnostic and treatment implications. *European Journal of Oral Science, 105*, 377–383.

De Gagne, T. A., Mikail, S. F., & D'Eon, J. L. (1995). Confirmatory factor analysis of a 4-factor model of chronic pain evaluation. *Pain, 60*, 195–202.

Derogatis, L. (1983). *The SCL–90–R: II: Administration, scoring and procedure*. Baltimore, MD: Clinical Psychometric Research.

Dworkin, R. H., Richlin, D. M., Handlin, D. S., & Brand, L. (1986). Predicting treatment response in depressed and non-depressed chronic pain patients. *Pain, 24*, 343–353.

Epker, J., & Block, A. R. (2001). Presurgical psychological screening in back pain patients: A review. *Clinical Journal of Pain, 17*, 200–205.

Eysenck, H. J., & Eysenck, S. B. G. (1975). *The manual of the Eysenck Personality Questionnaire*. London: Hodder & Stoughton.

Fairbank, J. C. T., Couper, J., Davies, J. B., & O'Brien, J. P. (1980). The Oswestry Low Back Pain Disability Questionnaire. *Physiotherapy, 66*, 271–273.

Folstein, M. F., Folstein, S. E., & McHugh, P. R. (1975). "Mini-Mental State": A practical method for grading the cognitive of patients for the clinician. *Journal of Psychiatric Research, 12*, 189–198.

Gatchel, R. J. (2001). A biopsychosocial overview of pretreatment screening of patients with pain. *Clinical Journal of Pain, 17*, 192–199.

Hart, R. P., Martelli, M. F., & Zasler, N. D. (2000). Chronic pain and neuropsychological functioning. *Neuropsychology Review, 10*, 1231–1249.

Hathaway, S. R., & McKinley, J. C. (1967). *The Minnesota Multiphasic Personality Inventory manual*. New York: Psychological Corporation.

Hathaway, S. R., McKinley, J. C., & Butcher, J. N. (1989). *The Minnesota Multiphasic Personality–2: Manual for administration*. Minneapolis: University of Minnesota Press.

Inman, T. H., & Berry, D. T. R. (2002). Cross-validation of indicators of malingering. A comparison of nine neuropsychological tests, four tests of malingering, and behavioral observations. *Archives of Clinical Neuropsychology, 17*, 1–23.

Jackson, D. N. (1989). *The Basic Personality Inventory: BPI manual* (pp. 1–80). Port Huron, MI: Research Psychologists Press.

Jensen, M. P., Karoly, P., & Huger, R. (1987). The development and preliminary validation of an instrument to assess patients' attitudes toward pain. *Journal of Psychosomatic Research, 31*, 393–400.

Jensen, M. P., Turner, J. A., Romano, J. M., & Lawler, B. K. (1994). Relationship of pain-specific beliefs to chronic pain adjustment. *Pain, 57*, 301–309.

Jensen, M. P., Romano, J. M., Turner, J. A., Good, A. B., & Wald, L. H. (1999). Patient beliefs predict patient functioning: Further support for a cognitive-behavioral model of chronic pain. *Pain, 81*, 95–104.

Keefe, F. J., Williams, D. A., & Smith, S. J. (2001). Assessment of pain behaviors. In D. C. Turk & R. Melzack (Eds.), *Handbook of pain assessment* (2nd ed., pp. 170–190). New York: Guilford Press.

Kerns, R. D., Turk, D. C., & Rudy, T. E. (1985). The West Haven–Yale Multidimensional Pain Inventory (WHYMPI). *Pain, 23*, 345–356.

Kolbison, D. A., Epstein, J. B., & Burgess, J. A. (1996). Temporomandibular disorders, headaches, and neck pain following motor vehicle accidents and the effects of litigation: Review of the literature. *Journal of Orofacial Pain, 10*, 101–125.

Linton, S. J. (1997). A population-based study of the relationship between sexual abuse and back pain: Establishing a link. *Pain, 73*, 47–53.

Lofland, K. R., Semenchuk, E. M., & Cassisi, J. E. (1995, November). *The Multidimensional Pain Inventory and symptom exaggeration in chronic low back pain patients.* Paper presented at the 14th Scientific Meeting of the American Pain Society, Los Angeles.

Mayfield, D., McLeod, G., & Hall, P. (1987). The CAGE questionnaire. *American Journal of Psychiatry, 131*, 1121–1123.

Melzack, R. (1975). The McGill Pain Questionnaire: Major properties and scoring methods. *Pain, 1*, 277–299.

Mendelson, G. (1986). Chronic pain and compensation: A review. *Journal of Pain and Symptom Management, 1*, 135–144.

Merskey, H. (1986). International Association for the Study of Pain, Subcommittee on Taxonomy, chronic pain syndromes and definitions of pain terms. *Pain, Suppl 3*, S1–S226.

Mikail, S. F., DuBreuil, S., & D'Eon, J. L. (1993). A comparative analysis of measures used in the assessment of chronic pain patients. *Psychological Assessment: Journal of Consulting and Clinical Psychology, 5*, 111–120.

Mikail, S. F., Henderson, P. R., & Tasca, G. A. (1994). An interpersonally based model of chronic pain: An application of attachment theory. *Clinical Psychology Review, 14*, 1–16.

Nelson, D. V., Kennington, M., Novy, D. M., & Squitieri, P. (1996). Psychological selection criteria for implantable spinal cord stimulators. *Pain Forum, 5*, 93–103.

Novy, D. M., Nelson, D. V., Berry, L. A., & Averill, P. M. (1995). What does the Beck Depression Inventory measure in chronic pain? A reappraisal. *Pain, 61*, 261–270.

Pfingsten, M., Hildebrandt, J., Leibing, E., Carment, F., & Saur, P. (1997). Effectiveness of a multimodal treatment program for chronic low-back pain. *Pain, 73*, 77–85.

Piotrowski, C. (1998). Assessment of pain: A survey of practicing clinicians. *Perceptual and Motor Skills, 86*, 181–182.

Pincus, T., Callahan, L. F., Bradley, L. A., Vaughn, W. K., & Wolfe, F. (1986). Elevated MMPI scores for hypochondriasis, depression, and hysteria in patients with rheumatoid arthritis reflect disease rather than psychological status. *Arthritis and Rheumatism, 29*, 1456–1466.

Poole, G. D., & Craig, K. D. (1992). Judgments of genuine, suppressed, and faked expressions of pain. *Journal of Personality and Social Psychology, 63*, 797–805.

Prager, J., & Jacobs, M. (2001). Evaluation of patients for implantable pain modalities: Medical and behavioral assessment. *Clinical Journal of Pain, 17*, 206–214.

Richards, J. S., Nepomuceno, C., Riles, M., & Suer, Z. (1982). Assessing pain behavior: The UAB Pain Behavior Scale. *Pain, 14*, 393–398.

Robinson, J. P., Turk, D. C., & Aulet, M. R. (2002). Impairment Impact Inventory (I^3): Preliminary psychometric evaluation. *Journal of Pain, 3*(suppl. 1), 657.

Robinson, M. E., O'Connor, P. D., Riley, J. L., Kvaal, S. A., & Shirley, F. R. (1994). Variability of isometric and isotonic leg exercise: Utility for detection of submaximal efforts. *Journal of Occupational Rehabilitation, 4*, 163–169.

Robinson, M. E., & Riley, J. L. III. (2001). Presurgical psychological screening. In D. C. Turk & R. Melzack (Eds.), *Handbook of pain assessment* (2nd ed., pp. 385–399). New York: Guilford Press.

Robinson, R. C., Gatchel, R. J., Polatin, P., Deschner, M., Noe, C., & Gajraj, N. (2001). Screening for problematic prescription opioid use. *Clinical Journal of Pain, 17*, 220–228.

Rohling, M. L., Binder, L. M., & Langhinrichsen-Rohling, J. (1995). Money matters: A meta-analytic review of the association between financial compensation and the experience and treatment of chronic pain. *Health Psychology, 14*, 537–547.

Rosenstiel, A. K., & Keefe, F. J. (1983). The use of coping strategies in low-back pain patients: Relationship to patient characteristics and current adjustment. *Pain, 17*, 33–40.

Schade, V., Semmer, N., Main, C. J., Hora, J., & Boos, N. (1999). The impact of clinical, morphological, psychosocial and work-related factors on the outcome of lumbar discectomy. *Pain, 80*, 239–249.

Schofferman, J., Anderson, D., Hines, R., Smith, G., & White, A. (1992). Childhood psychological trauma correlates with unsuccessful lumbar spine surgery. *Spine, 17*(6 suppl.), S138–144.

Slosar, P. J., Reynolds, J. B., Schofferman, J., Goldthwaite, N., White, A. H., & Keaney, D. (2000). Patient satisfaction after circumferential lumbar fusion. *Spine, 25*, 722–726.

Spanier, G. B. (1976). Measuring dyadic adjustment: New scales for assessing the quality of marriage and similar dyads. *Journal of Marriage and the Family, 38*, 15–28.

Stone, A. A., Briderick, J. E., Porter, L. S., & Kaell, A. T. (1997). The experience of rheumatoid arthritis pain and fatigue: Examining momentary reports and correlates over one week. *Arthritis Care and Research, 10*, 185–192.

Tait, R. C., Chibnall, J. T., & Krause, S. (1990). The Pain Disability Index: Psychometric properties. *Pain, 40*, 171–182.

Turk, D. C. (1990). Customizing treatment for chronic patients who, what, and why. *Clinical Journal of Pain, 6*, 255–270.

Turk, D. C. (1996a). Biopsychosocial perspective on chronic pain. In R. Gatchel & D. C. Turk (Eds.), *Psychological approaches to chronic pain management: A practitioners' handbook* (pp. 3–33). New York: Guilford Press.

Turk, D. C. (1996b). Clinician attitudes about prolonged use of opioids and the issue of patient heterogeneity. *Journal of Pain and Symptom Management, 11*, 218–230.

Turk, D. C. (1997). Transition from acute to chronic pain: Role of demographic and psychosocial factors. In T. S. Jensen, J. A. Turner, & Z. Wiesenfeld-Hallin (Eds.), *Proceedings of the 8th World Congress on Pain, Progress in pain research and management* (pp. 185–213). Seattle, WA: IASP Press.

Turk, D. C. (2002). Clinical effectiveness and cost effectiveness of treatments for chronic pain patients. *Clinical Journal of Pain, 18*, 355–365.

Turk, D. C., & Melzack, R. (Eds.). (2001). *Handbook of pain assessment* (2nd ed.). New York: Guilford Press.

Turk, D. C., & Monarch, E. S. (2002). Biopsychosocial perspective on chronic pain. In D. C. Turk & R. J. Gatchel (Eds.), *Psychological approaches to chronic pain management: A practitioners' handbook* (2nd ed., pp. 3–29). New York: Guilford Press.

Turk, D. C., Monarch, E. S., & Williams, A. D. (2002). Psychological evaluation of patients diagnosed with fibromyalgia syndrome: Comprehensive approach. *Rheumatic Disease Clinics of North America, 28,* 219–233.

Turk, D. C., & Okifuji, A. (2002). Psychological factors in chronic pain: Evolution and revolution. *Journal of Consulting and Clinical Psychology, 70,* 678–690.

Turk, D. C., Okifuji, A., Sinclair, J. D., & Starz, T. W. (1998a). Interdisciplinary treatment for fibromyalgia syndrome: Clinical and statistical significance. *Arthritis Care and Research, 11,* 186–195.

Turk, D. C., Okifuji, A., Sinclair, J. D., & Starz, J. D. (1998b). Differential responses by psychosocial subgroups of fibromyalgia syndrome patients to an interdisciplinary treatment. *Arthritis Care and Research, 111,* 397–404.

Turk, D. C., Robinson, J. R., & Aulet, M. R. (2002). Impairment Impact Inventory (I^3): Comparison of responses by treatment-seekers and claimants undergoing independent medical examinations. *Journal of Pain, 3*(suppl. 1), 1 [602].

Turk, D. C., Robinson, J. R., Cocchiarella, L., & Hunt, S. (2001). Pain. In L. Cocchiarella & S. Lord (Eds.), *Master the AMA Guides 5th, A medical and legal transition to the Guides to the Evaluation of Permanent Impairment* (pp. 277–325). Chicago: AMA Press.

Turk, D. C., & Rudy, T. E. (1988). Toward an empirically-derived taxonomy of chronic pain patients: Integration of psychological assessment data. *Journal of Consulting and Clinical Psychology, 56,* 233–238.

Turk, D. C., & Rudy, T. E. (1990). Robustness of an empirically derived taxonomy of chronic pain patients. *Pain, 43,* 27–36.

Turk, D. C., Rudy, T. E., Kubinski, J. A., Zaki, H. S., & Greco, C. M. (1996). Dysfunctional TMD patients: Evaluating the efficacy of a tailored treatment protocol. *Journal of Consulting and Clinical Psychology, 64,* 139–146.

Turk, D. C., Sist, T. C., Okifuji, A., Miner, M. F., Florio, G., Harrison, P., Massey, J., Lema, M. L., & Zevon, M. A. (1998). Adaptation to metastatic cancer pain, regional/local cancer pain and non-cancer pain: Role of psychological and behavioral factors. *Pain, 74,* 247–256.

von Korff, M. (1992). Epidemiologic and survey methods: Chronic pain assessment. In D. C. Turk & R. Melzack (Eds.), *Handbook of pain assessment* (pp. 391–408). New York: Guilford Press.

Waddell, G., McCulloch, J. A., Kummel, E., & Venner, R. M. (1980). Nonorganic physical signs in low-back pain. *Spine, 5,* 117–125.

Williams, D. A., & Thorn, B. E. (1989). An empirical assessment of pain beliefs. *Pain, 36,* 351–358.

Williams, J. (1998). The malingering of memory disorder. In C. Reynolds (Ed.), *Detection of malingering during head injury litigation* (pp. 127–143). New York: Plenum Press.

9

Psychological Interventions for Acute Pain

Stephen Bruehl
Ok Yung Chung
Department of Anesthesiology,
Vanderbilt University School of Medicine

The importance of optimizing the clinical management of acute pain has been increasingly recognized (Carr & Goudas, 1999). For example, in the context of surgery, providing adequate acute pain control minimizes length of stay and improves outcomes (Kiecolt-Glaser, Page, Marucha, MacCallum, & Glaser, 1998; Ballantyne et al., 1998). Several factors may account for these beneficial effects. Postsurgical pain and associated psychological stress can have negative effects on the immune system and endocrine function that impact on recovery (Kiecolt-Glaser et al., 1998). Moreover, uncontrolled nociceptive input may over time result in pathological changes in the central nervous system that could contribute to pain chronicity (e.g., Gracely, Lynch, & Bennett, 1992). This central sensitization phenomenon may help explain findings that greater acute pain severity predicts transition to chronic pain (Murphy & Cornish, 1984), and that earlier aggressive management of acute pain may reduce the incidence of postsurgical chronic pain (Senturk et al., 2002). Overall, the results just described underscore the fact that effective management of acute postsurgical pain can have a significant impact on outcomes. Adequacy of pain control may also be an important issue to consider with regard to less invasive painful medical procedures. Optimal acute pain control in this latter context may increase tolerability of necessary procedures and impact on willingness to engage in similar procedures in the future (e.g., Wardle, 1983).

Although some clinical acute pain stimuli clearly call for pharmacological intervention due to their severity (surgery), for other clinical sources of acute pain, such as injections and painful diagnostic procedures, exclusive reliance on pharmacological interventions may not be considered necessary or desirable given the brief duration of the pain, risk of side effects, or need for patients' conscious awareness (e.g., Faymonville et al., 1995). Various psychologically based pain management interventions have been described for use in common clinical situations that result in acute pain (e.g., burn debridement, labor, medical diagnostic procedures, venipuncture, dental procedures, and surgery). Although not intended to be an exhaustive review of the literature, this chapter describes a number of the techniques available and will overview evidence for their efficacy based on controlled clinical trials. Studies examining use of these interventions in comparison to or in conjunction with pharmacological analgesia will be summarized. Finally, issues involved in the practical use of such interventions in the clinical setting will be addressed.

TYPES OF INTERVENTIONS

Substantial research following the gate control theory of pain described by Melzack and Wall (1965) has confirmed the presence of descending neurophysiological pathways through which psychological states can either exacerbate or inhibit afferent nociceptive input and the experience of pain. Although extreme emotional distress may be associated with stress-induced analgesia (Millan, 1986), at less extreme levels, greater emotional distress is generally associated with increased acute pain intensity (Graffenreid, Adler, Abt, Nuesch, & Spiegel, 1978; Litt, 1996; Sternbach, 1974; Zelman, Howland, Nichols, & Cleeland, 1991). Psychological strategies for managing acute pain therefore often intervene at the cognitive and physiological level to reduce distress and arousal that may lead to heightened experience of acute pain (Bruehl, Carlson, & McCubbin, 1993). In addition, the simple fact that a specific pain management technique has been provided is likely to increase patients' perceived sense of control, which also appears to be an important factor in reducing negative responses to painful stimuli (Litt, 1988; Weisenberg, 1987). Available psychological techniques for management of acute pain can be broadly categorized into information provision, relaxation and related techniques, and cognitive strategies (e.g., VanDalfsen & Syrjala, 1990). Although some interventions, such as information provision, are primarily preemptive and designed to minimize pain by preparing the patient for what will be experienced, others such as relaxation techniques may be useful both preemptively and for reducing acute pain as the patient is experiencing it. Common psychological pain management techniques are summarized in Table 9.1.

TABLE 9.1
Psychological Interventions for Acute Pain

Type of intervention	Intervention	Comments
Information provision	Sensory information Procedural information	Intended to reduce unrealistic anxiety-provoking expectations that increase pain. Effectively administered by videotape.
Relaxation related	Breathing relaxation	Simplest relaxation technique to implement.
	Progressive muscle relaxation	Effective but may require repeated training/practice sessions.
	Imagery	Can use scripted, patient-developed, or memory-based relaxing imagery. Most effective if it involves multiple senses.
	Hypnosis	Combines elements of relaxation and imagery + suggestions of analgesia or sensory transformation.
Cognitive	Positive coping self-statements (e.g., "I can handle this, it will be over soon, just relax")	Focused on reducing catastrophic cognitions that lead to elevated distress and pain.
	Distraction	Includes visual or auditory stimuli, or mental and behavioral tasks that divert attention away from pain. Easy to implement routinely.
	Sensory focus	Encourages focus on the sensations of the procedure being experienced. Prevents activation of emotional schema that may increase pain sensation.

Information Provision

Two common information provision strategies target the sensations (e.g., "stinging," "sharp") and the specific procedures that patients will experience during the painful stimulus. Both strategies are based on a presumption that providing accurate information in advance regarding the sensations and procedures that will be experienced will prevent development of inaccurate and fearful expectations that would otherwise elicit excessive anxiety and lead to increased pain sensations (Ludwick-Rosenthal & Neufeld, 1988). Frequently, such interventions are conducted via videotape. For example, videotaped information provision interventions may portray the process of a real patient undergoing and coping well with the medical procedure of interest (Doering et al., 2000; Shipley, Butt, & Horwitz, 1979). Scripted in-person presentations may also be used to describe the procedures and sensations the patient will be undergoing (Reading, 1982). To be effective, information provision interventions must be specific to the particular clinical procedure that the patient will be undergoing.

Relaxation and Related Techniques

A variety of relaxation-related techniques are available that may have a positive impact on the pain experience. Although these techniques may be used to reduce anticipatory distress prior to the onset of pain and thereby diminish subsequent pain responsiveness, they are most effective when patients are able to practice them successfully during exposure to the painful stimulus. If training and practice time are too limited, clinical experience indicates that anxiety and acute pain itself may interfere with patient's ability to utilize the intervention. Various relaxation-related interventions differ in the amount of preparation time required.

Deep, slow, and/or patterned breathing is one of the simplest methods of relaxation, and is designed to decrease somatic input (e.g., muscle tension), autonomic arousal, and anxiety (Cogan & Kluthe, 1981; Harris et al., 1976). For example, patients may receive instruction in use of breath counting as a means of pacing respiration to a lower rate (e.g., six breaths per minute; Bruehl et al., 1993). Slowing respiration rate has been shown to diminish autonomic arousal and anxiety (Harris et al., 1976). Adoption of an abdominal breathing pattern rather than a high chest pattern is also often incorporated into this type of relaxation strategy. Breathing-focused relaxation has the advantage of being brief and easy for patients to learn.

Other traditional relaxation techniques may require more instruction and practice time to be effective. Progressive muscle relaxation (PMR) has been shown to be a useful technique for reducing physiological arousal and anxiety, and appears to be effective even in somewhat abbreviated form (Carlson & Hoyle, 1993). PMR, which can be provided in person or using an audiotaped protocol, involves systematic and sequential tensing and releasing of specific muscle groups throughout the body (Jacobson, 1938). An initial in-person session of PMR training with follow-up practice using audiotaped PMR procedures appears to be an efficient and effective means of providing this intervention (Carlson & Hoyle, 1993). For example, three sessions of PMR lasting approximately 25 minutes per session (one in person and two audiotaped) have been shown to be sufficient to permit individuals to apply the relaxation technique and successfully reduce physiological responses under stress (McCubbin et al., 1996). Interestingly, this latter work indicates that PMR may exert its stress buffering effects in part through endogenous opioid mechanisms, which may also be associated with analgesia (McCubbin et al., 1996; Millan, 1986).

Another option for inducing a relaxed state is imagery-based interventions. As with PMR, a guided imagery intervention can be conducted using audiotaped instructions. Imagery instructions are usually designed to help patients develop a detailed mental image of a relaxing place on which to focus their attention during the painful procedure. The imagery can be provided by the therapist, or patients may be assisted in developing their own unique imagery, with the latter technique preferable. Imagery is likely to be most effective at eliciting relaxation when it incorporates multiple senses (i.e., visual, auditory, olfactory, tactile; Turk, Meichenbaum, & Genest, 1983). A related relaxation strategy is the use of memory-based positive emotion induction procedures (Bruehl et al., 1993). This brief technique anchors a patient's imagery in a memory of a specific event that is associated with a positive emotional state, and also involves as many senses as possible. All imagery-based strategies are likely to incorporate aspects of distraction as well as producing a relaxed, positive emotional state.

Various hypnotic techniques have also been applied to management of acute pain. These techniques incorporate aspects of both traditional relaxation procedures and imagery training, in combination with suggestions. Suggestions may be intended to induce analgesia ("your hand is insensitive, like a piece of rubber") or to transform the pain to a non-painful sensation, such as warmth or heaviness (Farthing, Venturino, Brown, & Lazar, 1997; Wright & Drummond, 2000). Hypnotic interventions are generally administered by a trained therapist rather than by audiotape. Nursing and other staff can be trained to administer this type of intervention, although a significant initial investment in time may be required, including classroom instruction, role playing, and supervised practice (Lang et al., 2000).

Cognitive Strategies

Several acute pain management interventions derive from cognitive behavioral theory (Turk et al., 1983). Catastrophizing cognitions regarding pain (e.g., "I can't stand it!" or "This is horrible!") have been shown to be associated with greater perceived pain intensity (Buckelew et al., 1992; Jacobsen & Butler, 1996; Sullivan, Rodgers, & Kirsch, 2001). Recent research on pain expectancies suggests that catastrophizers tend a priori to underestimate the level of acute pain they will experience, possibly as a means of minimizing anticipatory distress (Sullivan et al., 2001). One mediator of the relationship between catastrophizing and pain may therefore be that this underestimation of the impending pain stimulus results in a failure to mobilize coping resources in advance of pain onset (Sullivan et al., 2001). This may result in an excessive focus on the unexpectedly intense pain sensations when they are experienced (Sullivan et al., 2001). Another mediator of the relationship between catastrophizing and pain is presumed to be the increased emotional distress elicited by catastrophizing cognitions (Buckelew et al., 1992; Rosenstiel & Keefe, 1983). By altering appraisal of the pain-provoking situation through use of coping self-statements both prior to and during the pain stimulus, catastrophic and magnifying cognitions that increase pain, distress, and arousal can be reduced or prevented. Coping self-statement interventions educate patients regarding the negative impact of catastrophizing cognitions, and teach as an alternative the conscious engagement in positive coping self-statements during acute pain (e.g., "I can handle this," "The discomfort will go away quickly," "Just relax").

Sensory focus is another cognitive strategy that has been applied to acute pain. This strategy is based on theoretical work indicating that the cognitive schema used in interpreting pain stimuli can be either sensation focused or emotion focused, with activation of the latter type of schema more likely to lead to a more intense pain experience (Leventhal, Brown, Shacham, & Enquist, 1979). Based on this theory, sensory focus interventions encourage patients to focus exclusively on the sensations they are experiencing, thereby preventing activation of the emotional schema and resulting in a less intense pain experience (Logan, Baron, & Kohut, 1995).

Distraction is another common cognitive strategy used for management of acute pain. Distraction techniques may include listening to music (Lee et al., 2002; Fratianne, Presner, Huston, Super, & Yowler, 2001), attending to distracting visual stimuli such as a kaleidoscope (Cason & Grissom, 1997; Frere, Crout, Yorty, & McNeil, 2001), immersion in a virtual reality environment (Hoffman, Patterson, & Carrougher, 2000; Hoffman, Patterson, Carrougher, & Sharar, 2001), or engaging in any other distracting activity, such as blowing on a party blower, finger tapping, or playing a video game (Cogan & Kluthe, 1981; Corah, Gale, & Illig, 1979; Manne et al., 1990). Distraction techniques consume part of an individual's limited capacity for attention, thereby reducing the attentional resources that can be directed at the painful stimulus (McCaul & Malott, 1984). Review of the distraction literature indicates that it is more likely to be effective for brief and lower intensity pain, and become less effective as the stimulus becomes longer lasting or more intense (McCaul & Malott, 1984). Moreover, distraction techniques that require more attentional capacity appear to inhibit the experience of pain more than techniques requiring less attentional capacity (McCaul & Malott, 1984). For brief clinical pain of relatively low intensity, regular implementation of distraction techniques may be pragmatically appealing, given the low degree of effort required to provide them.

CONTROLLED TRIALS

Laboratory Studies

Studies using controlled laboratory stimuli as an analog of acute clinical pain have evaluated the efficacy of psychological acute pain interventions presumably under ideal conditions—intervention procedures are well standardized with no limitations on amount of time and effort that can be invested in implementing the techniques. Laboratory studies indicate that specific psychological interventions including distraction (Clum, Luscomb, & Scott, 1982; Fanurik, Zeltzer, Roberts, & Blount, 1993; Farthing et al., 1997), relaxation (Anseth, Berntzen, & Gotestam, 1985; Clum et al., 1982; Cogan & Kluthe, 1981), positive emotion induction (Bruehl et al., 1993; Zelman et al., 1991), and positive coping self-statements (Avia & Kanfer, 1980) can reduce responsiveness to acute pain. Early qualitative reviews of the efficacy of various psychological techniques under controlled laboratory conditions indicate that there is at least modest support for the efficacy of such interventions (Tan, 1982; Weisenberg, 1987). Definitive conclusions from this literature are limited by the variety of interventions, acute pain stimuli used (e.g., cold pressor, ischemic, finger pressure), and different outcome measures employed (Tan, 1982). Although laboratory studies suggest that psychological interventions *can* be effective for reducing acute pain, they may tell little about whether these interventions *will* be effective in the clinical context due to the limited generalizability of laboratory analog studies. Selection of interventions for use in the clinical environment should therefore be based primarily on results of clinical trials.

Clinical Trials in Adults

Empirically supported generalizations regarding the efficacy of specific psychological interventions for clinical acute pain are made difficult by the number of different techniques used alone or in a variety of combinations, the multitude of clinical acute pain stimuli differing substantially in intensity, and the relatively small number of studies examining any one technique for use with any given type of clinical situation. For these and a variety of methodological reasons, truly integrative reviews of the clinical literature have been limited. For example, a qualitative review of randomized controlled trials (RCTs) of relaxation techniques (limited to those studies in which relaxation was not combined with other techniques) for use in postsurgical and procedural acute pain settings identified only seven such studies that reported on pain outcomes (Seers & Carroll, 1998). An equal number of studies were found that reported only on distress-related outcomes, which do not necessarily correspond directly with pain outcomes

(Seers & Carroll, 1998). Results of this review indicated only weak evidence for efficacy of relaxation techniques in such settings, with only three of seven studies detecting significant pain-reducing effects of relaxation training (Seers & Carroll, 1998). Negative results do not appear to be unique to relaxation interventions, given that work examining combined interventions incorporating relaxation, distraction, and imagery (for knee arthrogram pain) has also described negative results (Tan & Poser, 1982). An important conclusion drawn from the review by Seers and Carroll (1998) is that small sample sizes are a common problem in relaxation-related RCTs, a conclusion that aptly describes the broader literature on psychological interventions as well. Therefore, lack of statistical power may often account for the negative results obtained. Despite findings such as those just described that might suggest that psychological interventions for acute pain are of questionable efficacy, other RCTs suggest that psychological interventions may be useful for some types of acute clinical pain. Results of several RCTs are next reviewed, organized by type of clinical setting.

Labor Pain

One of the earliest clinical applications of psychologically based interventions for acute pain was the use of the Lamaze technique for labor pain. The Lamaze approach incorporates elements of sensory and procedural information provision in addition to training in controlled breathing for purposes of relaxation and distraction. Controlled trials indicate that this technique is effective for reducing the pain associated with delivery (Leventhal, Leventhal, Shacham, & Easterling, 1989; Scott & Rose, 1976), and that it reduces analgesic requirements during childbirth (Scott & Rose, 1976). Work by Leventhal et al. (1989) indicates that repeated encouragement to focus on the sensations of labor contractions (a sensory focus intervention) may also contribute to reduced pain and distress during childbirth.

Burn Management

Studies in patients undergoing burn debridement, which can be associated with intense pain, suggest that very different psychological interventions may be effective (Fratianne et al., 2001; Wright & Drummond, 2000). An intervention combining music distraction with controlled breathing instructions resulted in significant reductions in self-reported pain during debridement relative to a same-subject control condition (Fratianne et al., 2001). Similarly, a hypnotic intervention including elements of relaxation, imagery, and suggestions of analgesia resulted in significantly lower ratings of pain during burn debridement compared to a "usual care" control group (Wright & Drummond, 2000). The significant treatment effects in the latter study were obtained even though the "rapid induction analgesia" intervention required only a single 15-minute session to implement (Wright & Drummond, 2000). In both of the studies just mentioned, routine analgesic medications (e.g., morphine sulfate) were administered to all patients prior to debridement. Results such as these indicate that even when acute pain is relatively intense, brief combined psychological interventions may have significant pain-reducing effects beyond that provided by standard analgesic regimens.

Physical therapy in burn patients may also be associated with significant acute pain. A novel application of virtual reality (VR) for pain reduction during physical therapy in such patients has recently been described (Hoffman et al., 2000, 2001). Although results to date are based on only a small number of patients, this technique appears to be encouraging. For example, a randomized crossover trial in 12 burn patients revealed that patients experienced significantly less pain during physical therapy while immersed in a computer-generated VR environment than when not experiencing VR (Hoffman et al., 2000). The magnitude of this effect was notable, with reductions in pain-related cognitions during physical therapy from 60/100mm (on a visual analog scale) in the no-intervention condition to 14/100mm during VR (Hoffman et al., 2000). Other similar work by these researchers (in seven burn patients) has confirmed the efficacy of this VR intervention, and further suggests that its efficacy does not diminish significantly with repeated use (Hoffman et al., 2001). As access to VR technology improves, these promising results suggest that further investigation of VR interventions may be worthwhile.

Nonsurgical Medical Procedures

Psychological interventions have demonstrated some evidence in RCTs of utility for controlling the acute pain associated with several medical diagnostic procedures. In one such study, an audiotaped relaxation intervention resulted in significantly lower self-reported pain intensity and significantly less analgesic medication requested during femoral angiography compared to both no-treatment controls and a music distraction control group (Mandle et al., 1990). Pain ratings for the music distraction group in this study were no different than those reported by no-intervention controls (Mandle et al., 1990). An RCT conducted in patients undergoing painful electromyographic examination also indicated that relaxation training (combining PMR and deep breathing), a positive coping statement intervention, and the combination of these interventions resulted in significantly lower pain, distress, and physiological arousal than exhibited by patients in a no-treatment control condition (Kaplan, Metzger, & Jablecki, 1983). This study indicated that both the relaxation and coping statement interventions were equally effective (Kaplan et al., 1983).

Acute pain that is less severe and of briefer duration, such as that associated with phlebotomy, may also be amenable to modification with simple
psychological interventions. Cason and Grissom (1997) reported that simple distraction through use of a kaleidoscope was sufficient to reduce the
intensity of phlebotomy-associated pain significantly compared to a no-
intervention control group.

Other studies of pain associated with medical procedures reveal mixed
results. Although no effect was observed on pain intensity, results of an
RCT of a combined music distraction/relaxation intervention for patients
undergoing colonoscopy indicated that the intervention resulted in significantly less self-administration of sedative medication compared to a group
receiving self-administered medication alone (Lee et al., 2002). In contrast, a
relatively large-scale RCT reported by Gaston-Johansson et al. (2000) revealed no apparent beneficial effects of psychological intervention for pain
associated with autologous bone marrow transplantation. A combined intervention including information provision, relaxation, imagery, and positive coping self-statements demonstrated no significant effects on pain or
distress compared to a no-intervention control condition (Gaston-Johansson et al., 2000). These negative results occurred despite having a sample
size larger than in many such studies (total $n = 110$). Moreover, results were
negative despite what appears to be a thorough intervention, including in-
person relaxation and imagery training, information provision, and use of
an audiotape for home relaxation practice, all provided well before the
scheduled procedure to allow adequate practice time (Gaston-Johansson et
al., 2000). The fact that fatigue and nausea were both significantly reduced
by the intervention suggest that the lack of effect on pain experienced was
not due to failure to utilize the intervention. In light of the generally positive
results of other RCTs, the lack of efficacy of the combined intervention in
this study is somewhat surprising. These results indicate that interventions
that should be effective sometimes fail for unclear reasons, possibly related
to the specific nature of the acute pain stimulus, patient population (i.e.,
breast cancer patients in this study) or an interaction of the type of intervention with patient variables (see below).

Dental Procedures

Psychological interventions for acute pain have also been applied to the
discomfort associated with dental procedures. As in other clinical settings,
relaxation techniques and distraction interventions (playing videogames)
have been shown in RCTs to reduce the discomfort associated with dental
procedures (Corah et al., 1979; Corah, Gale, Pace, & Seyrek, 1981). Other
types of interventions may have efficacy in dental patients as well. Croog
and colleagues (Croog, Baume, & Nalbandian, 1994) conducted a controlled

trial of patients undergoing repeated periodontal surgery. A coping self-statement intervention designed to increase perceived control over the aversive sequelae of the surgery resulted in significantly lower reports of pain following surgery relative to a no-intervention control group (Croog et al., 1994). Other work indicates that provision of sensory information about dental procedures, but not a visual distraction intervention, resulted in significantly decreased discomfort during "routine dental treatment" compared to a no-intervention control group (Wardle, 1983).

Other types of psychological interventions may have utility in the dental arena as well. Logan et al. (1995) and Baron, Logan, and Hoppe (1993) reported that a sensory focus intervention resulted in significantly reduced pain during root canal procedures compared to no-intervention controls. Provision of procedural information alone did not result in decreased pain intensity (Logan et al., 1995). A similar RCT by these researchers examined the efficacy of a combined intervention, including controlled breathing, videotaped modeling of successful coping, and control-enhancing statements, finding that the intervention resulted in lower pain levels compared to a neutral videotape control condition in patients undergoing various dental procedures (Law, Logan, & Baron, 1994). It is important to note that the pain-ameliorating effects in each of these three studies occurred only among patients with a high desire for control and a low level of perceived control (Baron et al., 1993; Law et al., 1994; Logan et al., 1995).

Postsurgical Pain

Of the various clinical sources of acute pain described in this chapter, interventions focused on postsurgical pain may have the potential for the greatest health impact. Even minor surgery can be perceived as a highly threatening experience (Kiecolt-Glaser et al., 1998), and the often intense acute pain accompanying surgical procedures is a major source of stress for recovering patients. Inadequately controlled pain and stress during the postsurgical period may interfere significantly in the recovery process (Ballantyne et al., 1998; Carr & Goudas, 1999; Kiecolt-Glaser et al., 1998). RCTs of psychological interventions suggest that such interventions may have beneficial effects in some post-surgical settings.

Several studies have examined the use of psychological interventions for the pain associated with colorectal surgery. An RCT of an audiotaped intervention including relaxation instructions and positive coping imagery/suggestions indicated that the intervention significantly reduced pain, distress, and analgesic use in patients undergoing colorectal surgery (Manyande et al., 1995). In a similar study, an audiotaped intervention combining relaxing imagery with calming music reportedly result in a nonsignificant trend (p .07) towards decreased pain relative to standard care among patients undergoing colorectal surgery (Renzi, Peticca, & Pescatori, 2000). Duration of exposure to the intervention may be one key to successful use of such techniques. Tusek and colleagues (Tusek, Church, & Fazio, 1997) reported that in a sample of colorectal surgery patients, an audiotaped intervention combining relaxing imagery with calming music, which was provided 3 days preoperatively, intraoperatively, and 6 days postoperatively, resulted in a significant reduction in postoperative pain intensity and a nearly 50% decrease in analgesic requirements during the postoperative period compared to a standard care group.

Interventions that prove effective for one type of surgical situation are not necessarily always effective for other surgical situations. In contrast to the positive results above regarding colorectal surgery, RCTs of interventions including relaxation techniques, distraction, and coping self-statements suggest that such techniques are of limited benefit in patients undergoing coronary artery bypass graft surgery (Ashton et al., 1997; Miller & Perry, 1990; Postlethwaite, Stirling, & Peck, 1986). Result of these studies revealed significant reductions in analgesic requirements in only one of the three studies (Ashton et al., 1997), and no differences in rated pain intensity in any study compared to no-intervention controls (Ashton et al., 1997; Miller & Perry, 1990; Postlethwaite, Stirling, & Peck, 1986). An RCT of an audiotaped relaxation intervention in patients undergoing total knee or hip replacement revealed similar negative results, producing no decrease in reported pain or analgesic requirements compared to patients getting surgical education information (Daltroy, Morlino, Eaton, Poss, & Liang, 1998). The authors of this latter study noted problems in being able to provide patients with the relaxation instructions sufficiently in advance of surgery to allow practice of the skills: Only 65% of patients reported practicing the technique at least once prior to surgery (Daltroy et al., 1998). This level of noncompliance may be a common occurrence in surgical situations in which minimally supervised audiotaped interventions are used.

Results of several RCTs in various other surgical settings do provide some support for use of adjunctive psychological interventions for acute pain. For example, a large-scale RCT ($n = 500$) comparing audiotaped relaxation (jaw relaxation and controlled breathing), music, and combined relaxation/music to a no-intervention control among patients undergoing major abdominal surgery reported positive results (Good et al., 1999). Patients in all three treatment groups reported lower pain intensity and distress than controls across both postsurgical days examined (Good et al., 1999). In another large-scale study ($n = 241$), patients undergoing percutaneous vascular and renal surgical procedures who received a combined intervention including relaxing imagery, muscle relaxation, and positive coping self-statements reported significantly less pain and used significantly less analgesic medication than did standard care controls (Lang et al., 2000). The intervention in the Lang et al. (2000) study was administered in person during the procedure by trained therapists, rather than through audiotaped instructions alone as in the Good et al. (1999) study. It may be of clinical relevance that both interventions significantly reduced pain despite differing substantially in the amount of staff time required. RCTs of patients undergoing various other types of surgery (e.g., cholecystectomy, herniorrhaphy, nephrectomy, laparotomy, hysterectomy) further confirm that various relaxation techniques (muscle relaxation, controlled breathing, relaxing imagery) can reduce postoperative pain and analgesic consumption (Daake & Gueidner, 1989; Flaherty & Fitzpatrick, 1978; Miro & Raich, 1999).

In contrast to the numerous studies of relaxation-related and cognitive interventions in the surgical context, information provision interventions have received fewer controlled tests with regard to postsurgical pain outcomes. However, similar results have been reported in two such RCTs (Doering et al., 2000; Reading, 1982). An information provision intervention (sensory and procedural) delivered in person to patients undergoing gynecological laparoscopic surgery did not reduce pain levels postsurgically compared to no-intervention controls (Reading, 1982). Despite this lack of effect on pain reports, a behavioral effect was observed, with intervention-group patients requesting significantly fewer analgesic medications (Reading, 1982). More recently, Doering and colleagues examined the efficacy of a procedural information videotape intervention in patients undergoing hip replacement surgery (Doering et al., 2000). Results of this RCT also revealed no significant effects on pain intensity ratings, although like the Reading (1982) study, significant reductions in analgesic requirements were observed (Doering et al., 2000). Results of studies such as these indicate some potential postsurgical benefit of information provision interventions.

Clinical Trials in Children

Although not a primary focus of this chapter, it is important to note that psychological interventions appear to have benefit in the control of acute pain associated with medical procedures in children as well as adults. A meta-analysis (total of 19 studies) of the effects of techniques including distraction, relaxation, and imagery on acute pain experienced during medical procedures in children indicated a significant overall clinical effect, with children receiving interventions on average reporting pain levels 0.6 standard deviations below those reported by no-intervention controls (Kleiber & Harper, 1999).

Children required to undergo repeated lumbar punctures or bone-marrow aspirations as part of cancer treatment have been the focus of a number of the available RCTs. These studies indicate the efficacy of combined interventions, including breathing relaxation, imagery, and distraction, for reducing the pain associated with such procedures (Jay, Elliott, Katz, & Siegel, 1987; Jay, Elliott, Woody, & Siegel, 1991; Jay, Elliott, Fitzgibbons, Woody, & Siegel, 1995; Kazak et al., 1996; Kazak, Penati, Brophy, & Himelstein, 1998). These pain reductions appear to be clinically meaningful: Children receiving such a combined intervention reported 25% less pain than children in an attentional control group (Jay et al., 1987).

Psychological interventions may also be effective for less intense but more common sources of acute clinical pain in children. For example, a simple distraction intervention (use of a kaleidoscope) resulted in significantly reduced pain and distress associated with venipuncture relative to a group given simple comforting responses by clinicians (Vessey, Carlson, & McGill, 1994). Despite positive results such as these, other studies examining distraction and controlled breathing interventions for venipuncture pain indicate selective effects, reducing emotional distress during venipuncture but not affecting pain intensity significantly (Blount et al., 1992; Manne et al., 1990). As a whole, controlled trials in children do suggest some benefit to the use of psychological interventions for acute pain.

COMPARISONS WITH PHARMACOLOGICAL PAIN MANAGEMENT

The results of several of the outcome studies just reviewed indicate that psychological interventions used in conjunction with pharmacological approaches may reduce the amount of such analgesic medications required (Ashton et al., 1997; Doering et al., 2000; Lang et al., 2000; Lee et al., 2002; Mandle et al., 1990; Manyande et al., 1995; Reading et al., 1982; Scott & Rose, 1976; Tusek et al., 1997). Direct comparisons of psychological to pharmacological techniques for acute pain management are rare and frequently suffer from methodological limitations, making interpretation difficult (Geden, Beck, Anderson, Kennish, & Mueller-Heinze, 1986; Kolk, van Hoof, & Dop, 2000; Schiff, Holtz, Peterson, & Rakusan, 2001).

In the context of relatively mild acute pain associated with venipuncture, evidence for the benefits of distraction interventions compared to topical anesthetic interventions is mixed. Work by Arts et al. (1994) indicated that children receiving a cream containing a eutectic mixture of local anesthetics (EMLA) reported significantly lower pain than did children receiving a music distraction intervention. A similar study also suggested no specific benefit (in terms of pain ratings) for a distraction intervention compared to a "standard care" condition, which frequently included EMLA cream (Kleiber, Craft-Rosenberg, & Harper, 2001). Other findings have been more positive. For children all of whom were provided with a distraction intervention, no differences in pain ratings were reported between those receiving EMLA versus those receiving placebo cream, suggesting no additive benefit of EMLA beyond distraction (Lal, McClelland, Phillips, Taub, & Beattie, 2001). Lack of statistical power does not account for the differences between these studies, as the study with the largest sample size ($n = 180$) reported the most negative results (Arts et al., 1994). These studies do not indicate whether other psychological strategies, such as brief relaxation or imagery, may have been more effective than distraction relative to the pharmacological approach. However, these studies suggest that for brief, low-intensity procedures in which simple pharmacological interventions with minimal side effects (e.g., EMLA) are likely to be effective, the incremental benefit of brief psychological techniques alone or in combination with pharmacological interventions appears questionable.

Several of the most methodologically sound controlled trials, all conducted in children, comparing psychological interventions with a pharmacological intervention have been reported by Jay and colleagues (1987, 1991, 1995). In the first such study (Jay et al., 1987), children undergoing repeated bone-marrow aspirations, serving as their own controls, underwent these procedures receiving a randomized sequence of three interventions: attention control, 0.3 mg/kg Valium only, and psychological intervention only (combining emotional imagery, breathing relaxation, and modeling of positive coping). Results indicated that the psychological intervention resulted in lower pain, distress, and physiological arousal than either the Valium or control conditions (Jay et al., 1987). A similar follow-up RCT by these researchers revealed identical effects on pain and arousal whether patients received a psychological intervention alone or in combination with Valium (Jay et al., 1991). Jay et al. (1995) also compared this same psychological intervention to light general anesthesia (halothane and nitrous oxide) in children undergoing repeated bone-marrow aspirations. Results indicated that general anesthesia was associated with less procedural distress, but no differences between interventions were observed regarding self-ratings of pain provided postprocedure. Subjects, all of whom received both types of pain intervention in the within-subject design, did not indicate a significant preference for one versus the other type of intervention, and it was noted that the psychological intervention required less time (Jay et al., 1995). As a whole, results of these well-controlled studies indicate that psychological interventions are of at least comparable efficacy to standard pharmacological approaches for management of the pain associated with bone-marrow aspiration in children.

It is important to note that such findings are not likely to generalize to all types of clinical acute pain. Clearly, procedures associated with more intense acute pain, such as even "minor" surgery, require pharmacological analgesia. However, the results reported earlier indicate that combining psychological and pharmacological approaches may have significant benefits to patients. This recommendation is consistent with controlled work by Kazak et al. (1996, 1998) suggesting that a behavioral intervention including breathing, distraction, and imagery combined with standard pharmacological interventions resulted in significantly reduced distress compared to standard pharmacological treatment alone in children undergoing repeated lumbar punctures or bone-marrow aspirations.

MODERATORS OF RESPONSES
TO PSYCHOLOGICAL INTERVENTIONS

Spontaneous Coping Strategies

Many individuals implement their own spontaneous pain coping strategies when faced with acute pain (Spanos et al., 1984; Zelman et al., 1991). The possibility that externally imposed interventions may interfere with patients' implementation of effective pain control strategies already in their behavioral repertoire cannot be ruled out. Although some studies suggest that these spontaneous coping strategies may be effective for pain reduction (Spanos et al., 1984), other controlled laboratory work suggests that structured interventions may be more effective than these spontaneous strategies (Bruehl et al., 1993).

Coping Style

Patients' preferred style of coping with stress, whether Monitoring or Blunting in character, may be relevant to understanding the efficacy of specific psychological acute pain interventions. Monitors, also referred to as Sensitizers or Vigilants, prefer to cope with stressful situations by seeking out information about the stimulus, and by monitoring and trying to mitigate their responses to the stimulus (Schultheis, Peterson, & Selby, 1987). Blunters, also termed Repressors, Avoiders, Distractors, or Deniers, prefer to cope with stressful situations through avoidance and by denial of the stressor (Schultheis et al., 1987).

A number of studies have hypothesized that psychological acute pain interventions work best if they match an individual's naturally preferred coping style. For example, providing a sensory focus intervention to a Blunter would be considered a mismatched intervention, whereas a relaxing imagery strategy would be considered a matched intervention for such an individual (Fanurick et al., 1993). Laboratory acute pain studies have provided some evidence indicating that interventions matched to preferred coping style result in more effective reductions in acute pain responsiveness (e.g., Fanurick et al., 1993; Rokke & al'Absi, 1992).

Clinical studies regarding this issue are mixed, but generally negative. Shipley and coworkers (Shipley et al., 1979) examined interactions between coping style and an information provision intervention for patients undergoing gastrointestinal endoscopy. Although there were no interaction effects regarding pain experienced during the procedures, Monitors were found to experience less distress in the information provision condition whereas Blunters experienced greater distress (Shipley et al., 1979). These results are consistent with the matching hypothesis. Studies performed in the context of more severe acute clinical pain, on the other hand, are more negative. In a study of general surgery patients, efficacy of information provision, relaxation, and no intervention was compared as a function of Monitoring and Blunting coping styles (Scott & Clum, 1984). Blunters reported less pain and used less analgesics when provided with no intervention, which appear at least not inconsistent with the matching hypothesis. However, contrary to the matching hypothesis, Monitors appeared to do best with breathing relaxation as opposed to information provision (Scott & Clum, 1984). Work by Wilson (1981) also in general surgery patients found that Blunters did not experience exacerbated pain following an information provision intervention, again failing to support the matching hypothesis. More recent work in surgical patients also indicated that efficacy of a relaxation intervention did not differ depending on the degree to which patients preferred a Monitoring coping style (Miro & Raich, 1999). Differences in the measures used to assess coping style, types of interventions employed, and other procedural details make comparisons across studies more difficult. However, clinical support for a coping style by intervention type matching hypothesis is at best weak. Moreover, the absence of validated clinical procedures for determining preferred coping style for purposes of selection of intervention type (e.g., empirically validated cutoffs on specific measures) makes coping style by intervention-type interactions more of an academic than a clinical issue.

Other Potential Moderators

As noted previously, there is evidence from several studies that interventions including sensory focus, breathing relaxation, and use of control-enhancing statements reduce the discomfort of dental procedures only among those with a high desire for control and a low level of perceived control prior to intervention (Baron et al., 1993; Law et al., 1994; Logan et al., 1995). Given the importance of perceived control in determining satisfaction with acute pain management (Pellino & Ward, 1998), these findings suggest that if resources for providing psychological acute pain interventions are limited, it may be most appropriate to focus these resources on individuals who express a desire for greater control over the acute pain experience.

Other authors have suggested that hypnotizability may also be an important moderator of treatment efficacy. Laboratory acute pain research has indicated that imagery, analgesia suggestions, and distraction were effective for reducing acute pain only among individuals high in hypnotizability (Farthing et al., 1997). This might not be considered surprising given that individuals high in hypnotizability may be more capable of developing vivid mental imagery (Farthing et al., 1997). As with coping style, validated clinical criteria for making treatment decisions based on assessment of hypnotizability are not available. Therefore, the practical clinical utility of this moderator variable is questionable.

BARRIERS TO EFFECTIVE CLINICAL USE OF PSYCHOLOGICAL INTERVENTIONS FOR ACUTE PAIN

If psychological interventions for acute pain can be clinically useful in some circumstances, as appears to be the case, what are the barriers to their use? A study by Jiang and colleagues (Jiang, Lagasse, Ciccone, Jakubowski, & Kitain, 2001) of hospital acute pain management practices indicated widespread underutilization of nonpharmacological techniques. A primary factor contributing to this underutilization was resource availability (Jiang et al., 2001). With the current focus on reduction of health care costs nationwide, cost containment becomes a major barrier to providing the trained personnel and staff time to implement many psychological pain management strategies in situations in which they have proven effective. Clearly, as described earlier, there are potential risks associated with inadequate control of acute post-surgical pain (e.g., delayed recovery, development of chronic pain; Kiecolt-Glaser et al., 1998; Murphy & Cornish, 1984; Senturk et al., 2002). Provision of psychologically based interventions in the context of an overall program for management of postsurgical pain may therefore be cost-effective in the long term. However, the short-term nature of the distress and pain associated with brief but painful medical and dental procedures may simply not be viewed as justifying the time and personnel costs needed to implement many psychological interventions for acute pain (Ludwick-Rosenthal & Neufeld, 1988). Moreover, the absence of a psychiatric diagnosis to justify provision of a psychological intervention, which is typically a requirement for purposes of insurance reimbursement, may be a practical barrier to having psychological acute pain interventions be administered by psychologically trained staff. Brief and simple techniques that can be implemented quickly either through automated procedures (e.g., audio or videotapes) or by staff already interacting with the patient (e.g., nursing staff) are those most likely to be of use clinically. For example, a memory-based positive emotion induction requiring less than 5 minutes of time has been shown to diminish acute pain sensitivity and pain-related physiological arousal, and could be carried out by nursing staff with limited training (Bruehl et al., 1993). Distraction techniques also require little effort to implement, and therefore may be more widely useful.

Our clinical experience indicates that unless significant skills acquisition and practice time are available prior to exposure to the acute pain situation, the benefits of using more elaborate interventions (e.g., progressive muscle relaxation training) are likely to be modest. Ideally, there would be sufficient contact time with the patient on a separate day prior to exposure to the pain stimulus for mutual selection of an acceptable intervention, for the intervention to be taught, and for patients to practice the skills on their own prior to the pain (using taped intervention instructions if appropriate). Such a situation may unfortunately be rare. If less time is available, it is important to select interventions that are reasonable for the patient to learn and practice adequately in the time that is available. Information provision and distraction interventions are most amenable to limited practice time, followed in (approximate) ascending order of difficulty by coping self-statement interventions, breathing relaxation, imagery techniques, hypnosis, progressive muscle relaxation, and combined approaches.

Patient acceptance and adherence may be another barrier to effective use of psychological interventions. Passive distraction techniques such as listening to relaxing music are likely to be accepted easily by patients. However, unless patients are provided with a compelling rationale for use of interventions that require active practice (e.g., relaxation training), they are unlikely to utilize the intervention approach during acute pain exposure even if training is provided. Even when intervention skills have been learned, results of a large-scale efficacy study of relaxation for postsurgical pain indicate that reminders to practice the technique are required for beneficial effects to be achieved (Good et al., 1999).

CONCLUSIONS

Results of controlled clinical trials testing the efficacy of psychological interventions for acute pain associated with burn management, labor, medical diagnostic procedures, venipuncture, dental procedures, and surgery suggest that these interventions are often effective for pain reduction and do not appear to be harmful. However, controlled trials have rarely tested the efficacy of individual strategies, but rather have examined various combinations of information-provision, relaxation-related, and cognitive strategies. It is therefore not possible to make determinations as to the clinical superiority of one type of intervention over another based on available trials. Audiotaped relaxation-related interventions do appear to be effective in some situations, although "live" intervention delivery by trained staff for the initial session is likely to optimize results if time and resources permit. There is little evidence to justify the use of psychological interventions as an alternative to standard pharmacological approaches, although there is much evidence that they have significant clinical utility in conjunction with pharmacological approaches. Although there are some indications that individual difference variables may impact on efficacy of various types of psychological interventions, there are insufficient data available to use individual difference variables for selection of optimal intervention types in routine clinical decision-making. Given the limitations of the available research, factors such as time constraints, resources, and patient preference are likely to be the most useful in selection of interventions.

ACKNOWLEDGMENT

The authors gratefully acknowledge the assistance of Pamela Ward in the preparation of this chapter.

REFERENCES

Anseth, E., Berntzen, K., & Gotestam, G. (1985). A comparison of the effects of flupentixol and relaxation on laboratory pain: An experimental study. *Acta Neurologica Scandinavica, 71*, 20–24.

Arts, S. E., Abu-Saad, H. H., Champion, G. D., Crawford, M. R., Fisher, R. J., Juniper, K. H., & Ziegler, J. B. (1994). Age related response to lidocaine–prilocaine (EMLA) emulsion and effect of music distraction on the pain of intravenous cannulation. *Pediatrics, 93*, 797–801.

Ashton, C., Whitworth, G. C., Seldmridge, J. A., Shapiro, P. A., Weinberg, A. D., Michler, R. E., Smith, C. R., Rose, E. A., Fisher, S., & Oz, M. C. (1997). Self hypnosis reduces anxiety following coronary bypass surgery. *Journal of Cardiovascular Surgery, 38*, 69–75.

Avia, M. D., & Kanfer, F. H. (1980). Coping with aversive stimulation: The effects of training in a self-management context. *Cognitive Therapy and Research, 4*, 73–81.

Ballantyne, J. C., Carr, D. B., deFerranti, S., Suarez, T., Lau, J., Chalmers, T. C., Angelillo, L. F., & Mosteller, F. (1998). The comparative effects of postoperative analgesic therapies on pulmonary outcome: Cumulative meta-analyses of randomized controlled trials. *Anesthesia and Analgesia, 86*, 598–612.

Baron, R. S., Logan, H., & Hoppe, S. (1993). Emotional and sensory focus as mediators of dental pain among patients differing in desired and felt dental control. *Health Psychology, 12*, 381–389.

Blount, R. L., Bachanas, P. J., Powers, S. W., Cotter, M. W., Franklin, A., Chaplin, W., Mayfield, J., Henderson, M., & Blount, S. D. (1992). Training children to cope and parents to coach them during routine immunizations: Effects on child, parent, and staff behaviors. *Behavior Therapy, 23*, 689–705.

Bruehl, S., Carlson, C. R., & McCubbin, J. A. (1993). Two brief interventions for acute pain. *Pain, 54*, 29–36.

Buckelew, S. P., Conway, R. C., Shutty, M. S., Lawrence, J. A., Grafing, M. R., Anderson, S. K., Hewett, J. E., & Keefe, F. J. (1992). Spontaneous coping strategies to manage acute pain and anxiety during electrodiagnostic studies. *Archives of Physical Medicine and Rehabilitation, 73*, 594–598.

Carlson, C. R., & Hoyle, R. H. (1992). Efficacy of abbreviated progressive muscle relaxation training: A quantitative review of behavioral medicine research. *Journal of Consulting and Clinical Psychology, 61*, 1059–1067.

Carr, D. B., & Goudas, L. C. (1999). Acute pain. *Lancet, 353*, 2051–2058.

Cason, C. L., & Grissom, N. L. (1997). Ameliorating adults' acute pain during phlebotomy with distraction intervention. *Applied Nursing Research, 10*, 168–173.

Clum, G. A., Luscomb, R. L., & Scott, L. (1982). Relaxation training and cognitive redirection strategies in the treatment of acute pain. *Pain, 12*, 175–183.

Cogan, R., & Kluthe, K. B. (1981). The role of learning in pain reduction associated with relaxation and patterned breathing. *Journal of Psychosomatic Research, 25*, 535–539.

Corah, N. L., Gale, E. N., & Illig, S. J. (1979). The use of relaxation and distraction to reduce psychological stress during dental procedures. *Journal of the American Dental Association, 98*, 390–394.

Corah, N. L., Gale, E. N., Pace, L. F., & Seyrek, S. K. (1981). Relaxation and musical programming as means of reducing psychological stress during dental procedures. *Journal of the American Dental Association, 103*, 232–234.

Croog, S. H., Baume, R. M., & Nalbandian, J. (1994). Pain response after psychological preparation for repeated periodontal surgery. *Journal of the American Dental Association, 125*, 1353–1360.

Daake, D. R., & Gueldner, S. H. (1989). Imagery instruction and the control of postsurgical pain. *Applied Nursing Research, 2*, 114–120.

Daltroy, L. H., Morlino, C. I., Eaton, C. I., Poss, R., & Liang, M. H. (1998). Preoperative education for total hip and knee replacement patients. *Arthritis Care and Research, 11*, 469–478.

Doering, S., Katzberger, F., Rumpold, G., Roessler, S., Hofstoetter, B., Schatz, D. S., Behensky, H., Krismer, M., Luz, G., Innerhofer, P., Benzer, H., Saria, A., & Schuessler, G. (2000). Videotape preparation of patients before hip replacement surgery reduces stress. *Psychosomatic Medicine, 62*, 365–373.

Fanurik, D., Zelter, L. K., Roberts, M. C., & Blount, R. L. (1993). The relationship between children's coping styles and psychological interventions for cold pressor pain. *Pain, 52*, 213–222.

Farthing, G. W., Venturino, M., Brown, S. W., & Lazar, J. D. (1997). Internal and external distraction in the control of cold pressor pain as a function of hypnotizability. *International Journal of Clinical Experimental Hypnosis, 45*, 433–446.

Faymonville, M. E., Fissette, J., Mambourg, P. H., Roediger, L., Joris, J., & Lamy, M. (1995). Hypnosis as adjuct therapy in conscious sedation for plastic surgery. *Regional Anesthesia, 20*, 145–151.

Flaherty, G. G., & Fitzpatrick, J. J. (1978). Relaxation technique to increase comfort level of postoperative patients: A preliminary study. *Nursing Research, 27*, 352–355.

Fratianne, R. B., Presner, J. D., Huston, M. J., Super, D. M., & Yowler, C. J. (2001). The effect of music based imagery and musical alternate engagement on the burn debridement process. *Journal of Burn Care and Rehabilitation, 22*, 47–53.

Frere, C. L., Crout, R., Yorty, J., & McNeil, D. W. (2001). Effects of audiovisual distraction during dental prophylaxis. *Journal of the American Dental Association, 132*, 1031–1038.

Gaston-Johansson, F., Fall-Dickson, J. M., Nanda, J., Ohly, K. V., Stillman, S., Krumm, S., & Kennedy, M. J. (2000). The effectiveness of the comprehensive coping strategy program on clinical outcomes in breast cancer autologous bone marrow transplantation. *Cancer Nursing, 23*, 277–285.

Geden, E. A., Beck, N. C., Anderson, J. S., & Kennish, M. E. (1986). Effects of cognitive and pharmacologic strategies on analogued labor pain. *Nursing Research, 35*, 301–306.

Good, M., Stanton-Hick, M., Grass, J. A., Anderson, G. C., Choi, C., Schoolmeesters, L. J., & Salman, A. (1999). Relief of postoperative pain with jaw relaxation, music and their combination. *Pain, 81,* 163–172.

Gracely, R. H., Lynch, S. A., & Bennett, G. J. (1992). Painful neuropathy: Altered central processing maintained dynamically by peripheral input. *Pain, 51,* 175–194.

Graffenried, B., Adler, R., Abt, K., Nuesch, E., & Spiegel, R. (1978). The influence of anxiety and pain sensitivity on experimental pain in man. *Pain, 4,* 253–263.

Harris, V. A., Katkin, E. S., Lick, J. R., & Habberfield, T. (1976). Paced respiration as a technique for the modification of autonomic response to stress. *Psychophysiology, 13,* 386–390.

Hoffman, H. G., Patterson, D. R., & Carrougher, G. J. (2000). Use of virtual reality for adjunctive treatment of adult burn pain during physical therapy: A controlled study. *Clinical Journal of Pain, 16,* 244–250.

Hoffman, H. G., Patterson, D. R., Carrougher, G. J., & Sharar, S. R. (2001). Effectiveness of virtual reality-based pain control with multiple treatments. *Clinical Journal of Pain, 17,* 229–235.

Jacobson, E. (1938). *Progressive relaxation.* Illinois: University of Chicago Press.

Jacobsen, P. B., & Butler, R. W. (1996). Relation of cognitive coping and catastrophizing to acute pain and analgesic use following breast cancer surgery. *Journal of Behavioral Medicine, 19,* 17–29.

Jay, S. M., Elliott, C. H., Fitzgibbons, L., Woody, P., & Siegel, S. (1995). A comparative study of cognitive behavioral therapy versus general anesthesia for painful medical procedures in children. *Pain, 62,* 3–9.

Jay, S. M., Elliott, C. H., Katz, E., & Siegel, S. E. (1987). Cognitive-behavioral and pharmacologic interventions for children's distress during painful medical procedures. *Journal of Consulting and Clinical Psychology, 55,* 860–865.

Jay, S. M., Elliott, C. H., Woody, P. D., & Siegel, S. E. (1991). An investigation of cognitive behavior therapy combined with oral Valium for children undergoing medical procedures. *Health Psychology, 10,* 317–322.

Jiang, H. J., Lagasse, R. S., Ciccone, K., Jakubowski, M. S., & Kitain, E. M. (2001). Factors influencing hospital implementation of acute pain management practice guidelines. *Journal of Clinical Anesthesia, 13,* 268–276.

Kaplan, R. M., Metzger, G., & Jablecki, C. (1983). Brief cognitive and relaxation training increases tolerance for a painful clinical electromyographic examination. *Psychosomatic Medicine, 45,* 155–162.

Kazak, A. E., Penati, B., Boyer, B. A., Himelstein, B., Brophy, P., Waibel, M. K., Blackall, G. F., Daller, R., & Johnson, K. (1996). A randomized controlled prospective outcome study of a psychological and pharmacological intervention protocol for procedural distress in pediatric leukemia. *Journal of Pediatric Psychology, 21,* 615–631.

Kazak, A. E., Penati, B., Brophy, P., & Himelstein, B. (1998). Pharmacologic and psychologic interventions for procedural pain. *Pediatrics, 102,* 59–66.

Kiecolt-Glaser, J. K., Page, G. P., Marucha, P. T., MacCallum, R. C., & Glaser, R. (1998). Psychology influences on surgical recovery. *American Psychologist, 52,* 1209–1218.

Kleiber, C., & Harper, D. C. (1999). Effects of distraction on children's pain and distress during medical procedures: A meta-analysis. *Nursing Research, 48,* 44–49.

Kleiber, C., Craft-Rosenburg, M., & Harper, D. C. (2001). Parents as distraction coaches during IV insertion: A randomized study. *Journal of Pain and Symptom Management, 22,* 851–861.

Kolk, A. M., van hoof, R., & Dop, M. J. C. F. (2000). Preparing children for venepuncture. The effect of integrated intervention on distress before and during venepuncture. *Child: Care, Health and Development, 26,* 251–260.

Kuttner, L. (1989). Management of young children's acute pain and anxiety during invasive medical procedures. *Pediatrician, 16,* 39–44.

Lal, M. K., McClelland, J., Phillips, J., Taub, N. A., & Beattie, R. M. (2001). Comparison of EMLA cream versus placebo in children receiving distraction therapy for venepuncture. *Acta Paediatrica, 90,* 154–159.

Lang, E. V., Benotsch, E. G., Fick, L. J., Lutegendorf, S., Berbaum, M. L., Berbaum, K. S., Logan, H., & Spiegel, D. (2000). Adjunctive non-pharmacological analgesia for invasive medical procedures: A randomised trial. *Lancet, 355*, 1486–1490.

Law, A., Logan, H., & Baron, R. S. (1994). Desire for control, felt control, and stress inoculation training during dental treatment. *Journal of Personality and Social Psychology, 67*, 926–936.

Lee, D. W. H., Chan, K., Poon, C., Ko, C., Chan, K., Sin, K., Sze, T., & Chan, A. C. W. (2002). Relaxation music decreases the dose of patient-controlled sedation during colonoscopy: A prospective randomized controlled trial. *Gastrointestinal Endoscopy, 55*, 33–36.

Leventhal, E. A., Leventhal, H., Shacham, S., & Easterling, D. V. (1989). Active coping reduces reports of pain from childbirth. *Journal of Consulting and Clinical Psychology, 57*, 365–371.

Leventhal, H., Brown, D., Shacham, S., & Enquist, G. (1979). Effect of preparatory information about sensations, threat of pain and attention on cold pressor distress. *Journal of Personality and Social Psychology, 37*, 688–714.

Litt, M. D. (1988). Self-efficacy and perceived control: Cognitive mediators of pain tolerance. *Journal of Personality and Social Psychology, 54*, 149–160.

Litt, M. D. (1996). A model of pain and anxiety associated with acute stressors: Distress in dental procedures. *Behavioral Research Therapy, 34*, 459–476.

Logan, H. L., Baron, R. S., & Kohout, F. (1995). Sensory focus as therapeutic treatments for acute pain. *Psychosomatic Medicine, 57*, 475–484.

Ludwick-Rosenthal, R., & Neufeld, R. W. J. (1988). Stress management during noxious medical procedures: An evaluative review of outcome studies. *Psychological Bulletin, 104*, 326–342.

Mandle, C. L., Domer, A. D., Harrington, D. P., Laserman, J., Bozadjian, E. M., Friedman, R., & Benson, H. (1990). Relaxation response in femoral angiography. *Radiology, 174*, 737–739.

Manne, S. L., Redd, W. H., Jacobsen, P. B., Gorfinkle, K., Schorr, O., & Rapkin, B. (1990). Behavioral intervention to reduce child and parent distress during venipuncture. *Journal of Consulting and Clinical Psychology, 58*, 565–572.

Manyande, A., Berg, S., Gettins, D., Stanford, S. C., Phil, D., Mazhero, S., Marks, D. F., & Salmon, P. (1995). Preoperative rehearsal of active coping imagery influences subjective and hormonal responses to abdominal surgery. *Psychosomatic Medicine, 57*, 177–182.

McCaul, K. D., & Malott, J. M. (1984). Distraction and coping with pain. *Psychological Bulletin, 95*, 516–533.

McCubbin, J. A., Wilson, J. F., Bruehl, S., Ibarra, P., Carlson, C. R., Norton, J. A., & Colclough, G. (1996). Relaxation training and opioidergic inhibition of blood pressure response to stress. *Journal of Consulting and Clinical Psychology, 64*, 593–601.

Melzack, R., & Wall, P. D. (1965). Pain mechanisms: A new theory. *Science, 150*, 971–979.

Millan, M. J. (1986). Multiple opioid systems and pain. *Pain, 27*, 303–347.

Miller, K. M., & Perry, P. A. (1990). Relaxation technique and postoperative pain in patients undergoing cardiac surgery. *Heart and Lung, 19*, 136–146.

Miro, J., & Raich, R. M. (1999). Effects of a brief and economical intervention in preparing patients for surgery: Does coping style matter? *Pain, 83*, 471–475.

Murphy, K. A., & Cornish, R. D. (1984). Prediction of chronicity in acute low back pain. *Archives of Physical Medicine and Rehabilitation, 65*, 334–337.

Pellino, T. A., & Ward, S. E. (1998). Perceived control mediates the relationship between severity and patient satisfaction. *Journal of Pain and Symptom Management, 15*, 110–116.

Postlethwaite, R., Stirling, G., & Peck, C. L. (1986). Stress inoculation for acute pain: A clinical trial. *Journal of Behavioral Medicine, 9*, 219–227.

Powers, S. (1999). Empirically supported treatments in pediatric psychology: Procedure-related pain. *Journal of Pediatric Psychology, 24*, 131–145.

Reading, A. E. (1982). The effects of psychological preparation on pain and recovery after minor gynecological surgery: A preliminary report. *Journal of Clinical Psychology, 38*, 504–512.

Renzi, C., Peticca, L., & Pescatori, M. (2000). The use of relaxation techniques in the perioperative management of proctological patients: Preliminary results. *International Journal of Colorectal Disease, 15,* 313–316.

Rokke, P. D., & al'Absi, M. (1992). Matching pain and coping strategies to the individual: A prospective validation of the cognitive coping strategy inventory. *Journal of Behavioral Medicine, 15,* 611–625.

Rosenstiel, A. K., & Keefe, F. J. (1983). The use of coping strategies in chronic low back pain patients: Relationship to patient characteristics and current adjustment. *Pain, 17,* 33–44.

Schiff, W. B., Holtz, K. D., Peterson, N., & Rakusan, T. (2001). Effect of an intervention to reduce procedural pain and distress for children with HIV infection. *Journal of Pediatric Psychology, 26,* 417–427.

Schultheis, K., Peterson, L., & Shelby, V. (1987). Preparation for stressful medical procedures and person x treatment interactions. *Clinical Psychology Review, 7,* 329–352.

Scott, J. R., & Rose, N. B. (1976). Effect of Psychoprophylaxis (Lamaze preparation) on labor and delivery in primiparas. *New England Journal of Medicine, 27,* 1205–1207.

Scott, L. E., & Clum, G. A. (1984). Examining the interaction effects of coping style and brief interventions in the treatment of postsurgical pain. *Pain, 20,* 279–291.

Seers, K., & Carroll, D. (1998). Relaxation techniques for acute pain management: A systemic review. *Journal of Advanced Nursing, 27,* 466–475.

Senturk, M., Ozcan, P. E., Tal, G. K., Kiyan, E., Camci, E., Ozyalcin, S., Dilege, S., & Pembeci, K. (2002). The effects of three different analgesia techniques on long-term post-thoracotomy pain. *Anesthesia and Analgesia, 94,* 11–15.

Shipley, R. H., Butt, J. H., & Horwitz, E. A. (1979). Preparation to reexperience a stressful medical examination: Effect of repetitious videotape exposure and coping style. *Journal of Consulting and Clinical Psychology, 47,* 485–492.

Spanos, N. P., Hodgins, D. C., Stam, H. J., & Gwynn, M. (1984). Suffering for science: The effects of implicit social demands on response to experimentally induced pain. *Journal of Personality and Social Psychology, 46,* 1162–1172.

Sternbach, R. A. (1974). *Pain patients: Traits and treatment.* New York: Academic Press.

Sullivan, M. J., Rodgers, W. M., & Kirsch, I. (2001). Catastrophizing, depression, and expectancies for pain and emotional distress. *Pain, 91,* 147–154.

Sullivan, M. J., Thorn, B., Haythornthwaite, J. A., Keefe, F., Martin, M., Bradley, L. A., & Lefebvre, J. C. (2001). Theoretical perspectives on the relation between catastrophizing and pain. *Clinical Journal of Pain, 17,* 52–64.

Tan, S. (1982). Cognitive and cognitive-behavioral methods for pain control: A selective review. *Pain, 12,* 201–228.

Tan, S., & Poser, E. G. (1982). Acute pain in a clinical setting: Effects of cognitive-behavioural skills training. *Behavioral Research and Therapy, 20,* 535–545.

Turk, D. C., Meichenbaum, D., & Genest, M. (1983). *Pain and behavioral medicine.* New York: Guilford Press.

Tusek, D., Church, J. M., & Fazio, V. W. (1997). Guided imagery as a coping strategy for perioperative patients. *AORN Journal, 66,* 644–649.

VanDalfsen, P. J., & Syrjala, J. L. (1990). Psychological strategies in acute pain management. *Critical Care Clinics, 6,* 421–431.

Vessey, J., Carlson, K. L., & McGill, J. (1994). Use of distraction with children during an acute pain experience. *Nursing Research, 43,* 369–372.

Wardle, J. (1983). Psychological management of anxiety and pain during dental treatment. *Journal of Psychosomatic Research, 27,* 399–402.

Weisenberg, M. (1987). Psychological intervention for the control of pain. *Behavioral Research and Therapy, 25,* 301–312.

Wilson, J. F. (1981). Behavioral preparation for surgery: Benefit or harm? *Journal of Behavioral Medicine, 4,* 79–102.

Wright, B. R., & Drummond, P. D. (2000). Rapid induction analgesia for the alleviation of procedural pain during burn care. *Burns, 26,* 275–282.

Zelman, D. C., Howland, E. W., Nichols, S. N., & Cleeland, C. S. (1991). The effects of induced mood on laboratory pain. *Pain, 46,* 105–111.

10

Psychological Interventions and Chronic Pain

Heather D. Hadjistavropoulos
Department of Psychology
University of Regina

Amanda C. de C. Williams
INPUT Pain Management Unit,
St. Thomas' Hospital, London

The use of psychological interventions in the management of nonmalignant chronic pain, such as low back pain, headaches, and arthritis, is no longer considered treatment of last resort. Previously, psychologists were involved only after other biologically based methods had failed (Turk & Flor, 1984). Today, psychological interventions are often delivered concurrently with many biologically based interventions, such as physiotherapy and exercise therapy. Treatment can be offered within a multidisciplinary context, but also as an independent or separate service. Treatment may occur as an outpatient or inpatient and may be offered individually or in a group context with or without the involvement of family members or significant others.

Therapy goals are highly variable and at times may be poorly specified by the patient beyond pain reduction and returning to abandoned activities and roles. Comprehensive assessment may reveal multiple treatment targets of interest, such as pain or symptom management (e.g., development of active coping strategies, reduction of pain behavior and avoidance, motivation enhancement, improved sleep habits, medication adherence), stress and psychological symptom management (e.g., resolution of anxiety, depression, anger, medical uncertainty, fear of pain), and/or resolution of interpersonal (e.g., family conflict, sexual difficulties, communication problems) and vocational concerns (e.g., job stress, job dissatisfaction, vocational planning). Goals of the patient, referrer, and staff who deliver the treatment may diverge or conflict, as may those of the employer, family, or others in the patient's environment. Goals at times will depend on the treatment approach that is taken—for instance, whether it is operant, respondent, cognitive, cognitive-behavioral, family, or psychodynamic therapy.

The purpose of this chapter is to provide a succinct overview of psychological approaches commonly used among chronic pain patients. Empirical evidence pertaining to their efficacy (e.g., comparison of outcomes between intervention and a control condition) and effectiveness (e.g., examination of social and clinical benefits in naturalistic settings) is highlighted. Comparisons among psychological interventions are made when appropriate, although this is complicated by the fact that the interventions have overlapping features and are often offered in combination within the context of multidisciplinary treatment. Very little research is available comparing psychological interventions to biologically based interventions, such as surgery, physiotherapy, and exercise therapy.

OPERANT CONDITIONING

Background and Description

Fordyce (1976) was the first to describe the application of operant conditioning to chronic pain and proposed that observable pain behaviors, such as medication consumption, limping, grimacing, and resting, although likely initially triggered by an antecedent event (e.g., injury, disease), are governed by their contingent consequences. He asserted that overt pain behaviors are maintained through systematic positive reinforcement (e.g., attention) and/or avoidance of negative consequences (e.g., unpleasant work) (Turner & Chapman, 1982a). He recommended that operant conditioning be used with chronic pain patients to reduce one or more overt pain behaviors (e.g., use of medication, bed rest) or to facilitate increase in those more adaptive well behaviors (e.g., activity). Fordyce appears to have been reacting to the then dominant psychogenic pain models that assumed that pain signals that resulted with little or no associated pathology were the result of psychological disturbance (see Fordyce, 1973). Treatment was characteristically offered within a controlled inpatient environment in order to provide consistent contingencies. A multidisciplinary team typically delivered treatment, with patients also attending sessions with physicians, vocational counselors, physical therapists, occupational therapists, and others.

In a relatively recent review chapter, Sanders (1996) summarized the essential elements of the operant approach. The first component begins prior to the initiation of treatment and involves a functional behavioral analysis to identify relevant overt pain and well behaviors, and, as far as possible, antecedent stimuli and contingent consequences contributing to pain behavior. At this stage, patients are frequently encouraged to monitor and record their behavior (e.g., up and down time, walking, medication). Thereafter, operant treatment is described as involving several ingredients including: (a) response prevention for escape/avoidance behaviors; (b) positive and negative reinforcement (e.g., encouragement) to increase well behaviors from baseline (e.g., physical exercise, up time), with gradual reduction in this to a variable schedule once well behaviors are on the rise; (c) shaping or gradual change of well behaviors, which includes exercising to quota rather than exercising to tolerance; (d) elimination or reduction of factors that may maintain the overt pain behaviors outside the treatment environment, such as economic reinforcers, social attention, and avoidance of responsibilities; and (e) time-contingent delivery of medication while reducing the amount of medication per day.

With respect to medication, the physician determines the drug needs. The psychologist, however, may play an important role in monitoring these needs. According to Fordyce (1973), medications are at first provided to patients on a prescribed-as-needed (PRN) basis for 2 to 4 days to establish the medication baseline. Baseline doses are then delivered on a fixed time schedule such that if patients had previously requested medication every 5 hours, medication would be delivered instead every 4 hours. With this method, medication is not contingent on soreness and therefore does not serve as positive reinforcer for pain or pain behavior; gradually over time medication is ultimately withdrawn. The role of the psychologist in time-contingent medication is to assist with monitoring of medication prior to adjustment and then with positive reinforcement and encouragement of adherence to the regimen.

The operant methods are applied to each overt pain and well behavior across as many different conditions as possible, and when possible the patient and family are encouraged to directly apply operant conditioning methods to behavior change (Sanders, 1996). Unique to operant conditioning, the operant treatment principles are applied by all health care providers involved in care, not exclusively the psychologist (van Tulder et al., 2000).

Evidence

The earliest evidence in support of operant conditioning for chronic pain came, not surprisingly, from Fordyce and colleagues in the form of a case study (Fordyce, Fowler, Lehmann, & DeLateur, 1968). In 1973, Fordyce and colleagues (Fordyce et al., 1973) described pre–post treatment findings based on operant conditioning with 36 chronic pain patients. In their study, pain medications were provided on a time-contingent rather than PRN basis in order to decrease the association of pain behavior and relief. Furthermore, nursing staff withheld social reinforcement when patients displayed pain behaviors, and provided extensive praise when patients showed well behaviors. Positive treatment effects were observed following the inpatient program and at 22-month follow-up, including report of increased activity level and exercise tolerance, and decreased medication usage and pain ratings.

Since the time of these earliest observations, several studies have been conducted along with reviews of operant therapy that have generally been encouraging (e.g., Fordyce, Roberts, & Sternbach, 1985; Keefe & Bradley, 1984; Linton, 1982, 1986; Turner & Chapman, 1982a; van Tulder et al., 2000). In an effort to improve the practice of psychotherapy, a number of task forces have reviewed the research literature and identified empirically supported treatments. Chambless and Ollendick (2001) summarized the work of these task forces and reported that operant behavior therapy for heterogeneous chronic pain patients has category II support, meaning that there is at least one RCT supporting the treatment, showing it as superior to a control condition or an alternative treatment.

Our review of this area of research generally reveals that there are few research studies that address operant conditioning directly, and those that are carried out do not often follow the prototypical approach advocated by Fordyce (1976). Although there are a number of studies that address cognitive-behavioral treatment, or behavioral treatment that also includes relaxation training, randomized control studies focused exclusively on operant conditioning are rare. Furthermore, because the operant approach involves numerous components it is difficult to clarify the extent to which psychological intervention is crucial versus other components such as occupational therapy and physiotherapy (Turk & Flor, 1984).

Commentary

The lack of studies addressing operant conditioning alone is perhaps a reflection of our own direct experiences that, in practice, in clinical settings the prototypical operant approach is rarely used. Although this observation is not made explicitly in the literature, systematic attempts at assessment of well behaviors and illness behaviors as well as contingencies between overt pain behaviors and positive and negative reinforcers are infrequent in practice. Instead, clinicians routinely assume that certain pain behaviors are positive (e.g., exercising, distraction, positive coping self-statements) and others are negative (e.g., guarding) (LaChapelle, Hadjistavropoulos, & McCreary, 2001). Furthermore, it is often assumed that certain contingencies are always negative (e.g., disability benefits, medical staff attention, family support). Evidence is emerging that even some of the apparently simple relationships that were previously observed between pain behavior and spouse solicitous behavior and facilitative behavior (Romano et al., 1992) are more complex than was previously understood (Romano et al., 1995). Romano and colleagues (1995) reported, for instance, that spouse solicitous responses are predictive of pain behavior only among patients with high levels of pain and low mood.

With respect to treatment protocol, in practice, we also expect that ethical considerations largely prevent extensive use of response prevention for escape/avoidance behaviors. Treatment requires the full cooperation of the patient. It is a mistaken belief that operant conditioning methods can be used to modify the behavior of the most resistant patients without their cooperation (Keefe & Bradley, 1984). Furthermore, although positive and negative reinforcement may be used to increase supposed well behaviors and decrease pain behaviors, we question the degree to which this is employed as systematically as recommended by Fordyce (1976). This may in part be because staff members feel uncomfortable with the approach, but also because of the time demands that exist in a busy clinical setting. The elimination of factors that are hypothesized to maintain pain (e.g., economic incentive, family support) is also not as realistic as the treatment descriptions provided by Sanders (1996) suggest and may have serious decremental consequences for the patient's quality of life. Finally, although it is stated that operant methods should be applied across as many overt and well behaviors as possible, in practice this is most commonly applied to the extent that it is important and relevant to the patient.

It is misleading to assume that operant conditioning, as proposed by Fordyce, is routinely employed in practice. In reality, some operant conditioning strategies are used with other psychological interventions and physical/medical treatments within a multidisciplinary treatment program. What appears to be one of the most useful aspects of the operant approach is the identification of a broad range of behaviors that are associated with pain, rather than a focus on simply pain intensity (Keefe, Dunsmore, & Burnett, 1992). Furthermore, as a result of operant conditioning approaches, it appears that there has been much greater attention on reducing inactivity, and the negative side effects associated with it, and on goal setting in general (Fordyce, 1988). Finally, the operant approach also has served to emphasize that chronic pain occurs in a social context (Fordyce, 1976). As such, therapists today are more likely to involve family members in treatment (Keefe et al., 1992) and also to recognize a role for other health care providers in the administration of psychological treatment strategies (van Tulder et al., 2000).

RESPONDENT THERAPY

Background and Description

Diverse pain management strategies deriving from the respondent formulation of pain are commonly used to treat chronic pain, such as progressive muscle relaxation and biofeedback. The rationale identifies the pain–tension cycle as contributing to the pain experience, and thus reduction of muscle tension is the characteristic goal of treatment (Linton, 1982). Central to this view is that pain elicits a response of increased muscle tension, which itself produces more pain, and contributes directly to secondary problems such as sleep disturbance, immobilization, and depression (Linton, 1982). Therapy includes educating patients regarding the association between tension and pain, and learning to replace muscle tension with an incompatible response, namely, relaxation (Turk & Flor, 1984).

Relaxation therapy involves teaching patients to achieve a physiological sense of relaxation. Beyond physically reducing muscle tension, and thus pain, relaxation can have other aims, including anxiety reduction, assisting with sleep disturbance and fatigue, increasing well-being, and perhaps most importantly improving a sense of control. Progressive muscle relaxation is undoubtedly the most common form of relaxation training, and involves systematically tensing and the relaxing major muscle groups throughout the body (Turner & Chapman, 1982b).

Biofeedback also involves relaxation of muscles, but is achieved through monitoring bodily responses, typically through a computer or apparatus, and providing patients visual or auditory feedback about their physiological responding. With intense scrutiny and examination, it is hoped that the patient will be able to learn how to control certain physiological responses related to pain (Arena & Blanchard, 1996). Many forms of biofeedback exist, but electromyographic (EMG) feedback, aimed to reduce muscle tension, is by far the most common with chronic pain patients. The focus has also largely been on headaches, although other conditions such as low back pain (Arena & Blanchard, 1996; van Tulder et al., 2000) and temporomandibular joint pain (Crider & Glaros, 1999) have also been treated with biofeedback.

At times, relaxation and biofeedback strategies are used on their own, but most commonly they are used in combination with each other as well as with the other treatment approaches described in this chapter. The exception to this is with headache sufferers where biofeedback and relaxation are not infrequently used as sole treatment strategies (Arena & Blanchard, 1996). Treatment is most often offered on an outpatient basis in a group or individual format (Blanchard, 1992). These techniques help the patient to recognize and alter pain behavior patterns. As such responsibility for treatment rests largely with the patient (Keefe & Bradley, 1984). Home practice is often encouraged with these techniques, as is application to stressful situations and events. One interesting finding that has emerged with respect to headache is that home practice appears to be important with relaxation, but not necessarily with biofeedback (Blanchard, 1992).

In addition to relaxation strategies and biofeedback, imagery and hypnosis are also used to achieve similar effects with chronic pain patients

(Arena & Blanchard, 1996). To the extent that they rely on effective relaxation, respondent theory is relevant to them. Imagery involves the purposeful use of visual images to strengthen distraction and/or to transform aspects of the pain experience. Hypnosis involves suggestion for decreasing discomfort or transforming or altering pain into less noxious sensations (Syrjala & Abrams, 1996).

Evidence

A number of reviews of the effects of relaxation therapy and biofeedback have been carried out with headache (e.g., Blanchard, 1992; Compas, Haaga, Keefe, Leitenberg, & Williams, 1998), low back pain (e.g., van Tulder et al., 2000), temporomandibular joint pain (e.g., Crider & Glaros, 1999; Sherman & Turck, 2001), and mixed chronic pain patients (Chambless & Ollendick, 2001; Morley, Eccleston, & Williams, 1999). There is evidence in support of both biofeedback and relaxation therapy. The research, however, is hampered by a number of problems, including differences among studies related to procedures, patient groups, and duration of treatment (Turk & Flor, 1984).

Relaxation therapy alone has been found to be effective for headache (Blanchard, 1992; Compas et al., 1998), temporomandibular disorders (Sherman & Turk, 2001), low back pain (van Tulder et al., 2000), and mixed chronic pain patients (Morley et al., 1999). It is not easy to separate specific effects of biofeedback from those of relaxation, with which it is used in treatment. Despite the encouraging reviews just cited, there are some negative studies that led Compas et al. (1998) to conclude that biofeedback cannot be classified as an efficacious treatment for chronic pain patients, except for headache. Turner and Chapman (1982b) suggested that much of the interest in biofeedback has resulted from the efforts of commercial equipment suppliers. From an efficiency perspective alone, relaxation therapy is often preferred.

With respect to imagery, although there is significant research support for usage of this technique with acute pain patients (e.g., Fernandez & Turk, 1989), much less research exists on the effects of imagery with chronic pain. Nevertheless, these techniques are commonly part of treatment of chronic pain patients. Similarly, much of the evidence that is used to support the usage of hypnosis (e.g., Patterson, Everett, Burns, & Marvin, 1992; Tan & Leucht, 1997) rests with acute pain (see chap. 9, this volume), and there are few controlled studies on the use of hypnosis with chronic pain (Haythornthwaite & Benrud-Larson, 2001). Perhaps some preliminary support for use of hypnosis with chronic pain patients comes from a study by Haanen et al. (1991). This group of researchers compared hypnosis with physical therapy (but primarily massage and relaxation therapy) for patients suffering from fibromyalgia, and reported that the former treatment resulted in greater reductions in pain, sleep difficulties, and fatigue than the latter.

Commentary

In general, although there is evidence in support of respondent techniques with patients, the evidence in support of the respondent theory itself is much lower. There is very little evidence for muscle tension under voluntary control causing pain (e.g., Knost, Flor, Birbaumer, & Schugens, 1999). On the other hand, there is evidence for greater muscle activity in the sites distal to the primary pain location among patients compared to healthy controls (Flor, Birbaumer, Schugens, & Lutzenberger, 1992). For instance, Flor and colleagues (1992) used anxiety or personally relevant stress induction techniques with healthy controls and individuals with chronic pain conditions (including low back pain, temporomandibular pain, and tension-type headache), and found significantly increased activity in the musculature specific to the person's pain complaints among pain patients as compared to healthy controls. There is also research on simple back movements like bending forward. This research shows very slow return to baseline of muscles after they have tensed, making for a painful and effortful movement (Watson, Booker, Main, & Chen, 1997). Finally, centrally mediated deep muscle tension around the spine has been found to occur in response to pain and instability; this then puts unmanageable demands on superficial muscle, and these mechanisms are hard to bring under voluntary control (Simmonds, 1999). The respondent theory has been criticized most strongly for being an oversimplification of the nature of chronic pain problems and especially the involvement of psychological factors in pain (Turner & Chapman, 1982b).

Self-efficacy appears crucial to understanding the effects of respondent techniques, especially relaxation and biofeedback. Holroyd and colleagues (Holroyd et al., 1984) conducted one of the most compelling studies in this regard. This research group demonstrated that it makes little difference whether subjects learn to increase or decrease their muscle tension in terms of experiencing improvements in chronic head pain. On the other hand, participants who were told that they were successful in their attempts to alter their muscle tension, whether they were increasing or decreasing it, reported greater improvement in headache compared to those who were told they were only moderately successful with the technique. Blanchard and his group (Blanchard, Kim, Hermann, & Steffek, 1993) found similar results with relaxation procedures among chronic headache sufferers. In other words, those who perceive themselves to be successful with relaxation report greater improvement in their headaches, whether they are in actual fact successful or not.

COGNITIVE-BEHAVIORAL THERAPY

Background and Description

Cognitive-behavioral therapy (CBT) for chronic pain evolved from the behavioral interventions described above, but with the addition of cognitive methods. Both the focus and some of the behavioral techniques have changed since the early 1980s when CBT was first described (Turk, Meichenbaum, & Genest, 1983). The early formulations drew substantially on stress management methods from mainstream psychological treatment, and this was compatible more with respondent and relaxation methods than with operant programs. The model emphasized the reciprocal influence of cognitive content (schemata and beliefs), cognitive processes (automatic thoughts, appraisals of control), behavior, and its interpersonal consequences; all were the proper target of intervention. Although Beck's work was cited (e.g., Beck, 1976), the psychological intervention did not approximate to cognitive therapy along Beckian lines, with only very brief mention of affect; instead, early CBT was concerned with self-control and the acquisition of coping skills. Some cognitive strategies such as distraction and relabeling were imported from successful use in acute (particularly procedural) pain, although never satisfactorily demonstrated to be effective for moderate to severe chronic pain.

In a 1992 review, Keefe and colleagues (Keefe et al., 1992) identified improved outcome methodology and the first preventive programs as recent advances, but no other notable innovations in treatment were noted. In contrast, they identified spouse behavior (Romano et al., 1991) and the identification of the mediation of the pain–depression link by impact of pain (Rudy, Kerns, & Turk, 1988) as two of the most important contributions in the field. They also pointed out the confusion developing in the cognitive arena due to multiple overlapping instruments measuring overlapping constructs that are studied using correlation and thus cast little light on causal processes. A contemporaneous review, Turk and Rudy (1992), used an information-processing model to describe patients with low expectations of control over pain or their situations, and as thereby inactive and demoralized. Emotion was an implicit rather than explicit target of intervention.

Since these reviews in 1992, there have been exciting developments in cognitive therapy, with some concepts, predominantly catastrophizing, emerging as key variables from diverse studies in several countries (e.g., Eccleston & Crombez, 1999; Jensen, Turner, & Romano 2001; Sullivan et al.,

2001). There has also been a recent reformulation of fear and avoidance (Lethem, Slade, Troup, & Bentley, 1983) by Vlaeyen and colleagues (Vlaeyen & Linton 2000) that is securely grounded in psychological theory of fear and phobia, and accompanied by careful modeling of change. This takes over from broader (and unsatisfactory) concepts of control and coping. The interest is now in specific fear rather than general neuroticism/anxiety, and avoidance as a purposeful strategy rather than an incidental event for managing fears of pain and injury. There is also a more confident approach to emotion and to intervention in emotion using Beckian and other techniques, and revised models are under development (e.g., see Pincus & Morley, 2001).

CBT programs today are diverse and (unsurprisingly) none of the descriptions of "ingredients" coincides exactly with practice. In the absence of demonstration that each is essential to outcome (this question and attempts to answer it are addressed later with efficacy), one might reasonably expect each ingredient to be based securely either in theory or in mainstream psychology practice, but it is not always so. The following are generally regarded as core components of CBT:

• Education on pain, the distinction of chronic from acute pain, the dissociation of the pain experience from physical findings accessible to current investigations, the integral place of psychology and behavior in the pain experience, and the rationale for the pain management or rehabilitation model used in treatment may be delivered by medical or psychology personnel, or others. Education aims to combat demoralization and feelings of victimization and to motivate patients to take an active role in treatment (Turk & Rudy, 1989).

• Exercise and fitness training, to reverse deconditioning due to reduced activity, and to address directly patients' fears about certain movements or physical demands on their bodies, is usually guided by physiotherapists. Programs differ in the extent to which they attempt corrective hands-on physiotherapy, with some explicitly teaching nothing that the patient cannot do him- or herself at home or in a suitable sports facility.

• Most CBT programs focus on skills acquisition and rehearsal (Bradley, 1996). Relaxation, described earlier, is a core component of this and may be integrated to a greater or lesser extent with physical rehabilitation, and/or with management techniques described later, such as activity pacing, attention diversion, and stress management; it may also be applied to sleep problems.

• Behavioral change by contingency management—operant methods—was described earlier. Many programs describe contingent relationships and encourage patients to self-reinforce "well behaviors" and to involve those close to them in similar selective reinforcement. However, this is far from the carefully observed and formulated consistent contingency management described by Fordyce. A particular aspect of behavioral change addressed in many programs is the reduction of analgesic drug use, but targets and endpoints vary considerably. Although some programs substitute nonopioid for opioid analgesics, and supply antidepressants, others aim to reduce all drug intake to nil (Keefe et al., 1992).

• Goal setting, by the patient with varying degrees of guidance by staff, identifies short- and long-term goals, skills deficits, and methods for achieving those goals. Most involve activity scheduling, or pacing, where, starting from a modest baseline of any challenging or demanding physical activity or position, patients build by small increments their blocks of activity, interspersed with rest and/or change of position or activity. Blocks of activity may be defined by time or another quantum, and for many patients, taking regular breaks requires that they challenge previously unquestioned rules and standards by which they lived.

• Cognitive therapy is the cornerstone of CBT, but the most variable in content and extent of all the components. It can involve any or all of the attention diversion methods (see Fernandez & Turk 1989), and often is used with relaxation, problem-solving strategies, and cognitive restructuring familiar to cognitive therapists. Although this is sometimes described in terms of coping skills training (Keefe et al., 1996), it is in fact cognitive therapy, in that it addresses patients' elicited concerns, addresses emotional material, and teaches the identification of catastrophizing cognitions and the means to challenge and change them. By contrast, some programs offer such brief intervention, apparently mostly didactic, that although described as cognitive therapy, it cannot be deemed to approximate it.

• Generalization and maintenance are increasingly emphasized, with many studies referring to the relapse prevention model (Marlatt & Gordon, 1980), although it is far harder to identify a state of relapse when multiple behaviors are involved and are only loosely connected. Identification of vulnerable states or situations (e.g., increased depression or pain), and preparation to deal effectively with them, are widely practiced. Essentially, patients are encouraged to anticipate setbacks and plan for good management.

• Like operant and respondent treatment, CBT is often delivered to groups, over a fixed time and number of sessions, with in-session and between-session rehearsal and application to individual goals (Keefe et al., 1996). Patients with chronic pain, even if they all differ in site of pain and history of previous treatments, share sufficient problems in managing pain that groups can be mixed or have a single condition. Many programs also provide additional individual sessions for specific psychological problems, for individual applications (such as work), or for unspecified reasons. Given that the format of the groups involves didactic teaching, sharing of experience, and experiential learning, it is not clear to what extent the processes of group therapy, and its benefits, apply. Nevertheless, on a practical basis, group sharing serves to normalize the experience of isolated patients; it validates both their difficulties and their efforts to manage them; and it provides vicarious learning as other group members start to use pain management methods taught. In CBT groups it may be more difficult to elicit emotional material from members of the group if they are not a cohesive group, but there is still the opportunity for learning from the disclosures of those who are more forthcoming with emotionally charged experiences.

Multicomponent programs necessitate a range of professionals with appropriate training; key members are physicians, clinical psychologists, and physiotherapists or physical therapists; occupational therapists, and therapists with particular focus on vocational concerns may also be involved. A little-addressed aspect of multidisciplinary treatment is the extent to which the team members of different disciplines really work in an integrated way, or alternatively operate independently, and potentially with incompatibilities between them. Treatment on an outpatient basis provides the greatest opportunities for the patient to apply and generalize pain management techniques learned on the program to his or her own environments, but intensive (usually inpatient) programs may be required to enable change in more severely disabled and distressed patients (Williams et al., 1996).

Evidence

The Division of Clinical Psychology of the American Psychological Association (APA) published a list of 25 empirically validated psychological treatments for various disorders (APA, Division of Clinical Psychology, 1995). CBT for chronic pain was included in this list, based mainly on evidence examined by Keefe et al. (1992). A recent systematic review and meta-analysis of 25 randomized control trials (RCTs) of CBT for chronic pain except headache by Morley et al. (1999) concluded that the available data demonstrate that CBT is effective across a range of outcomes when compared with minimal control conditions (waiting list and treatment as usual) and as good as or better than other active psychological treatments. Effect sizes were modest (many around 0.5), but respectable in terms of psychological treatment of an intractable problem, and many studies were underpowered, risking Type 1 error. This summary represents an optimistic picture, qualified somewhat by concerns that these RCTs probably represented the better end of the spectrum of treatment, and by the recognition of enormous diversity among them, to the extent that subgroup analyses or dose-response effects could not be addressed despite the large *n*.

Two other systematic reviews have appeared since, both concerned only with chronic low back pain. van Tulder et al. (2000) found on meta-analysis good outcome from seven studies comparing CBT with minimal control conditions in pain and in "behavioral" outcomes that included cognitive and emotional measures, but not in function (i.e., disability). For the comparison of CBT with alternative treatment (such as physical therapy), six studies showed no significant improvement in any of the three outcome areas. Guzmán, Esmail, Karjalainene, Irvin, and Bombardier (2001) concluded from 10 studies that only intensive (longer, rather than brief) multidisciplinary treatment with a CBT approach reduced pain and improved function when all were compared with treatment as usual (a conclusion also borne out by Williams et al., 1996). They thus recommended careful attention to treatment content by referrers. A recent narrative review (Compas et al., 1998) adds to this and suggests some treatment variability among conditions. Among patients with rheumatoid arthritis, CBT was the only form of psychological intervention that was found to be efficacious; among patients with headache, CBT was actually no more effective than simpler respondent techniques (Compas et al., 1998).

Only one study appears to have addressed the question of inpatient versus outpatient treatment. Williams et al. (1996) found that both inpatient and outpatient CBT results in improvement, but that at 1-year follow-up patients receiving inpatient CBT maintained gains better and used less health care than those who received treatment on an outpatient basis.

The research literature to date has not been able to answer the question of whether CBT adds significantly to medical interventions provided in multidisciplinary pain clinics. Although overall there is considerable evidence for the effectiveness of multidisciplinary pain clinics, at this time it is not possible to identify or isolate active ingredients within the pain clinics that contribute to outcomes (Fishbain, 2000).

There is disappointingly little research to guide the practitioner on size and constitution of CBT groups, or on process (Keefe, Jacobs, & Underwood-Gordon, 1997). Group versus individual treatment is not a major research issue, given the efficacy of CB group programs and the increased costs of treating patients individually. There is a move toward patient-led and self-management groups, of which the work of Lorig and colleagues (Lorig, Lubeck, Kraines, Seleznick, & Holman, 1985) is an important early example. They trained lay leaders, who then led large groups of arthritic patients (and family or friends where they wished to attend) in largely experiential learning for six weekly 2-hour groups. Gains in pain and activity frequency were comparable to those from similar CBT programs; changes in depression, low at the outset, were modest, and there were none in self-rated disability. Although this is now a widely replicated model, and there are doubtless deficits in knowledge and strategies to be remedied among chronic pain patients, the model cannot be extrapolated unquestioningly to populations of patients who are frequent users of health care and are significantly distressed and disabled. Although it has been demonstrated by some control conditions (e.g. Bradley et al., 1987; Nicholas, Wilson, & Goyen, 1992) that a sympathetic group that shares experience but has no expert introduction of information and pain management methods can produce high satisfaction ratings, and some short-term improvement in subjective state, there are typically no gains in function. Attending support groups over a 1-year period shows no enhanced treatment gains in terms of sick leave, function, and pain (Linton, Hellsing, & Larsson, 1997). Together the just cited studies suggest support groups may have a place as an adjunct approach among chronic pain patients, but provide evidence against reducing the level of expertise and time and resources put into CBT group pain management programs.

Commentary

In 1992, Keefe and colleagues expressed widely held hopes that research using larger sample sizes would demonstrate the "active ingredients" of CBT treatment packages; discover how to improve maintenance of treatment gains; and extend CBT to other patient groups, such as those with osteoarthritis, rheumatoid arthritis, and sickle-cell disease. The intervening 10 years have perhaps only met the last prediction. Meanwhile, extensive CBT programs have been subject to cost cutting, thereby reducing the quality and quantity of established treatment facilities. Research has been limited largely to small volunteer studies, making it particularly hard to model change in treatment (and maintenance after treatment) or to carry out studies with sufficient sample size to do justice to the many interacting variables affecting outcome.

The questions identified by many clinicians and researchers (Turk, 1990), and to which some anticipate answers from large treatment studies or meta-analyses, are, "Which are the right and wrong patients?" and "Which are the right and wrong treatment components?" Unfortunately, the proper prospective tests on patient selection—where all are assessed and all treated—can never be done. Meanwhile, no consistent findings have emerged from many component dismantling trials (see Morley et al., 1999, Morley & Williams, 2002). This is not so remarkable given that all investigations are subject to local peculiarities of referral, funding, and acceptance and rejection criteria. We can, however, draw some practical suggestions from mainstream psychology: People with major depressive disorder are unlikely to engage or participate until they have more hope and sense of a tolerable future, so immediate treatment of depression is indicated; phobias of groups or health care settings may preclude common methods and settings for delivery.

As for "essential ingredients," the implicit model of component dismantling studies of additive, independent, and specific component-outcome relationships is too far from reality to provide an adequate model for analysis. One can no more ask which are the essential ingredients of a cake—butter, sugar, flour, or eggs. The absence of any, or serious compromises of quality, will result in a different and inedible end product; minor variations in one or another or the addition of cocoa or currants does not render it inedible. The interaction of components (the mixing and cooking process) is crucial, yet team processes and program integration are rarely described. At a risk of stretching the analogy too far, the skills of the cook are also relevant, and cost-cutting pressures on programs are likely to reduce efficacy. As NASA engineers profess: "Faster (briefer), better, cheaper: you can have any two of these, but not all three."

The classification of components of CBT used earlier is a simplification of the components derived from 30 treatment studies included in the systematic review by Morley et al. (1999). What is curious is the extent to which discontinuities were evident (beyond those included in the systematic review) in studies' rationales, treatment methods, and outcomes chosen. Almost all study introductions invoke costs and demands on health care and loss of work; few measure either. At least half do not make clear whether they expect pain ratings to change, although these are universally measured and reported. Perhaps because of editorial restrictions, the factors affecting the choice of components, their order, timing, and processes, are rarely described. The use of manuals is still very rare. Whether these apparent confusions in accounts of treatment reflect real contradictions embedded in treatment methods and processes is an open question. It is of some concern that beyond its basic assumptions—that thoughts, emotions and behavior influence one another, that behavior is determined both by the interaction of individual and his or her environment, and that individuals can change their thoughts, emotion, and behavior (Keefe et al., 1997)—the variety of methods by which those basic assumptions are realized has not led to the evolution of demonstrably better practice.

What are some of the issues requiring clarification? On education, arguably, psychologists and their colleagues unnecessarily restrict themselves to the initial gate control model (Melzack & Wall, 1965), underusing the rich neurophysiological research which has resulted from the initial proposal of that model. There is a dearth of models described in terms that are accessible to the lay public of central nervous system plasticity developing subsequent to pain, and of the nonconscious psychological processes that influence the processing of pain at spinal and supraspinal levels. Emotion is still poorly integrated with this, perhaps because of the lack of adequate overall models and the shortage of data on nonconscious processes (Keefe et al., 1997).

The findings of sophisticated and large-scale studies of cognitive therapy in mainstream psychology (Chambless & Ollendick, 2001) are rarely addressed in the pain field, yet they provide testable models for particular components of treatment and for more examination of processes of change. To an extent, we are constrained by our measurement instruments: For instance, cognitive strategies are measured in terms of frequency, which may be important for some but neglects appropriateness of content and timing, which are crucial in a more integrated model of mind and body. Well-focused study of particular mechanisms (see Vlaeyen & Linton, 2000, review) offers more secure building blocks for examining multicomponent treatment than do components as currently described.

Another area is the determination of goals. Patients may be overambitious or overcautious in identifying them, or restrict themselves to duties to the exclusion of more pleasant and reinforcing activities; the experience of staff can enrich the range of goals and increase the likelihood of estimating an appropriate time span and size of increment. However, a patient's goals (and that of those close to him or her) may differ substantially from those of treatment staff and of the funders and referrers who impress their expectations on staff. Return to (unsatisfying) work, foregoing compensation due after accidental injury, abstinence from all analgesic and psychotropic drug use, and taking regular exercise are areas where more seems to be expected of pain patients than is achieved by the general (pain-free) population, and staff and patient may differ on what is a reasonable goal. Although prosaic, it could be that failure to maintain treatment gains lies partly in the choice of goals, and the extent to which they express the patients' desires and hopes. Further issues in maintenance and generalization may concern the extent to which patients feel "expert" at the end of treatment. Traditional therapeutic relationships can counteract the development of patients' confidence in their own expertise, rather than respect for staff members' knowledge and skills. Although booster sessions are often invoked as the solution, none has shown lasting benefit (Turk, 2001). We still know very little about the processes that undermine treatment gains, given that they are probably as diverse and complex as are patients' circumstances, and the use of mean data at follow-up (following an implicit model of natural decay of treatment gains) is unlikely to disclose any.

There remain also hints of the pejorative terminology and patronizing representation of pain patients, explicit in early studies and descriptions of chronic pain populations, and now expressed more in the implication that they have no skills, take no responsibility, and aspire only to recline in the bosom of their enslaved families for their remaining decades. It is notable, but rarely commented on, that although in all other areas of health and illness social support is identified (by theoretical and empirical work) as a potent factor promoting health, help provided to pain patients by those around them is often characterized as contributing to disability. A study by Feldman, Downey, and Schaffer-Neitz (1999) is a notable exception, and found social support to have both main and buffering effects against distress associated with pain; an unrelated study by Jamison and Virts (1990) showed good family support (as reported by the patient) to be associated with better outcome of rehabilitation. Most of the work under the rubric of social support comes from patient–spouse interaction and largely correlational studies. These were originally thought to support the operant formulation, by demonstrating the association of spouse solicitousness and patient disability. However, even these studies and further replications show relationships between patient and spouse behavior to be mediated by gender, state of the relationship, and mood: The picture is substantially more complicated than suggested by the dominant study paradigms and measures of the 1980s and 1990s (Newton-John & Williams, 2000).

FAMILY AND MARITAL THERAPY

Background and Description

Family and or marital therapy is also used as an adjunct to the treatment of chronic pain in adults, and more directly in relation to pain and related behavior in children and adolescents, but much less is written regarding the topic (Kerns & Payne, 1996). The interest in treating the family of the chronic pain patient comes from recognition that not only the patient but also the spouse and other family members suffer the impact of pain. All family members are likely to experience reductions in leisure activities, changes in responsibilities and roles, and changes in how emotions are expressed (Turk et al., 1983).

Family therapy can take on many different forms. Some therapists take a traditional family systems approach and focus on how the family may or may not be using or developing resources and capacities to meet the demands of chronic pain (Patterson & Garwick, 1994). With this approach, the therapist attempts to restore a comfortable balance in the family system in light of the pain (Moore & Chaney, 1985). Alternatively, a family therapist may take an operant approach as described earlier. Fordyce (1976) in his early writings recommended that in some cases patients be refused treatment without spouse involvement, although today this would be regarded as ethically unacceptable. In this approach, the focus is on how pain behaviors are maintained by contingent social reinforcement (Fordyce, 1976) and draws on evidence showing that pain behavior can be influenced by spousal reactions to pain (e.g., Block, Kremer, & Gaylor, 1980). Family members are encouraged to withhold pain-contingent attention and instead reinforce well behaviors. Still other therapists take a CBT approach. Central to this approach is the belief that family members help patients understand the painful condition, and make judgments about the family and patient's ability to meet the challenge of the condition. The family develops beliefs about pain, disability, and emotional responses, which in turn influence how the patient and family members deal with the challenges of chronic pain (Kerns & Weiss, 1994). With this treatment approach, family members and the patient are encouraged to identify and develop strategies for coping with the effects of pain (Moore & Chaney, 1985), and to express the patient's needs directly and verbally, rather than indirectly and through pain behaviors—hence, the teaching of assertion skills and the recognition of the need to negotiate for help and exchange of favors, rather than one-way helping, which ultimately benefits neither patient nor family caregivers.

Evidence

Despite strong clinical assumptions that the family is important in determining response to chronic pain (e.g., Kerns, 1994), there has been little empirical research directed toward the benefits of family therapy for chronic pain (Radojevic, Nicassio, & Weisman, 1992), especially from a family systems point of view. Moore and Chaney (1985) evaluated the efficacy of outpatient group treatment of chronic pain and the effect of the spouse involvement in treatment; they randomly assigned patients to couples group treatment, patient-only group treatment, or waiting list control. In this study, both groups were treated from a CBT perspective. Both groups showed improvement on several measures, including pain behavior and functioning, marital satisfaction, and health care utilization. Improvements were no greater for those receiving couples group treatment compared to the patient-only group treatment. The study is not without limitations, including small sample size and the fact that the spousal involvement did not appear to be clearly delineated. Radojevic et al. (1992) drew similar conclusions. They examined a larger sample of rheumatoid arthritis patients and contrasted four groups: (a) behavior therapy with family involvement (e.g., family members taught to prompt and reinforce pain coping responses); (b) behavior therapy with no family involvement; (c) educational support group with the involvement of a family member; and (d) no-treatment control group. It should be noted that the behavioral conditions followed more of a CBT approach than a pure behavioral approach, in that treatment involved a cognitive component along with instruction in relaxation and operant conditioning. At immediate follow-up the behavioral intervention with family involvement was superior to all other conditions on disease activity measures, but did not differ from the behavior therapy group without family support at 2-month follow-up.

In terms of marital therapy, the research in this area is even more scant. Saaraijarvi (1991) provided some support for couples therapy using a systems approach, but not necessarily in terms of impact on pain and disability. In this study, chronic low back pain patients were randomized to either a control group or a couples therapy treatment group. At follow-up 12 months later, couples in the therapy group reported improved marital communication compared to those in the control group; no differences between the groups on health beliefs were observed, however.

Commentary

More questions than answers exist in this area, and there is a strong need for further research, especially given strong clinical assumptions regarding the importance of family. Would a traditional family systems approach be as effective as an operant or CBT approach involving the spouse? With the described CBT approaches, would more attention to family issues that do not revolve around pain assist with outcomes? Would clinical work with individual families be of greater benefit than family group treatment? Should issues or family interactions that are independent of illness-specific family issues also be addressed in therapy? What outcomes are of greatest interest in the treatment of families, individual cognitive and behavioral outcomes, or transactions with family members?

Much of this research has been undertaken with surprisingly little reference to the psychological literature on couples and families, as if all usual interactions are rendered unimportant by the presence of pain. When questioned or tested, the assumptions made about transactions are not well supported, such as the many interactions that don't fit the widely used categories of the Multidimensional Pain Inventory, which captures only responses by spouses that are solicitous, punishing, or distracting (see Newton-John & Williams, 2000). Further, as described earlier, in other fields of health and illness, social support is demonstrated to be a resource for health (e.g., Spanier & Allisson, 2001), whereas in pain it is frequently portrayed as an operant reinforcer of disability. Some changes to this view are apparent in the literature (e.g., Jamison & Virts, 1990, found that chronic pain patients who perceived their family as supportive as compared to nonsupportive, at 1-year follow-up reported better outcomes), but have not necessarily been incorporated in treatment programs.

PSYCHODYNAMIC PSYCHOTHERAPY

Background and Description

The final psychological treatment approach that merits mention with respect to chronic pain is psychodynamic therapy. In general, psychodynamic psychotherapy is not considered to be treatment of choice, but rather is regarded by some as a final treatment option for those who have not responded to other forms of psychological intervention or have not maintained treatment gains (Grzesiak, Ury, & Dworkin, 1996). It has been speculated that this form of treatment is appropriate for those individuals who have had early experiences (e.g., trauma, loss, abandonment) that lay a foundation for vulnerability to suffering and pain proneness; these experiences are hypothesized to lie dormant only to be triggered and expressed when a genuine organic painful condition is present. Others have elaborated that this form of therapy is appropriate for those who demonstrate certain psychological characteristics such as marked dependency, passivity, masochism, denial, regression, repressed anger, overt hostility, or neuroticism (Lakoff, 1983).

Few extended discussions of psychodynamic therapy for chronic pain exist. Central to psychodynamic therapy, however, is the importance of influences on behavior of which the patient may not be aware (Perlman, 1996). Therapy involves gaining understanding of the patient's world, especially developmental history, on which a dynamic model of pain can be formulated (Lakoff, 1983). Pain appears by most therapists following this tradition to be understood as a "real" problem, not simply symbolic or metaphorical.

Numerous themes may arise in psychodynamic therapy and have been discussed in a recent chapter by Grzesiak et al. (1996). Themes can range from discussion of early childhood experiences, such as relationships with family or the experience of physical or sexual abuse, to discussion of the expression, or lack thereof, of emotion. In part, the therapist and patient work together to release affect and may explore pain as in part a metaphor for underlying conflicts (Perlman, 1996). Psychodynamic therapists at times focus on the therapeutic relationship, which may be particularly appropriate for those patients who tend to be unrealistically dependent in their relationship to caregiver. Therapy can utilize the patient–therapist relationship as a method of facilitating change; the therapist works to establish and sustain a relationship that enables patients to change.

The themes that emerge in psychodynamic therapy are not necessarily unique to this approach and emerge in other types of therapy as well. It is incorrect to imply that only psychodynamic treatment addresses emotional problems. The final outcome that is expected in psychodynamic therapy is similar to CB therapy, namely, a cognitive emotional shift. The therapist aims to help the patient accept his or her pain as important but not a defining aspect of the self, and as regrettable but nevertheless manageable. Through therapy the person becomes an individual with persistent pain, who is able to remove pain from the center of existence and find purpose instead of anguish (Grzesiak et al., 1996).

Evidence and Commentary

One of the main criticisms regarding the psychodynamic approach is that the ideas are not well formulated or comprehensive (Turk & Flor, 1984). There is very little data on the efficacy or effectiveness of psychodynamic therapy, and therefore one must question whether time and financial resources should be used for a therapy of no proven value. Evidence that exists is of very low quality (e.g., Bassett & Pilowsky, 1985; Guthrie, Creed, Dawson, & Tonenson, 1991; Lakoff, 1983), and no RCTs involving standardized treatment have yet been carried out (Compas et al., 1998). For psychodynamic therapy to warrant serious consideration, attention needs to be given to standardization of treatment protocols and randomized comparison to alternate treatment strategies. Given the higher cost involved in this typically longer term approach, it needs to show itself to be considerably more effective than other approaches.

PSYCHOLOGICAL INTERVENTION SECONDARY TO MEDICAL INTERVENTION

Although psychological treatment for chronic pain is no longer conceptualized as a treatment of last resort, and some suggest it as first resort (Loeser, 2000), there are few published accounts of its integration with medical treatment and much less research. The primary area where reference is made to the integration of psychologists on medical teams is in multidisciplinary pain clinics or programs (e.g., Becker, Sjogren, Bech, Olsen, & Eriksen, 2000). In this case, patients have been found to give higher ratings of treatment helpfulness to psychological and educational interventions than to physical and medical modalities (Chapman, Jamison, Sanders, Lyman & Lynch, 2000). Some attention has also been given to how psychologists can be part of a team in selecting patients for treatments of true last resort (e.g., insertion of morphine pumps) (Prager & Jacobs, 2001) and health care teams attempting to improve adherence to treatment, such as drug therapy and physiotherapy (Turk & Rudy, 1991). Meanwhile, there is a strong argument for maximizing the gains to be made from analgesic and surgical interventions by combining them with pain management methods.

Providing pain management components alongside analgesic or surgical or medical treatment can appear confusing to patients if pain management components are presented as managing pain that cannot be relieved, at the same time as medical treatment attempts to relieve it. In addition, the increased cost of providing both types of treatment does not recommend their combination to health care funders. Presented with an apparent choice, the patient understandably will invest in pain relief and take a rain check on pain management. The lack of adequate integrated models in delivering medically based interventions and pain management strategies, in medical as well as in lay minds, perpetuates this problem.

On adherence to drugs, commonsense models dominated early research but have been disappointing (Horne, 1998). Adherence is a set of behaviors, not a single behavior, and is weakly or not predicted by knowledge (of the aim of taking the drug, of its unwanted effects, of what to do in the event of a missed dose, etc.). Addressing the costs and benefits of taking the drug, and identifying the patient's beliefs about drug use in general and in the particular case, can be helpful, as can the physician's monitoring of the drug and the patient's progress. It is not at all unusual for patients to have major and unfounded fears concerning the risks of using particular drugs that mean that they use those drugs in a suboptimal way; this has been shown most clearly in relation to opioid non-use in cancer patients (Ward et al., 1993). The phenomenon of intelligent nonadherence, when the benefits are outweighed by the costs of taking the drug, must also be recognized and addressed, or the physician is rendered ineffective by the patient's incomplete account of his or her behavior. Physicians' and patients' estimates of the extent of barrier to use presented by particular adverse effects differ substantially. Therefore, eliciting the report of an adverse effect (such as dry mouth with tricyclic antidepressants) should be followed by investigation of its implications (such as avoiding social conversation).

The cognitive approach that estimates the personal costs and benefits of adherence to recommended physical exercises may also be useful, although the area presents some different problems. Physiotherapists often offer too much rather than too little information (so that desirable adherence is hard to measure) (Sluijs, Kerssens, van der Zee, & Myers, 1998), and enjoyment of the exercise may be an important factor in maintaining exercise regimens (Jones, Harris, & McGee, 1998). That would suggest that introducing the patient to as many as possible sports, exercise routines, and even energetic leisure activities, such as some types of dance, may encourage adherence by finding at least one that he or she enjoys. However, adherence to exercise by the healthy population is notoriously low over months, and practical issues of access to facilities play an important part (Sallis & Owen, 1998).

Adherence to pain management methods both during and after treatment programs is somewhat underresearched, and little evidence has so far accrued that can identify the extent of adherence necessary to ensure maintenance of treatment gains or improvement on them. Research evidence suggests that complete adherence is not necessary for a positive treatment outcome (Silver, Blanchard, Williamson, Theobold, & Brown, 1979), but rather that gains may be greater among those with the highest adherence (Parker et al., 1988). Causes of nonadherence to pain management programs have been investigated (Turk & Rudy, 1991), but measurement of nonadherence itself is complicated in that patients often adhere to some aspects of a program and not others (so cannot be simply divided into adherents and nonadherents for comparison). Results of this research suggest that adherence is generally low among patients (e.g., Sullivan, Allegrante, Peterson, Kovar, & MacKenzie, 1998). As noted by Turk and Rudy (1991), hundreds of variables have been studied in relation to adherence, and not surprisingly the results are inconsistent, with contributions to variance from components of treatment program, the injury, the provider–patient relationship, social support, and patient characteristics (see Turk & Rudy, 1991). In terms of patient characteristics, dysfunctional pain beliefs (e.g., Williams & Thorn, 1989) and low self-efficacy (Granlund, Brulin, Johansson, & Sojka, 1998; Taal, Rasker, Seydel, & Wiegman, 1993) have been found to predict nonadherence.

Given this evidence, psychologists can play an important role in promoting adherence to treatment regimens, whether the treatment is medication, physiotherapy, or other components of pain management. Four general strategies exist: (a) assisting the patient in modifying the environment to facilitate adherence (e.g., charts, reminders); (b) implementation of a reinforcement schedule for the desired behavior; (c) fostering self-control and self-efficacy (e.g., setting realistic goals, positive self-talk); and (d) identifying, exploring, and modifying beliefs that may interfere with adherence. Efforts to address at least some of these dimensions have resulted in improved outcomes (Holroyd et al., 1989; Linton, Hellsing, & Bergstroem, 1996).

The other area where psychologists at times assist is the selection and preparation of patients for surgery. Although there is lots of evidence for psychological preparation for surgery helping a range of outcomes (e.g., reduced negative affect, pain, pain medication, length of stay) (Contrada, Leventhal, & Anderson, 1994) selection of patients for surgery has received much less support. Carragee (2001) reviewed the literature and concluded that psychological screening prior to disc surgery is of limited value in many cases, and can be viewed as useful only when less pathology is present, there have been longer periods of disability, and economic issues are present.

There is considerable correlational research evidence to suggest that psychological functioning prior to surgery predicts outcome following surgery. de Groot et al (1997) found, for instance, that preoperative anxiety was associated with poorer short-term and long-term recovery from lumbar surgery. Similarly, Graver et al. (1995) found that lower anxiety and fewer psychosomatic distress symptoms before surgery predicted a better outcome of lumbar disc surgery. Other variables, such as internal locus of control and lower catastrophic cognitions, have also been associated with better outcomes, such as shorter time to achieve a straight leg raise following total knee replacement (Kendell, Saxby, Malcolm, & Naisby, 2001). The research is correlational in nature and does not rule out the possibility that patient anxiety reflects a realistic interpretation of the circumstances surrounding surgery. It is also possible, however, that anxiety serves to limit activity and thus reduces the probability of a positive outcome. In line with this interpretation, concurrent psychological intervention with surgery may serve to enhance surgical outcome. That is, psychological interventions specifically aimed at anxiety reduction and improving self-efficacy and control may serve to facilitate recovery in some patients. Supporting this supposition, Scherzer et al. (2001) recently found that goal setting and positive self-talk helped to facilitate rehabilitation following reconstruction of the anterior cruciate ligament (ACL). Cupal et al. (2001) similarly found that psychological skills can enhance outcome following ACL reconstruction. In particular, usage of imagery and relaxation strategies following surgery was associated with significantly greater knee strength, and less pain anxiety about reinjury. Overall, there appears to be increasing support for psychological interventions in improving outcomes following surgery, but clearly more research is needed in this area.

PAIN IN CHILDREN

Prior to concluding, it must be acknowledged that this chapter, due largely to space constraints, has focused on psychological interventions for adults with chronic pain. We recognize that psychological interventions are also used to manage pain among children and adolescents (McGrath & Hillier, 1996; see also chap. 5, this volume). Cognitive interventions with children typically focus on modifying thoughts and coping abilities related to pain (e.g., provision of information, distraction, guided imagery, hypnotic imaginative involvement, stress management), whereas behavioral interventions most often focus on assisting children in changing pain behaviors (progressive muscle relaxation, deep breathing, reinforcement). McGrath (1987), in particular, strongly advocated a multistrategy approach (both pharmacological and nonpharmacological) for optimal management of recurrent persistent pain that is tailored to the child and follows from the needs identified through a multidimensional pain assessment. The interested reader is encouraged to review Eccleston, Morley, Williams, Yorke, and Mastroyannopoulou (2002), who conducted a recent systematic review and meta-analysis that shows good efficacy, but only really for headache, and secondarily for abdominal pain and sickle cell where there has been some preliminary research. There is no controlled research on several major childhood chronic problems such as juvenile rheumatoid arthritis.

CONCLUSION

Although psychological treatments for chronic pain have been shown to be valuable, there is far greater support for CB interventions than any other form of treatment. Even with this form of treatment, however, there is a need for further research evaluations. A number of valuable recommendations in this regard have been made (e.g., Keefe et al., 1992; Turk, Rudy, & Sorkin, 1993). Morley and Williams (2002) most recently highlighted some of the issues that deserve reflection for those considering conducting and evaluating psychological treatments for chronic pain. A significant challenge, for instance, is to understand why patients vary in their response to treatment and to develop interventions that are sensitive to individual needs. They further noted that there are severe limits to the extensive testing of all the parameters of treatment such as length and intensity. In this regard, they suggested that the way to move forward is through articulation of theories of change, of both specific and process components, to guide research on efficacy and effectiveness of treatment. In the selection and development of outcome measures they suggested that we need to examine the needs of various stakeholders and that both qualitative and quantitative approaches to this research are required.

Schwartz and colleagues (Schwartz, Cheney, Irvine, & Keefe, 1997) cautioned that clinical research on psychosocial interventions has flourished in the past two decades, and that due to the wide availability of interventions, reliance on standard no-treatment control conditions is really no longer possible. A new design for randomized clinical trials is described by Schwartz's group (1997) that does not require a no-treatment control group, and that potentially identifies dose-response relationships between interventions and treatment outcomes. They proposed use of a three-arm variation of a standard crossover trial. In the first arm patients receive active treatment followed by standard care; in the second arm patients receive standard care followed by active treatment; and in the third arm, patients receive active treatment throughout, allowing also for the study of dose-response relationships. The design avoids ethical difficulties by ensuring all patients receive treatment and also in the final arm allows for study of the process of change. Sample size, however, will continue to be a challenge. Most studies are hopelessly underpowered for their aims, and the use of treatment rather than no-treatment controls (as recommended) will require even larger samples to show differences. This takes us beyond the resources of almost any single clinic.

Based on review of the research as it stands, it is apparent that many patients have benefited from the development of psychological interventions outlined here and are substantially better served than they were 40 years ago. There is now widespread acceptance for the role of psychological interventions in the treatment of chronic pain, and, in particular, it has been recommended that pain treatment facilities, in addition to physical therapy and education, include CBT on a routine basis (Fishbain, 2000). What are the implications of the review for the clinician? At the present time a CBT approach would appear to have the greatest support in working with patients. Within this approach, however, there is considerable variability in how this can be applied, and until further research is available, clinicians are likely to continue to tailor their approach to the needs of the patients. To maintain the rate of improvement we have achieved, a critical appreciation of where we are now is needed, as well as continued attempts to overcome methodological challenges in research already noted. Above and beyond improved research as described earlier, routine audit and publication of outcomes of existing clinical programs would be highly beneficial so that best practice can evolve from the widest possible clinical base.

REFERENCES

American Psychological Association, Division of Clinical Psychology, Task Force on Promotion and Dissemination of Psychological Procedures. (1995). Training in and dissemination of empirically-validated psychological treatments: Report on recommendations. *Clinical Psychologist, 48,* 3–23.

Arena, J. G., & Blanchard, E. B. (1996). Biofeedback and relaxation therapy. In R. J. Gatchel & D. C. Turk (Eds.), *Psychological approaches to pain management* (pp. 179–230). New York: Guilford Press.

Bassett, D. L., & Pilowsky, I. A. (1985). Study of brief psychotherapy for chronic pain. *Journal of Psychosomatic Research, 29,* 259–264.

Beck, A. T. (1976). *Cognitive therapy and emotional disorders.* New York: International Universities Press.

Becker, N., Sjogren, P., Bech, P., Olsen, A. K., & Eriksen, J. (2000). Treatment outcome of chronic non-malignant pain patients managed in a Danish multidisciplinary pain centre compared to general practice: A randomized controlled trial. *Pain, 84,* 203–211.

Blanchard, E. B. (1992). Psychological treatment of benign headache disorders. *Journal of Consulting and Clinical Psychology, 60,* 537–551.

Blanchard, E. B., Kim, M., Hermann, C., & Steffek, B. D. (1993). Preliminary results of the effects of headache relief of perception of success among tension headache patients receiving relaxation. *Headache Quarterly, 4,* 249–253.

Block, A. R., Kremer, E. F., & Gaylor, M. (1980). Behavioral treatment of chronic pain: The spouse as a discriminative cue for pain behavior. *Pain, 9,* 243–252.

Bradley, L. A. (1996). Cognitive-behavioral therapy for chronic pain. In R. J. Gatchel & D. C. Turk (Eds.), *Psychological approaches to pain management* (pp. 131–147). New York: Guilford Press.

Bradley, L. A., Young, L. D., Anderson, K. O., Turner, R. A., Agudelo, C. A., McDaniel, L. K., Pisko, E. J., Semble, E. L., & Morgan, T. M. (1987). Effects of psychological therapy on pain behaviour of rheumatoid patients: Treatment outcome and six-month follow-up. *Arthritis and Rheumatism, 30,* 1105–1114.

Carragee, E. J. (2001). Psychological screening in the surgical treatment of lumbar disc herniation. *Clinical Journal of Pain, 17,* 215–219.

Chambless, D. L., & Ollendick, T. H. (2001). Empirically supported psychological interventions. *Annual Review of Psychology, 52,* 685–716.

Chapman, S. L., Jamison, R. N., Sanders, S. H., Lyman, D. R., & Lynch, N. T. (2000). Perceived treatment helpfulness and cost in chronic pain rehabilitation. *Clinical Journal of Pain, 16,* 169–177.

Compas, B. E., Haaga, D. A., Keefe, F. J., Leitenberg, H., & Williams, D. A. (1998). Sampling of empirically supported psychological treatments from health psychology: Smoking, chronic pain, cancer, and bulimia nervosa. *Journal of Consulting and Clinical Psychology, 66,* 89–112.

Contrada, R., Leventhal, E., & Anderson, J. (1994). Psychological preparation for surgery: Marshalling individual and social resources to optimize self-regulation. *International Review of Health Psychology, 3,* 219–266.

Crider, A. B., & Glaros, A. G. (1999). A meta-analysis of EMG biofeedback treatment of temporomandibular disorders. *Journal of Orofacial Pain, 13,* 29–37.

Cupal, D. D., & Brewer, B. W. (2001). Effects of relaxation and guided imagery on knee strength, reinjury anxiety, and pain following anterior cruciate ligament reconstruction. *Rehabilitation Psychology, 46,* 28–43.

de Groot, K. I., Boeke, S., van den Berge, H. J., Duivenvoorden, H. J., Bonke, B., & Passchier, J. (1997). Assessing short- and long-term recovery from lumbar surgery with pre-operative biographical, medical and psychological variables. *British Journal of Health Psychology, 2,* 229–243.

Eccleston, C., & Crombez, G. (1999). Pain demands attention: A cognitive-affective model of the interruptive function of pain. *Psychological Bulletin, 125,* 356–366.

Eccleston, C., Morley, S., Williams, A., Yorke, L., & Mastroyannopoulou, K. (2002). Systematic review of randomised controlled trials of psychological therapy for chronic pain in children and adolescents, with a subset meta-analysis of pain relief. *Pain, 99,* 157–165.

Feldman, S. I., Downey, G., & Schaffer-Neitz, R. (1999). Pain, negative mood, and perceived support in chronic pain patients: A daily diary study of people with reflex sympathetic dystrophy syndrome. *Journal of Consulting & Clinical Psychology, 67,* 776–785.

Fernandez, E., & Turk, D. C. (1989). The utility of cognitive coping strategies for altering pain perception: A meta-analysis. *Pain, 38,* 123–135.

Fishbain, D. A. (2000). Non-surgical chronic pain treatment outcome: A review. *International Review of Psychiatry, 12,* 170–180.

Flor, H., Birbaumer, N., Schugens, M. M., & Lutzenberger, W. (1992). Symptom-specific psychophysiological responses in chronic pain patients. *Psychophysiology, 29,* 452–460.

Fordyce, W. E. (1973). An operant conditioning method for managing chronic pain. *Postgraduate Medicine, 53,* 123–138.

Fordyce, W. E. (1976). *Behavioural methods for chronic pain and illness.* St. Louis, MO: C. V. Mosby.

Fordyce, W. E. (1988). Pain and suffering. A reappraisal. *American Psychologist, 43,* 276–283.

Fordyce, W. E., Fowler, R., Lehmann, J., & DeLateur, B. (1968). An application of behaviour modification techniques to a problem of chronic pain. *Behaviour Research and Therapy, 6,* 105–107.

Fordyce, W. E., Fowler, R., Lehmann, J., DeLateur, B., Sand P., & Treischmann, R. (1973). Operant conditioning in the treatment of chronic pain. *Archives of Physical Medicine and Rehabilitation, 54,* 399–408.

Fordyce, W. E., Roberts, A. H., & Sternbach, R. A. (1985). The behavioural management of chronic pain: A response to critics. *Pain, 22,* 113–125.

Granlund, B., Brulin, C., Johansson, H., & Sojka, P. (1998). Can motivational factors predict adherence to an exercise program for subjects with low back pain? *Scandinavian Journal of Behaviour Therapy, 27,* 81–96.

Graver, V., Ljunggren, A. E., Malt, U. F., Loeb, M., Haaland, A. K., Magnaes, B., & Lie, H. (1995). Can psychological traits predict the outcome of lumbar disc surgery when anamnestic and physiological risk factors are controlled for? Results of a cohort study. *Journal of Psychosomatic Research, 39,* 465–476.

Grzesiak, R. C., Ury, G. M., & Dworkin, R. H. (1996). Psychodynamic psychotherapy with chronic pain patients. In R. J. Gatchel & D. C. Turk (Eds.), *Psychological approaches to pain management* (pp. 148–178). New York: Guilford Press.

Guthrie, E., Creed, F., Dawson, D., & Tonenson, B. (1991). A controlled trial of psychological treatment for irritable bowel syndrome. *Gastroneterology, 100,* 450–457.

Guzmán, J., Esmail, R., Karjalainen, K., Irvin, E., & Bombadier, C. (2001). Multidisciplinary rehabilitation for chronic low back pain: Systematic review. *British Medical Journal, 322,* 511–516.

Haanen, H. C. M., Hoenderdos, H. T. W., van Romunde, L. K. J., Hop, W. C. J., Malle, C., Terwiel, J. P., & Hekster, G. B. (1991). Controlled trial of hypnotherapy in the treatment of refractory fibromyalgia. *Journal of Rheumatology, 18,* 72–75.

Haythornthwaite, J. A., & Benrud-Larson, L. M. (2001). Psychological assessment and treatment of patients with neuropathic pain. *Current Pain and Headache Reports, 5,* 124–129.

Holroyd, K. A., Cordingley, G. E., Pingel, J. D., Jerome, A., Theofanous, A. G., Jackson, D. K., & Leard, L. (1989). Enhancing the effectiveness of abortive therapy: A controlled evaluation of self-management training. *Headache, 29,* 148–153.

Holroyd, K. A., Penzien, D. B., Hursey, K. G., Tobin, L. R., Holm, J. E., Marcille, P. J., Hall, J. R., & Chila, A. G. (1984). Change mechanisms in EMG biofeedback training: Cognitive changes underlying improvements in tension headache. *Journal of Consulting and Clinical Psychology, 52,* 1039–1053.

Horne, R. (1998). Adherence to medication: A review of existing research. In L. B. Myers & K. Midence (Eds.), *Adherence to treatment in medical conditions* (pp. 285–310). London: Harwood.

Jamison, R. N., & Virts, K. L. (1990). The influence of family support on chronic pain. *Behaviour Research and Therapy, 28,* 283–287.

Jensen, M. P., Turner, J. A., & Romano, J. M. (2001). Changes in beliefs, catastrophizing, and coping are associated with improvement in multidisciplinary pain treatment. *Journal of Consulting and Clinical Psychology, 69,* 655–662.

Jones, F., Harris, P., & McGee, L. (1998). Adherence to prescribed exercise. In L. B. Myers & K. Midence (Eds.), *Adherence to treatment in medical conditions* (pp. 343–362). Amsterdam, Netherlands: Harwood.

Keefe, F. J., & Bradley, L. A. (1984). Behavioral and psychological approaches to the assessment and treatment of chronic pain. *General Hospital Psychiatry, 6,* 49–54.

Keefe, F. J., Dunsmore, J., & Burnett, R. (1992). Behavioral and cognitive-behavioral approaches to chronic pain: Recent advances and future directions. *Journal of Consulting and Clinical Psychology, 60,* 528–536.

Keefe, F. J., Jacobs, M., & Underwood-Gordon, L. (1997). Biobehavioral pain research: A multi-institute assessment of cross-cutting issues and research needs. *Clinical Journal of Pain, 13,* 91–101.

Keefe, F. J., Kashikar-Zuck, S., Opiteck, J., Hage, E., Dalrymple, L., & Blumenthal, J. A. (1996). Pain in arthritis and musculoskeletal disorders: The role of coping skills training and exercise. *Journal of Orthopedic Sports Physiotherapy, 21,* 279–290.

Kendell, K., Saxby, B., Farrow, M., & Naisby, C. (2001). Psychological factors associated with short-term recovery from total knee replacement. *British Journal of Health Psychology, 6,* 41–52.

Kerns, R. D. (1994). Families and chronic illness. *Annals of Behavioural Medicine, 16,* 107–108.

Kerns, R. D., & Payne, A. (1996). Treating families of chronic pain patients. In R. J. Gatchel & D. C. Turk (Eds.), *Psychological approaches to pain management* (pp. 283–304). New York: Guilford Press.

Kerns, R. D., & Weiss, L. H. (1994). Family influences on the course of chronic illness: A cognitive-behavioural transactional model. *Annals of Behavioural Medicine, 16,* 116–130.

Knost, B., Flor, H., Birbaumer, N., & Schugens, M. M. (1999). Learned maintenance of pain: Muscle tension reduces central nervous system processing of painful stimulation in chronic and subchronic pain patients. *Psychophysiology, 36,* 755–764.

LaChappelle, D. L., Hadjistavropoulos, H. D., & McCreary, D. R. (2001). Contribution of pain-related adjustment and perceptions of control to coping strategy use among cervical sprain patients. *European Journal of Pain, 5,* 405–413.

Lakoff, R. (1983). Interpretive psychotherapy with chronic pain patients. *Canadian Journal of Psychiatry, 28,* 650–653.

Lethem, J., Slade, P. D., Troup, J. D., & Bentley, G. (1983). Outline of a fear-avoidance model of exaggerated pain perception—I. *Behaviour Research & Therapy, 21,* 401–408.

Linton, S. J. (1982). A critical review of behavioural treatments for chronic benign pain other than headache. *British Journal of Clinical Psychology, 21,* 321–337.

Linton, S. J. (1986). Behavioral remediation of chronic pain: A status report. *Pain, 24,* 125–141.

Linton, S. J., Hellsing, A. L., & Bergstroem, G. (1996). Exercise for workers with musculoskeletal pain: Does enhancing compliance decrease pain? *Journal of Occupational Rehabilitation, 6,* 177–190.

Linton, S. J., Hellsing, A. L., & Larsson, I. (1997). Bridging the gap: Support groups do not enhance long-term outcome in chronic back pain. *Clinical Journal of Pain, 13,* 221–228.

Loeser, J. D. (2000). Pain and suffering. *Clinical Journal of Pain, 16*(2 Suppl.), S2–S6.

Lorig, K., Lubeck, D., Kraines, R. G., Seleznick, M., & Holman, H. R. (1985). Outcomes of self help education for patients with arthritis. *Arthritis and Rheumatism, 28,* 680–685.

Marlatt, G. A., & Gordon, J. R. (1980). Determinants of relapse: Implications for the maintenance of behavior change. In P. O. Davidson & S. M. Davidson (Eds.), *Behavioral medicine: Changing health lifestyles* (pp. 410–452). New York: Brunner/Mazel.

McGrath, P. A. (1987). The multidimensional assessment and management of recurrent pain syndromes in children and adolescents. *Behaviour Research and Therapy, 25,* 251–262.

McGrath, P. A., & Hillier, L. M. (1996). Controlling children's pain. In R. J. Gatchel & D. C. Turk (Eds.), *Psychological approaches to pain management* (pp. 331–370). New York: Guilford Press.

Melzack, R., & Wall, P. D. (1965). Pain mechanisms: A new theory. *Science, 150,* 971–979.

Morley, S., Eccleston, C., & Williams, A. C. de C. (1999). Systematic review and meta-analysis of randomized controlled trials of cognitive behaviour therapy and behaviour therapy for chronic pain in adults, excluding headache. *Pain, 80,* 1–13.

Morley, S., & Williams, A. C. (2002). Conducting and evaluating treatment outcome studies. In D. C. Turk & R. J. Gatchel (Eds.), *Psychological approaches to pain management: A practitioner's handbook* (2nd ed., pp. 52–68). New York: Guilford Press.

Moore, J. E., & Chaney, E. F. (1985). Outpatient group treatment of chronic pain: Effects of spouse involvement. *Journal of Consulting and Clinical Psychology, 53,* 326–334.

Newton-John, T. R., & Williams, A. C. de C. (2000). Solicitousness revisited: A qualitative analysis of spouse responses to pain behaviours. In M. Devor, M. C. Rowbotham, & Z. Wiesenfeld-Hallin (Eds.), *Proceedings of the 9th World Congress on Pain* (pp. 1113–1122). Seattle, WA: IASP Press.

Nicholas, M. K., Wilson, P. H., & Goyen, J. (1992). Comparison of cognitive-behavioral group treatment and an alternative non-psychological treatment for chronic low back pain. *Pain, 48,* 339–347.

Parker, J. C., Frank, R. G., Beck, N. C., Smarr, K. L., Buescher, K., Phillips, L. R., Smith, E. I., Anderson, S. K., & Walker, S. E. (1988). Pain management in rheumatoid arthritis: A cognitive-behavioural approach. *Arthritis & Rheumatism, 31*, 593–601.

Patterson, D. R., Everett, J. J., Burns, G. L., & Marvin, J. A. (1992). Hypnosis for the treatment of burn pain. *Journal of Consulting and Clinical Psychology, 60*, 713–717.

Patterson, J. M., & Garwick, A. W. (1994). The impact of chronic illness on families: A family systems perspective. *Annals of Behavioural Medicine, 16*, 131–142.

Perlman, S. D. (1996). Psychoanalytic treatment of chronic pain: The body speaks on multiple levels. *Journal of the American Academy of Psychoanalysis, 24*, 257–271.

Pincus, T., & Morley, S. (2001). Cognitive-processing bias in chronic pain: A review and integration. *Psychological Bulletin, 127*, 599–617.

Prager, J., & Jacobs, M. (2001). Evaluation of patients for implantable pain modalities: Medical and behavioral assessment. *Clinical Journal of Pain, 17*, 206–214.

Radojevic, V., Nicassio, P. M., & Weisman, M. H. (1992). Behavioural intervention with and without family support for rheumatoid arthritis. *Behaviour Therapy, 23*, 13–30.

Romano, J. M., Turner, J. A., Friedman, L. S., Bulcroft, R. A., Jensen, M. P., & Hops, H. (1991). Observational assessment of chronic pain patient–spouse behavioural interactions. *Behaviour Therapy, 22*, 549–568.

Romano, J. M., Turner, H. A., Friedman, L. S., Bulcroft, R. A., Jensen, M. P., Hops, H., & Wright, S. F. (1992). Sequential analysis of chronic pain behaviors and spouse responses. *Journal of Consulting & Clinical Psychology, 60*, 777–782.

Romano, J. M., Turner, J. A., Jensen, M. P., Friedman, L. S., Bulcroft, R. A., Hops, H., & Wright, S. F. (1995). Chronic pain patient-spouse behavioral interactions predict patient disability. *Pain, 63*, 353–360.

Rudy, T. E., Kerns, R. D., & Turk, D. C. (1988). Chronic pain and depression: Toward a cognitive-behavioral mediation model. *Pain, 35*, 129–140.

Saarijarvi, S. (1991). A controlled study of couple therapy in chronic low back pain patients: Effects on marital satisfaction, psychological distress and health attitudes. *Journal of Psychosomatic Research, 35*, 265–272.

Sallis, J. F., & Owen, N. (1998). Physical activity and behavioral medicine. *Behavioral Medicine & Health Psychology, 3*. Newbury Park, CA: Sage Publishing.

Sanders, S. H. (1996). Operant conditioning with chronic pain: Back to basics. In R. J. Gatchel & D. C. Turk (Eds.), *Psychological approaches to pain management* (pp. 112–130). New York: Guilford Press.

Scherzer, C. B., Brewer, B. W., Cornelius, A. E., Van Raalte, J. L., Petitpas, A. J., Sklar, J. H., et al. (1997). Psychological skills and adherence to rehabilitation after reconstruction of the anterior cruciate ligament. *Journal of Sport Rehabilitation, 10*, 165–172.

Schwartz, C. E., Chesney, M. A., Irvine, M. J., & Keefe, F. J. (1997). The control group dilemma in clinical research: Applications for psychosocial and behavioral medicine trials. *Psychosomatic Medicine, 59*, 362–371.

Sherman, J. J., & Turk, D. C. (2001). Nonpharmacologic approaches to the management of myofascial temporomandibular disorders. *Current Pain and Headache Reports, 5*, 421–431.

Silver, B., Blanchard, E., Williamson, D., Theobold, D. E., & Brown, D. (1979). Temperature biofeedback and relaxation training in the treatment of migraine headaches: One-year follow-up. *Biofeedback & Self Regulation, 4*, 359–366.

Simmonds, M. (1999). Physical function and physical performance in patients with pain: What are the measures and what do they mean? In *Pain 1999—An updated review* (pp. 127–136). Seattle, WA: IASP Press.

Sluijs, E. M., Kerssens, J. J., van der Zee, J., & Myers, L. B. (1998). Adherence to physiotherapy. In L. B. Myers & K. Midence (Eds.), *Adherence to treatment in medical conditions* (pp. 363–382). London: Harwood.

Spanier, P. A., & Allison, K. R. (2001). General social support and physical activity: An analysis of the Ontario Health Survey. *Canadian Journal of Public Health, 92*, 210–213.

Sullivan, M. J. L., Thorn, B., Haythornthwaite, J. A., Keefe, F., Martin, M., Bradley, L. A., & Lefebvre, J. C. (2001). Theoretical perspectives on the relation between catastrophizing and pain. *Clinical Journal of Pain, 17*, 53–61.

Sullivan, T., Allegrante, J. P., Peterson, M. G. E., Kovar, P. A., & MacKenzie, C. R. (1998). One-year followup of patients with osteoarthritis of the knee who participated in a program of supervised fitness walking and supportive patient education. *Arthritis Care & Research, 11*, 228–233.

Syrjala, K. L., & Abrams, J. R. (1996). Hypnosis and imagery in the treatment of pain. In R. J. Gatchel & D. C. Turk (Eds.), *Psychological approaches to pain management* (pp. 231–258). New York: Guilford Press.

Taal, E., Rasker, J. J., Seydel, E. R., & Wiegman, O. (1993). Health status, adherence with health recommendations, self-efficacy and social support in patients with rheumatoid arthritis. *Patient Education & Counseling, 20*, 63–76.

Tan, S. Y., & Leucht, C. A. (1997). Cognitive-behavioral therapy for clinical pain control: A 15-year update and its relationship to hypnosis. *International Journal of Clinical and Experimental Hypnosis, 45*, 396–416.

Turk, D. C. (1990). Customizing treatment for chronic pain patients: Who, what, and why. *Clinical Journal of Pain, 6*, 255–270.

Turk, D. C. (2001). Combining somatic and psychosocial treatment for chronic pain patients: Perhaps 1 + 1 does = 3. *Clinical Journal of Pain, 17*, 281–283.

Turk, D. C., & Flor, H. (1984). Etiological theories and treatments for chronic back pain: II. Psychological models and interventions. *Pain, 19*, 209–233.

Turk, D. C., Meichenbaum D., & Genest, M. (1983). *Pain and behavioural medicine: A cognitive-behavioural perspective*. New York: Guilford Press.

Turk, D. C., & Rudy, T. E. (1989). A cognitive-behavioral perspective on chronic pain: Beyond the scalpel and syringe. In C. D. Tollison (Ed.), *Handbook of chronic pain management* (pp. 222–236). Baltimore, MD: Williams & Wilkins.

Turk, D. C., & Rudy, T. E. (1991). Neglected topics in the treatment of chronic pain patients—Relapse, noncompliance, and adherence enhancement. *Pain, 44*, 5–28.

Turk, D. C., & Rudy, T. E. (1992). Cognitive factors and persistent pain: A glimpse into Pandora's box. *Cognitive Therapy & Research, 16*, 99–122.

Turk, D. C., Rudy, T. E., & Sorkin, B. A. (1993). Neglected topics in chronic pain treatment outcome studies: Determination of success. *Pain, 53*, 3–16.

Turner, J. A., & Chapman, C. R. (1982a). Psychological interventions for chronic pain: A critical review. Operant conditioning, hypnosis, and cognitive-behavioral therapy. *Pain, 12*, 23–46.

Turner, J. A., & Chapman, C. R. (1982b). Psychological interventions for chronic pain: A critical review. I. Relaxation training and biofeedback. *Pain, 12*, 1–21.

van Tulder, M. W., Ostelo, R., Vlaeyen, J. W., Linton, S. J., Morley, S. J., & Assendelft, W. J. (2000). Behavioral treatment for chronic low back pain: A systematic review within the framework of the Cochrane Back Review Group. *Spine, 25*, 2688–2699.

Vlaeyen, J. W., & Linton, S. J. (2000). Fear-avoidance and its consequences in chronic musculoskeletal pain: A state of the art. *Pain, 85*, 317–332.

Ward, S. E., Goldberg, N., Miller-McCauley, V., Mueller, C., Nolan, A., Pawlik-Plank, D., Robbins, A., Stormoen, D., & Weissman, D. E. (1993). Patient related barriers to management of cancer pain. *Pain, 52*, 319–324.

Watson, P. J., Booker, C. K., Main, C. J., & Chen, A. C. (1997). Surface electromyography in the identification of chronic low back pain patients: The development of the flexion relaxation ratio. *Clinical Biomechanics, 11*, 165–171.

Williams, A. C. de C., Richardson, P. H., Nicholas, M. K., Pither, C. E., Harding, V. R., Ridout, K. L., Palphs, J. A., Richardson, I. H., Justins, D. M., & Chamberlain, J. H. (1996). Inpatient vs. outpatient pain management: Results of a randomised controlled trial. *Pain, 66*, 13–22.

Williams, D. A., & Thorn, B. E. (1989). An empirical assessment of pain beliefs. *Pain, 36*, 351–358.

11

Psychological Perspectives on Pain: Controversies

Kenneth D. Craig
Department of Psychology,
University of British Columbia

Thomas Hadjistavropoulos
Department of Psychology,
University of Regina

Controversies abound concerning the role of psychological features of pain and their use in pain management. Although pain has been clearly identified as a psychological experience, one does not have to spend much time talking to people or reading the literature to discover disagreements about the nature of this experience. Contested issues include a willingness to dismiss the importance of patient thoughts and feelings, questions about the meaning of behavioral displays of pain, debates about the role of social contexts, disagreements about how one should assess pain, and whether and how one should attempt to control painful distress. Similar disagreements concerning pain mechanisms and intervention approaches are found when considering anthropological, nursing, pharmacological, surgical, neurophysiological, genetic, or any other perspective on pain; however, the focus here is on psychological processes.

Roots of dissension concerning models of pain and pain management are found in persistent and uncontrolled pain. Pain remains a very serious problem with highly debilitating and destructive consequences for large numbers of people. Almost everyone can anticipate episodes of poorly controlled acute pain in their future, and there are distressingly high numbers of patients with persistent or recurrent pain. Both signal the failures of current explanatory models and the inadequacies of current applications of treatment or palliative interventions, despite numerous advances in our understanding of biological, psychological, and social mechanisms in pain and

303

improved pain control strategies (Wall & Melzack, 2001). There should be urgency and contention in the field until a better measure of pain control is accomplished. Indeed, it seems surprising that the inadequacies of our understanding of pain and our limitations in controlling pain are not more widely understood or publicized, and that they are not greater sources of scientific, practitioner, and public unrest. Fortunately, there is reason for optimism. Recent decades have seen concerted efforts to provide an evidence-based understanding of pain, and to improve utilization of these understandings by practitioners. Many of the recent advances have resulted from the inspiration and leadership of John Bonica (1953; Loeser, Butler, Chapman & Turk, 2001), the integrative perspective and heuristic benefits of the gate control theory of pain (Melzack & Wall, 1965), and the organizational structure and impetus generated by the founding of the International Association for the Study of Pain in 1974 (http://www.iasp-pain.org/).

Many factors contribute to differences of opinion in our understanding of pain and pain management. Scholars from numerous disciplines, including the humanities and the biological, behavioral, and social sciences, as well as health care professionals with diverse education and commitments, all bring varied perspectives to the challenges of understanding a broad range of issues and untested concepts about the nature of pain and pain management. The tragedies of uncontrolled pain and suffering have engaged humans throughout evolutionary history in varied, and sometimes isolated, cultures around the globe; hence, varied views in different cultures and communities have emerged (Craig & Pillai, in press). Most of these views deserve respect, but no model has as yet proven wholly satisfactory. Nonetheless, the evidence-based perspective (McQuay, Moore, Moore, 1998) has great potential because methods of science are more effective in identifying valid concepts and useful interventions than are trial and error solutions.

In the developed world, there is a tendency to focus on technological understandings and answers, in part because of the unfettered promise of biological solutions. In addition, government agencies and the pharmaceutical industry provide generous resources to support this perspective. Although there have been celebrated successes in development of new analgesic pharmaceuticals, these often remain unavailable to the community at large, and sometimes the widespread potential of such discoveries appears exaggerated. Dissatisfaction with biomedical approaches is reflected in the major resurgence of interest in alternative and complementary medicine and the substantial market share of health expenditures this sector has been able to capture in providing services to chronic pain patients who have not benefited from conventional western medical care. Essentially, failures of Western approaches to health care and urgent need for relief from pain have led to free-market competition. This situation can be recognized as advantageous, as it encourages exploration of new ideas and diffusion of inno-vation on an essentially global basis.

The psychological perspective on pain offers considerable promise, and there have been substantial advances since Sternbach (1968) published the first book representing a synthesis in the area. Most major health problems (cardiovascular disease, musculoskeletal disorders, diabetes, obesity, HIV-AIDS, cancer) are largely due to psychosocial and lifestyle factors. The focus of medicine is on management of disease, with the medical profession not effectively addressing behavioral health issues or pain arising from many conditions. The well-being of patients would seem to dictate stronger alliances between primary care physicians, other health care professionals, and psychologists.

Our task in this chapter is to identify contentious issues, both those already recognized and others that became apparent as we surveyed the field. The task was not difficult. Having noted this, we recognize that this account represents a subjective perspective. Not everyone would recognize the same controversies, and we would encourage those who do not agree with our concerns to describe the issues that are problematic for them.

THE NATURE OF PAIN AND CONTROVERSIES ABOUT ITS DEFINITION

As amply demonstrated in the earlier chapters of this volume, concepts of pain have evolved dramatically throughout the last century. Sensory-specific models proved unable to explain many of the complexities of pain (see Melzack & Wall, 1996 for an overview) and yielded to multidimensional models that acknowledge pain as a complex synthesis of thoughts, feelings, and sensory input, as described in the chapter by Melzack and Katz in this volume as well as in the work of others. For example, Price (2000) showed that the cortico-limbic pathway in the brain integrates nociceptive input with contextual information and memory to provide cognitive mediation of pain affect. There is no need here to review the history or the basis for the advances in thinking, although the transformations in thinking have not fully pervaded the practice of working with pain patients.

While there would be agreement that considerable pain is suffered need-lessly (Melzack, 1988), one might generate the argument that not all pain is undesirable. Advocates of corporal punishment and those who practice vio-lence appear to perceive merit in inflicting pain to punish or modify the be-havior of others. Evidence of its limited effectiveness and the unfortunate consequences of misuse of punishment (Gershoff, 2002) do not seem to in-hibit its use. Others argue that personal experiences of pain have beneficial consequences. Few would disagree that pain serves to warn of injury and disease. The consequences of congenital insensitivity to pain are well known (Melzack, 1973): The injuries sustained and diseases not averted have the potential to cause early death. Anthropological literature reinforces the idea that pain is desirable under certain circumstances. In some religious perspectives, pain can be a source of divine experience and importance (Tu, 1980). The current popularity of tattooing, body piercing, and even self-inflicted branding signals a willingness to tolerate pain for personal outcomes. Pain during masochistic sexual rituals illustrates how social contextual factors can transform the pain experience. Religious penitents who subject themselves to flagellation, fire-walking, body piercing and mutilation, and even death (Glucklich, 2000) display a dramatic willingness to self-inflict pain. These examples illustrate the human capacity to override biological imperatives to avoid pain in the interests of personal values. These varying social contexts highlight the importance of value judgments in appraisals of the role of pain in human experience.

The widely used and accepted definition of pain created by the International Association for the Study of Pain (1979), has been a powerful influence in our understanding. The initial definition described pain as, "An unpleasant sensory and emotional experience associated with actual or potential tissue damage, or described in terms of such damage" (Merskey, 1991). The definition has served psychology well because it emphasizes the complexities of psychological experiences; however, limitations can be observed. The definition was criticized (e.g., Anand & Craig, 1996) because it defined pain as an experience that is either associated with tissue damage or can be *described* (emphasis added) in terms of such damage. Specifically, it was felt that nonverbal populations (e.g., infants, people with severe cognitive and neurological impairments) are unable to describe their pain. Although there is a possibility that someone else could describe it on their behalf, the unavailability of such an observer would reduce the probability of these individuals meeting the definitional criteria for pain. Responsive to these concerns, in 2001 IASP added the following note to its definition: "The inability to communicate in no way negates the possibility that an individual is experiencing pain and is in need of appropriate pain relieving treatment" (http://www.iasp-pain.org/terms-p.html). Although the note represents an improvement, we would argue that the phrase "inability to communicate" is not adequate. Consistent with the Communications Model of Pain (e.g., Hadjistavropoulos & Craig, 2002), the ability to communicate should be represented as a continuum. The vast majority of infants and other nonverbal populations are capable of some form of communication (e.g., paralinguistic vocalizations, facial expressions, guarding behaviors). Although such communications are often more difficult to decode than is verbal report, they are communication nonetheless. As such, we would prefer references to "limitations in ability to communicate" rather than to "inability to communicate" (e.g., Hadjistavropoulos, von Baeyer, & Craig, 2001). Representing an evolution in thinking, more recently, IASP added the word *verbally* to its note which now reads "The inability to communicate verbally does not negate the possibility that an individual is experiencing pain and is in need of appropriate pain-relieving treatment" (http://www.iasp-pain. org./terms-p.html).

One can also question whether the definition satisfactorily captures the key features of pain, as a definition should. Although it includes emotion and sensation as essential components, it does not acknowledge the role of cognition in the experience. Melzack and Casey (1968) made it clear that all pain is a multidimensional experience made up of a complex interaction of sensory, affective, and cognitive features within the central nervous system (see also Gagliese & Katz, 2000). People's interpretations of the meaning and implications of the experience, as determined by memory or perception of the immediate context, and their ongoing thoughts and coping strategies, are very important features (Turk, 1996). Turk and Okifuji (2002) provide a recent review of the importance of people's appraisals of their symptoms, their ability to self-manage pain, and their fears about pain and injury that motivate efforts to avoid exacerbation of symptoms and further injury. Cognition plays an important role in the human pain experience. This includes cognitive influences in the pain experience of infants and persons with cognitive impairments (i.e., there is always some awareness, and cognitive factors such as learning, attention, and anticipation play a role). Moreover, cognitive components such as attention, learning, and anticipation are also likely to be part of the pain experience of animals.

Omission of the cognitive component seems particularly important as it precludes attracting attention to powerful cognitive-behavioral therapeutic interventions (Keefe & Lefebvre, 1999; Turk & Okifuji, 1999). The definition does provide a foundation for interventions focusing on sensory input, thereby favoring pharmacological interventions. Unfortunately, this feeds into the tradition of many practitioners who continue to characterize pain as only a sensation, thereby limiting interventions to those designed to reduce the sensation. Fortunately, the recognition of emotional components in the definition encourages interventions designed to alleviate fear, depression, or other emotional states (Fernandez & Turk, 1992), domains in which psychological interventions have proven powerfully effective. It is acknowledged that the absence of reference to cognitive mechanisms in the definition has not inhibited growth of cognitive-behavioral interventions for pain (Norton, Asmundson, Norton, & Craig, 1999), but this area probably would be facilitated by acknowledgment of the role of cognitive processes.

Other difficulties arise from emphasis on pain as "subjective" experience. The IASP definition added in its notes, "Pain is always subjective." The term *subjective* is used in this context to emphasize the importance of the individual's personal experience when perceiving somatic states, rather than the tissue damage giving rise to the experience. It makes it explicit that one must infer the experience using whatever verbal and nonverbal information is available, in the contexts of the sufferer's life. Unfortunately, subjective experience can also be derided as "illusory" or "lacking in reality or substance," to use terms employed to define *subjective* in the *Merriam-Webster Collegiate Dictionary* (http://www.m-w.com/cgi-bin/dictionary). It is not unusual for people to refer to somebody's opinion as "so subjective as to be ridiculous," implying that it is speculative, likely to be biased, and not grounded in facts or reality. This feeds into propensities of some practitioners to belittle patients by referring to their pain as "all in their head," psychogenic, or psychological overlay. Gagliese and Katz (2000) provided a careful analysis and rejection of the supposition that chronic pain that is not medically explained represents psychopathology. The American Medical Association (AMA) Guides (AMA, 2000) pointed out that some physicians have a low threshold for terms such as "chronic pain syndrome" or "psychogenic" pain and tend to dismiss pain as a nonmedical phenomenon if there is not biological pathology available to account for such pain complaints and disability. The term *subjective* can be contrasted with the term *objective*, with the latter referring to tangible or material properties of the world that do not depend on the report of the individual. Thus, the term *subjective* can be misused to dismiss pain reports as having no basis in concrete, objective or physical reality, despite the potency of the distress experienced by the individual. It is important to rectify minimization of the value of subjective experience by emphasizing the importance of verbal, nonverbal, and physiological measures of pain. Careful psychometric validation of these measures has made powerful tools available, despite some limitations (Turk & Melzack, 2001).

Subjective reports also are frequently described as being amenable to personal or self-serving bias. This perspective or attitude contributes to suspicions that complaints without a substantial organic basis are not real, making it easy to dismiss them as exaggerated, or otherwise inaccurate. These reports of pain apparently unrelated to the magnitude of tissue damage are written off as imaginary, reflecting moral weakness, or malingering. The reality is that people invariably present themselves in a manner that they perceive as serving their best interests. Even the most sincere, credible, honest, and earnest person operates to maximize opportunities, even though this sometimes will be seen by others as self-sacrificing or unreasonably altruistic. Individuals' perceptions of their best interests are recognized as a key determinant of self-report. In this sense, complete "objectivity" cannot be accomplished. Nevertheless, it usually is to people's advantage to be as accurate and disclosive about internal distress as possible. People presenting with pain are usually in considerable distress and recognize their need for expert care; hence, at least during diagnostic examination, they will cooperate and work to provide the information an expert or professional requires. There undoubtedly is an incidence of pain fabrication or exaggeration. This usually is estimated to be relatively low, although external criteria for estimating the true incidence are not available. Fortunately, strategies are beginning to emerge for detection of deception and malingering (Craig, Hill, & McMurtry, 1999; Hill & Craig, 2002; Rogers, 1997).

The problem is compounded in practitioners heavily trained in the biomedical model, who focus on underlying physical pathology and largely ignore the important contributions of psychological and social factors to illness recognized in the biopsychosocial model. Although pain can arise automatically or reflexively as a result of tissue damage or stress, a considerable amount of pain presents without explainable medical pathology. Kroenke and Mangelsdorff (1980) reported a survey of over 1,000 patient records in an internal medicine clinic, finding that less than 16% of somatic complaints (e.g., chest pain, fatigue, dizziness, headache, back pain, numbness, cough, constipation) could be attributable to an organic cause. The fifth edition of the American Medical Association *Guides to the Evaluation of Permanent Impairment* (AMA, 2000) provides similar illustrations, pointing out that pain without an apparent underlying biological basis is commonplace, as is asymptomatic pathophysiology. It noted that "For example, in up to 85% of individuals who report back pain, no pain-producing pathology can be identified; conversely, some 30% of asymptomatic people have significant pathology on magnetic resonance imaging (MRI) and computed tomographic (CT) scans that might be expected to cause pain" (p. 566) As a further illustration, it observed that "Headache is another common disabling condition in which impairment must be assessed primarily on the basis of individuals' reports of pain rather than on tissue pathology or anatomic abnormality" (p. 577). The AMA *Guides* (AMA, 2000) provided an illustrative list of other well-established pain syndromes without significant, identifiable organ dysfunction capable of explaining the pain, including postherpetic neuralgia, tic douloureux, erythromelalgia, complex regional pain syndrome, type 1 (reflex sympathetic dystrophy), and any injury to the nervous system. It seems clear that practitioners whose focus is on identifying organic etiology and providing biologically oriented treatments will often fail to have satisfactory assessment methods or interventions available for the vast majority of their patients. The risk of iatrogenic factors compounding initial problems was observed by Kouyanou, Pither, and Wessely (1997), who reported overinvestigation, and inappropriate information and advice given to patients. The same researchers also observed misdiagnosis, overtreatment, and inappropriate prescription of medication in a group of 125 chronic pain patients. Given the inadequacies of medical investigations focusing exclusively on the organic basis of pain, psychological methods are increasingly employed in the assessment of the genuineness of pain complaints, although there are limitations (Rogers, 1997).

Neuroscience Questions

The neurosciences are working effectively and rapidly toward an understanding of biological substrates of pain that would account for the dynamic process whereby the individual's life history of past experiences with pain combined with current thoughts and feelings continuously interact with sensory input to determine the complex experience of pain. Understanding peripheral pathophysiological events is no longer sufficient because past experiences and current brain activity are capable of modifying neural input.

Pain experiences early in life have a potential for powerful structural and functional impact (Porter, Grunau, & Anand, 1999). Anand and Scalzo (2000) demonstrated that multiple exposures to unintended or culturally sanctioned pain may alter the biological systems that control pain. For example, these experiences could potentially dampen reactivity or produce hypersensitivity, among other possibilities. Grunau (2001) observed that repeated pain early in life affects how children interact with others. For example, children who are born early with low birth weights, and who are exposed frequently to pain in neonatal intensive care nurseries, become predisposed to increased somatization in interactions with their mothers (Grunau, Whitfield, Petrie, & Fryer, 1994). In adults, an appreciation of the substantial central modulation and plasticity of the nervous system has allowed us to begin to understand the basic mechanisms whereby acute pain evolves into chronic pain (Coderre, Katz, Vaccarino, & Melzack, 1993). Through numerous mechanisms, the brain is capable of attenuating, magnifying, and prolonging perception of noxious events. Phenomena of peripheral and central sensitization, increased adrenergic sensitivity in injured nociceptive fibers, accumulation of ion channels at sites of nerve injury, and other factors appear capable of producing severe pain in response to trivial stimulation (allodynia) (Covington, 2000). The AMA *Guides* (AMA, 2000, p. 568) reviewed neurophysiologic mechanisms of acquired hypersensitivity in peripheral and central neural systems that would account for persistent pain, independent of the initial disease or injury, including evidence that "the primary afferent discharge actually has the ability to injure or kill spinal inhibitory neurons (excitotoxicity), leading, to hyperexcitability due to disinhibition" and that "peripheral nerve injury can initiate evolving abnormalities in spinal cord neurons, which in turn generate abnormal responsiveness of thalamic neurons, which in turn generate cortical dysfunction" (p. 567). Melzack and Katz's chapter in this volume provides extensive discussion of related mechanisms. This work represents major advances that challenge explanations of pain that require strong correlations between peripheral pathology and subjective experiences of pain. Complementing an appreciation of the complexity are the current advances in imaging brain activity during painful events (Casey & Bushnell, 2000; Price, 2000). The diverse qualities of painful experience are reflected in the distributed processing of pain in the brain, leading to rejection of the proposition that there should be a "pain center" and further appreciation of the heterogeneity of painful experiences, despite common features. Variation in brain activation is reflected in studies demonstrating that psychological interventions, such as hypnoanalgesia, have a powerful impact on brain activity (Rainville, Carrier, Hofbauer, Duncan, & Bushnell, 1999). The research on central neuroplasticity and functional brain imaging is relatively uncontroversial, given the impeccable scientific controls that are introduced, and has created major changes in the thinking of theoreticians and practitioners.

Although our understanding of the role of the central nervous system during pain is rapidly developing, major questions remain concerning how neural activity relates to the experience of pain. This is "the big question" in philosophy and consciousness research: How do conscious experiences arise from biological activity? Chapman pursues these questions in his chapter in this volume. The role of consciousness has been particularly contentious in the study of pain in infants, as it has been proposed that newborns and infants roughly throughout the first year of life could not experience pain because they do not have a capacity to understand the nature of the experience (Derbyshire, 1996, 1999; Leventhal & Sherer, 1987). Anand and Craig's (1996) appeal for improved sensitivity and management of infant pain was met by a characterization of this position as "dangerous," because it promoted the use of potent analgesics early in life (Derbyshire, 1996). Similar unfortunate beliefs and positions seem pervasive among health care practitioners and the public. An example of these attitudes is found in a recently published and widely available book written by a neurosurgeon (Vertosick, 2000), *Why We Hurt: The Natural History of Pain*. This book was very favorably reviewed by *The Lancet, Journal of Neurosurgery*, and *New York Times Book Review*. The author asserted:

Technically, all we really need to perform painless surgery are two drugs: a paralytic agent to keep patients from yelling and wriggling about during the operation and an amnesic agent administered afterward to make them forget what a terrible thing we just did to them. Without any anesthesia save curare, paralyzed patients will be in silent agony during the operation itself, of course, since they will be feeling everything while incapable of moving a muscle in protest. The thought of having open-heart surgery while fully awake and totally paralyzed must rank as one of the most awful images the average intellect can conjure. Nevertheless, with the appropriate amnesic agent, we wouldn't remember any of it, so why should it matter? In fact, in certain select pediatric cases, anesthesiologists may use only drug-induced paralysis. They may not even use amnesic drugs afterward. . . . Babies can't remember anything anyway. I had a spinal tap without anesthesia as an infant and I don't recall a thing. I'm sure I screamed bloody murder at the time, but it hasn't affected me otherwise. (Vertosick, 2000, p. 215)

The author appears unaware of studies demonstrating destructive long-term consequences of early pain (Anand, 2000) and that infants as young as 1 day of age can anxiously anticipate pain and become hypersensitized to pain if they experience it repeatedly (Taddio, Shah, Gilbert-MacLeod, & Katz, 2002).

Social Determinants

It is widely appreciated that ethnic and other sociocultural factors have a substantial impact on the presentation of pain. The position that socialization in different families, communities and cultures would change the subjective experience of pain (Craig & Pillai, in press) is more contentious. Resistance to the latter proposition is most likely to come from those focusing on pain as a sensory experience. Nevertheless, there is evidence that suggests that contextual factors influence fundamental sensory, affective, and cognitive features of the experience of pain (Craig, 1986).

Study of social and cultural factors in pain receives little attention relative to the emphasis on biological mechanisms in pain. But one can mount a strong argument for shifts in emphasis. Pain undoubtedly has been conserved through the phylogenetic development, given its adaptive role. It protects and enhances survival by warning of real or impending tissue damage and by motivating avoidance of further harm and efforts to recuperate (Wall, 1999). Associated behavior can be observed in non-human animals, including mammals and non-human primates. The social parameters of pain receive less attention. These parameters are observable when pain displays are reliably followed by an observer's actions which promote recovery and survival, protection from danger, and assistance with life-sustaining requirements (Prkachin, 1997; Prkachin, Currie, & Craig, 1983). These behaviors are often observable in nonhuman species. For example, animals are frequently sensitive to alarm in other members of their species and use various signals communicating warning to engage in protective behavior. Certain bird species will fake injury to distract predators from searching for their nest. De Waal (1988) described a chimpanzee who would exaggerate injury by limping pitifully to avoid the brutality of an alpha male in the colony only when he was in that animal's field of vision. Evidence of physical dysfunction can have more complex social implications. Harris

(1995) provided the following anecdote from Goodall (1986) to illustrate the implications of sick role behavior in non-human species:

> A polio epidemic struck the chimpanzee troop that Goodall (1986) was observing, and a few of the animals became partially paralyzed. According to Goodall, "When the other chimpanzees saw these cripples for the first time, they reacted with extreme fear; as their fear decreased, their behavior (toward the cripples) became increasingly aggressive." (p. 330)

It is reasonable to speculate that in the course of evolution pain and its expression came to fulfill certain social functions over and beyond fundamental self-preservation. Pain became implicated in survival of the social group. The course of human adaptation to its current ecological niche required several million years in progenitor hominids, and perhaps 150,000 years in our species, *Homo sapiens*. The evolutionary process led to brains with unique mechanisms that allow for language, and a capacity to engage in the intricacies of complex social living that distinguish humans from other species. One can learn a great deal about pain by observing the behavior and biological mechanisms in nonhuman animals. It is noted that there is considerable cross-species consistency in behavior following injury (Walters, 1994). Nonetheless, a good understanding of human pain would be expected to take into account the evolved features of the human brain that have enabled uniquely human adaptations (Preuss, 2001). It must be understood that human biological predispositions (relating to pain) reflect natural selection pressures to be sensitive to social context (Williams, 2003) and to engage in flexible, adaptive behavior. They also demand integration in models of pain that acknowledge the roles of both nature and nurture as determinants of human pain and illness behavior.

The sociocommunications model of pain, described in chapter 4, and adapted to understand pain assessment (Hadjistavropoulos & Craig, 2002), facial expression of pain (Prkachin & Craig, 1995), and pain in infants and children (Craig, Lilley, & Gilbert, 1996; Craig, Prkachin, & Grunau, 2001), appears suited to describe both social complexities and biological predispositions to engage in certain types of pain reactions. It acknowledges key roles for life histories and the current social context as determinants of the suffering person's pain experience, patients' pain expression, observing persons' (e.g., caregivers') sensitivity and understanding of the expression, and the reactions of others to the person's distress. An appreciation of the role of pain in complex human organizations remains to be pursued.

Introduction of the operant model of pain (Fordyce, 1976; Fordyce, Fowler, Lehmann, & DeLateur, 1968) effectively transformed thinking about the meaning of pain behavior. This approach provided clear evidence that verbal and nonverbal behavior are not necessarily the automatic or reflexive product of tissue damage, but also may be under the control of external reinforcement contingencies in the form of sympathetic attention from others, release from aversive responsibilities, potent psychoactive medications, and avoidance of pain. Substantial evidence has accumulated describing the mechanisms and parameters of this perspective (e.g., Romano, Turner, Jensen, Friedman, Bulcroft, Hops, & Wright, 2000), although the intricacies remain poorly understood, as not all findings are consistent with operant predictions (Williamson, Robinson, & Melamed, 1997); more negative responses to pain behaviors of partners are associated with higher reported pain intensity (Summers, Rapoff, Varghese, Porter, & Palmer, 1991) and poorer physical functioning in patients (Schwartz, Slater, & Birchler, 1996). Also, there is often a neglect of the costs to the person who finds her or himself suspected of fictional complaint and is often undertreated (Williams, 2003). Nonetheless, the operant model has made a valuable contribution to a formulation of pain behavior recognizing the importance of social learning, contextual, and interactional factors, and it has led to innovations in clinical practice (Fordyce, 1976).

Despite its positive impact in our understanding of pain, the operant model has also led to controversies. The operant model is often misinterpreted as suggesting that people in pain purposefully seek insurance benefits, even though the model does not include suggestions about conscious deliberation (Badali, 2002; Williams, 2003). Studies of medically incongruous behavior (Reesor & Craig, 1988), or signs and symptoms of pain that could not have a basis in physical pathology given our current understanding anatomy and physiology (Waddell, Main, Morris, DiPaolo, & Gray, 1984) have similarly been misinterpreted. Waddell and his associates (Waddell, Pilowsky, & Bond, 1989) made specific efforts to ensure that such behavior is not construed as purposeful exploitation of opportunities, but instead is interpreted as expression of distress embedded in the history of the individual. Misinterpretation and misattribution of intent is most likely to emerge when observers have limited sophistication in psychosocial parameters of pain, or are unaware that virtually all theories of human behavior provide for behavior that is not under volitional control.

Further misunderstanding arose when the International Association for the Study of Pain (IASP) Task Force on Pain in the Workplace released a highly criticized report (Fordyce, 1995). The report, based on operant formulations, pointed out that disability compensation (i.e., construed as a reinforcer) was being granted with increasing frequency in cases where there was no known physical evidence of back injury and that research (Robertson & Keeve, 1983) showed that although the minimization of physical hazards reduces objectively verifiable injuries, subjective injury complaints can remain unaffected. The task force argued that assignment of disability status for low back pain can lead to debilitating consequences including excessive rest, potentially harmful treatments, and overprotection by significant others. It characterized workers with nonspecific low back pain as "activity intolerant" and recommended that wage replacement benefits be limited to 6 weeks unless credible physical evidence of injury could be identified (i.e., if there is a physical condition other than nonspecific low back pain).

The IASP Task force did not imply that those with nonspecific low back pain were malingering, but merely suggested that operant factors play a potent role in the maintenance of non-specific low back pain. Nonetheless, the IASP Task Force report led to a significant amount of controversy (e.g., Block, 1997; Craig, 1996; Fordyce, 1996; Loeser, 1996; Merskey, 1996a, 1996b). Specifically, it was argued that the implementation of the report's recommendations could lead to the financial hardship of many honest injured workers. Moreover, our ability to identify physical pathology is limited. For example, Giles and Crawford (1997) provided histopathological findings that are associated with pain, but that cannot be seen through imaging due to device limitations.

We take the position that use of the operant model by the IASP Task Force ignored other important considerations. Although operant factors appear responsible for many cases of disability, there are likely to be marked individual differences in the extent to which learning plays a role in nonspecific low back pain. Hadjistavropoulos (1999) presented a series of recommendations that could facilitate recovery from disability without the risks associated with the elimination of disability payments for nonspecific low back pain 6 weeks postinjury. Hadjistavropoulos's recommendations were as follows:

1. Health professionals can do more to encourage compensated and other injured persons to return to work given evidence (e.g., Catchlove & Cohen, 1982) that, when return to work during treatment is encouraged, outcomes are more favorable.
2. Given that job dissatisfaction can be a predictor of chronicity (Turk, 1997), employers can do more to address this issue in the workplace.
3. Given evidence that rates of incomplete and inaccurate pain-related diagnoses are very high (Hendler & Kozikowski, 1993), more can be done to enhance diagnostic accuracy.
4. Research designed to improve the clinical assessment of malingering and deception should continue.
5. Given evidence that specific patient characteristics can mediate the relation between treatment responsiveness and compensation status (Burns, Sherman, Devine, Mahoney, & Pawl, 1995), patient subtypes that may be especially susceptible to operant and compensation factors should be identified.

6. Given that countries with less adversarial compensation systems tend to accomplish better recovery rates (e.g., Walsh & Dumitru, 1988), modifications in the adversarial nature of North American compensation/ litigation systems should be considered.

In addition to the operant model, several psychological perspectives on pain have emerged which elaborate on socialization and developmental determinants of pain expression (Chambers, in press; Chambers, Craig & Bennett, 2002) and the role of evolution in social parameters of pain (Williams, in press). Greater attention to these social parameters of pain is likely to improve quality of life in currently contentious areas such end-of-life care and its relation to requests for euthanasia and physician assisted suicide.

CLINICAL ISSUES

There is no shortage of contentious issues concerning the role of psychology in the delivery of services to people suffering from pain. Practitioner/ patient communication invariably has implicit psychological dimensions that can be the focus of attention in efforts to improve quality of care. This is the case for all forms of conventional and alternative practice, whether addressing biomedical or psychosocial issues. For example, we (Pillai Riddell & Craig, 2003) recently noted a paucity of research consistent with strong advocacy and excellent arguments for postoperative analgesics on a time contingent as opposed to a PRN (as needed) basis. Similarly, one could debate elements of interventions delivered by psychologists who represent a variety of theoretical orientations.

There is wide-ranging recognition of the importance of recognizing, assessing, and controlling pain. The concept of "Pain: The Fifth Vital Sign" was developed by the American Pain Society (http://www.ampainsoc.org/ advocacy/fifth.htm) and is increasingly endorsed because it emphasizes the importance of pain control. In contrast to the usual vital signs assessed routinely in hospital (temperature, respiration rate, heart rate, and blood pressure), pain has no identifiably direct biological equivalent. It is a symptom, not a sign. Yet the misnomer is allowed because of the importance of controlling pain. In Canada, recognition of severe undermanagement of pain led the Canadian Pain Society to promulgate a "Patient Pain Manifesto" (http://www.canadianpainsociety.ca/manifesto/manifesto1.stm), a statement of patients' rights to control of their pain. These policies support major public campaigns designed to improve the quality of care provided to people suffering from poorly controlled pain. The manifesto declares patients' rights to have their pain controlled and notes the obligations of health care staff to treat their pain.

Measurement and assessment issues remain a major challenge (McGrath, 1996). Practitioners can deliver pain-specific services to the extent that they have access to sensitive and specific pain indexes that can be used in the context of comprehensive assessments. The field of pain assessment has developed substantially in recent decades and many standardized and practical measures with good psychometric properties are available (Turk & Melzack, 2001), although none provide the level of validity and accuracy that is ultimately desirable. Self-report was long represented as the gold standard for pain measurement. Nonetheless, questions have been raised as to whether this is the only acceptable means of understanding subjective experience, whereas others asserted that self-report must be believed (see, e.g., Engel, 1959; Meinhart & McCaffery, 1983; Melzack & Katz, 2001) in order to rectify the embarrassing trends of pain undermanagement among many patient populations (e.g., because of beliefs that their pain reports were exaggerated). This unqualified endorsement of self-report has been criticized because it fails to recognize limitations of self-report, including the difficulties people encounter reporting on the complexities of painful distress, the inevitability of selective reporting, the reflection of the individual's perception of his or her self-interests, and the advantages examiners or other interested persons gain when they consider observations of nonverbal behavior (Craig, 1992; Jensen & Karoly, 2001). Unfortunately, we have not been able to devise a measure of pain that is wholly credible. Virtually all measures delegated as indicative of pain are ambiguous. Self-report, nonverbal expression, and physiological measures all have shortcomings when used to assess pain (i.e., problems with specificity, subject to conscious distortion). There is little evidence of a specific pain reaction that would provide an ideal index of pain.

AMA *Guides* (AMA, 2000) noted, "a fundamental divide between a person who suffers from pain and an observer who attempts to understand that suffering. Observers tend to view pain complaints with suspicion and disbelief, akin to complaints of dizziness, fatigue, and malaise" (p. 566). The guides also quoted (p. 566) Scarry (1985), who observed, "To have great pain is to have certainty, to hear that another person has pain is to have doubt." This divide seems to become more severe when people are attempting to understand pain in others who differ from themselves in substantial ways. One can find numerous quotes referring to pain insensitivity or pain indifference in infants and young children, children with developmental disabilities, children with autism, adults with intellectual disabilities, and elderly persons with dementia. In contrast, fine-grained behavioral studies of the reactions of these people to invasive procedures (deemed painful by people capable of describing the experience) usually yield substantial reactions indicative of pain (e.g., Hadjistavropoulos, LaChapelle, MacLeod, Snider, & Craig, 2000; LaChapelle, Hadjistavropoulos, & Craig, 1999; Nader, Oberlander, Chambers, & Craig, in press). Examples of pain insensitivity exist with congenital insensitivity to pain, or among young adults suffering significant neurological impairment, but these appear to be exceptions (Oberlander, Gilbert, Chambers, O'Donnell, & Craig, 1999).

Although there appears to be a rough capability to observe and judge the severity of pain in others, such judgments often represent underestimates (Chambers, Reid, Craig, McGrath, & Finley, 1998; Romsing, Moller-Sonngergaard, Hertel, & Rasmussen, 1996; Sutherland et al., 1988), although some studies also report overestimation (Olden, Jordan, Sakima, & Grass, 1995). The general tendency toward underestimation may be explained through evolutionary theory, which would suggest that it would be to an observer's advantage to detect pain, but also to make judgments that would result in the least disadvantage to the observer. Williams (2003) observed that "the cost to health professionals of overestimating pain (and overprescribing treatment) is considerably higher, and then therefore more warranting conservatism, than for neutral onlookers." Badali (2002) observed, "In sum, observers' propensities for accurately detecting pain in another person and acting upon their judgments, must also be considered in context (i.e., the health care provider's desire to avoid negative consequences, such as litigation or harm to another, the suffering person's family's investment in that person, or the research volunteer's search for evidence of pain)" (p. 20). The study of judgments of pain in others, whether undertaken by clinicians, family members, or others, clearly requires work as proxy judgments appear to have serious limitations.

Credibility is a major issue. Efforts have been made to describe criteria clinicians should use to judge the credibility of people who represent themselves as being in pain. A prominent and influential attempt to do so, rather unsatisfactorily, is reflected in the American Medical Association *Guides to the Evaluation of Permanent Impairment* (AMA, 2000). This document provides several reasons why reports may lack credibility: "Some people appear unable to provide information that is sufficiently detailed for an examiner to assess pain-related impairment. The reasons for this are multiple, including psychosis, severe depression, memory deficits secondary to brain injury, and a lack of cooperation. Other individuals provide detailed information, but the validity of the information is questionable" (p. 571). This list reasonably extends credibility issues beyond voluntary misrepresentation to include questions about competence. Although some limited illustrations of this are provided (note a substantially more extended analysis of pain measurement in people with limited communication competence in Hadjistavropoulos et al., 1991), it is noteworthy that no guidance is provided as to when "validity of information is questionable."

One must also be concerned about the limited attention devoted to development of psychological, social, and other environmental interventions, relative to expenditures on pharmacological and surgical interventions. It seems almost self-evident that the latter approaches should receive the most attention. However, that may reflect our inability to contemplate interventions "outside the box" of thinking created by the biomedical model. Caudill, Schnable, Zuttermeister, Benson, and Friedman (1991) showed that participation in a psychosocial pain management program resulted in reductions in physician visits as well as decreases in depression, pain levels, anxiety, and pain-related activity interference. Arnstein, Caudill, Mandle, Norris, and Beasley (1999) demonstrated that beliefs in ability to manage and cope with pain (i.e., self-efficacy) influence the extent of pain-related depression and disability. Recent analyses of placebo effects indicate that the psychosocial parameters of any intervention are very powerful features, and responsible for some portion of the potency of any analgesic intervention (Wall, 1999). Certainly, patient and investigator expectancies are powerful determinants of the outcome of clinical trials of analgesics (Turner, Jensen, Warms, & Cardenas, 2002). Recent studies including controls for placebo effects have demonstrated that even sham arthroscopic surgery can substantially alleviate knee pain (Mosely et al., 2002). Ordinarily, placebos constitute the controls for active interventions, with investigators not interested in evaluating the magnitude of impact of the placebo itself and going to extraordinary lengths to rule this impact out. The reasons behind placebo effectiveness are not fully understood, however, and merit further investigation.

PUBLIC HEALTH AND POLICY ISSUES

There is growing evidence that chronic and acute pain are attracting the concerted attention of the public and public policy makers. Chronic pain represents a huge drain on the health care system. Okifuji, Turk, and Kalauokalani (1999) estimated that over 90 million Americans suffer from some form of persistent or recurrent pain. Health care expenditures and indirect costs associated with disability compensations and loss of productivity resulting from absenteeism represent enormous sums of money. Over $125 billion is estimated to be expended annually on health care to treat chronic pain sufferers! Concern for inadequacies in our understanding of pain and pain control led the U.S. Congress to designate the first decade of the 21st century "The Decade of Pain Control and Research."

One would hope there will be greater attention to the provision of psychological services for people suffering from pain, given the central role of psychosocial factors in pain and suffering. This lack of attention has long represented a problem; traditionally the health care community has emphasized medical aspects of patient care rather than psychological and social factors (Chambliss, 2000). Undermanagement of pain appears to be a particularly severe problem for special populations, or people with handicaps. There also appears to be a need for improvement in treatment of pain complaints and disabilities that do not have a clear explanation in physical pathology; these conditions must be recognized as serious problems. Many administrative agencies (compensation boards, insurance companies, etc.) require objective findings of biological dysfunction (or a causal link between an index injury and an individual's present symptoms and findings) if benefits are to the accorded to the person (AMA, 2000).

Fears of the impact of potent analgesics (e.g., addiction) often constrain their use or access to their use. The complex controls for evaluation and approval of drugs in the United States and Canada appear to be sensible. But the concerns of police authorities, legislators, and others about substance abuse has led to an unfortunate reluctance to prescribe these effective medications. Similarly, fears of the side effects of opioids (respiratory suppression in particular) led to great reluctance in their use with infants and young children and others. Fortunately, monitoring the impact of therapeutic opioids is readily accomplished and the risk of morbidity has been deemed minimal. Many now believe that there are greater risks associated with not administering opioids than those associated with their use under careful medical supervision. There is also a real problem with the diversion of prescription analgesics for illicit purposes. OxyContin, for example, is a time-release opioid. Drug dealers were successful in breaking the time-release barrier of this formulation and it became a favored street drug, despite the substantial risks of addiction and overdose. All these factors have contributed to physicians being subjected to high levels of surveillance of their prescription practices and risks of professional harassment when they prescribe opioids for nonmalignant pain. This situation has led to poor-quality pain management for large numbers of people suffering from chronic pain who would benefit from prescription opioids.

Various professional and scientific organizations (e.g., Canadian Pain Society, 1998) developed policies encouraging the use of opioids for people suffering chronic nonmalignant pain, following careful screening to minimize risk factors and to ensure other treatment modalities have not been neglected. It generally is recognized that opioids provide efficacious care with a low incidence of addiction and manageable side effects.

Throughout this chapter we have noted that ideological, professional, and financial self-interests have been powerful determinants of trends in understanding pain and in the development and application of interventions for the control of pain. This idea is illustrated at the level of care of the individual person suffering from pain. Parties responsible for disability adjudication (physicians, psychologists, insurance company adjudicators, and others) may be influenced by incentives to doubt or deny the reality of pain complaints (Hadjistavropoulos, 1999). Similarly, there are concerns about potential biases in contract, as opposed to investigator-driven, research, because of the disparate goals of industry and science. At broader levels, biomedical research approaches have dominated the scientific study of pain, and the pharmaceutical industry's marketing and advertising juggernaut can obscure the importance of psychological and social parameters in pain and their potential usefulness in generating efficacious pain control strategies. Fortunately, recent trends indicate that the more inclusive biopsychosocial model of pain is increasingly prominent in pain research (Norton, Asmundson, Norton, & Craig, 1999).

It is noteworthy that behavioral research has the potential to contribute to public policy debate and changes because it provides an informed basis for decision making. For example, behavioral research contributed to decisions by state courts in the United States to abandon judicial execution by electrocution because it represents cruel and unusual punishment (Price, 2002). Price (2002) marshaled evidence indicating the electrical charges coursing through the body would instigate pain through both central and peripheral stimulation. Behavioral signs of pain and suffering, such as moaning, screaming, gasping for air, and writhing movements in the chair, were recognized as classic signs of pain and suffering. Demonstration that facial expression during execution was consistent with scientific criteria for facial displays of pain (Craig et al., 2001) substantiated these observations.

CONCLUSIONS

In summary, we have identified many controversies that are particularly relevant to pain psychology. These relate to issues about the nature and definition of pain, the insufficient availability of psychosocial interventions designed to treat pain, the misuse of self-report as the gold standard in pain assessment, fears about the implementation of certain biomedical interventions, and others. Clearly, a lot remains to be done before the controversies can be resolved. At the same time, a few decades ago, the inclusion of psychology as a major player in the pain research and management was highly controversial. We have come a long way since, with our field having made major contributions to the development of the gate control theory of pain (and the neuromatrix model) and the wide acceptance of psychosocial pain treatment programs in research centers, hospitals, and pain clinics around the world. Much more will change and a greater understanding of the psychological determinants of pain and pain outcomes will lead to improved care and less controversy.

ACKNOWLEDGMENTS

The preparation of this chapter was supported in part by a Canadian Institutes of Health Research Senior Investigator Award to Kenneth D. Craig and by a Canadian Institutes of Health Research Investigator Award to Thomas Hadjistavropoulos.

REFERENCES

American Medical Association. (2000). *Guides to the evaluation of permanent impairment* (5th ed.). Chicago: Author.

American Psychiatric Association. (2000). *Diagnostic and statistical manual of mental disorders* (4th ed., text rev.). Washington, DC: Author.

Anand, K. J. S. (2000). Effects of perinatal pain and stress. *Progress in Brain Research, 122,* 117–129.

Anand, K. J. S., & Craig, K. D. (1996). Editorial: New perspectives on the definition of pain. *Pain, 67,* 3–6.

Anand, K. J. S., & Scalzo, F. M. (2000). Can adverse neonatal experiences alter brain development and subsequent behavior. *Biology of the Neonate, 77,* 69–82.

Arnstein, P., Caudill, M., Mandle, C. L., Norris, A., & Beasley, R. (1999). Self-efficacy as a mediator of the relationship between pain intensity, disability and depression in chronic pain patients. *Pain, 81,* 483–491.

Badali, M. A. (2002). *Sociality of pain behaviour: Audience effects.* Unpublished manuscript, University of British Columbia.

Block, A. (1997). Controlling the costs of pain-related disability. *Journal of Pain and Symptom Management, 13,* 1–3.

Bonica, J. (1953). *The management of pain.* Philadelphia: Lea & Febiger.

Burns, J. W., Sherman, M. L., Devine, J., Mahoney, N., & Pawl, R. (1995). Association between worker's compensation and outcome following multi-disciplinary treatment for chronic pain: Roles of mediators and moderators. *Clinical Journal of Pain, 11,* 94–102.

Canadian Pain Society. (1998). Use of opioid analgesics for the treatment of chronic noncancer pain—A consensus statement and guidelines from the Canadian Pain Society. *Pain Research and Management, 3,* 225–232.

Casey, K. L., & Bushnell, M. C. (Eds.). (2000). *Pain imaging.* Seattle, WA: IASP Press.

Catchlove, R., & Cohen, K. (1982). Effects of a directive return to work approach in the treatment of workman's compensation patients with chronic pain. *Pain, 14,* 181–191.

Caudill, M., Schnable, R., Zuttermeister, P., Benson, H., & Friedman, R. (1991). Decreased clinic use by chronic pain patients: Response to behavioral medicine intervention. *Clinical Journal of Pain, 7,* 305–310.

Chambers, C. T. (in press). The role of family factors in pediatric pain. In P. J. McGrath & G. A. Finley (Eds.), *Context of pediatric pain: Biology, family, culture.* Seattle, WA: IASP Press.

Chambers, C. T., Craig, K. D., & Bennett, S. M. (2002). The impact of maternal behavior on children's pain experiences: An experimental analysis. *Journal of Pediatric Psychology, 27,* 293–301.

Chambers, C. T., Reid, G. J., Craig, K. D., McGrath, P. J., & Finley, G. A. (1998). Agreement between child and parent reports of pain. *Clinical Journal of Pain, 14,* 336–342.

Chambliss, D. (2000). *Psychotherapy and managed care: Reconciling research and reality.* Boston: Allyn and Bacon.

Coderre, T. J., Katz, J., Vaccarino, A. L., & Melzack, R. (1993). Contribution of central neuroplasticity to pathological pain: Review of clinical and experimental evidence. *Pain, 52,* 259–285.

Covington, E. C. (2000). The biological basis of pain. *International Review of Psychiatry, 12,* 128–147.

Craig, K. D. (1986). Social modeling influences: Pain in context. In R. A. Sternbach (Ed.), *The psychology of pain* (2nd ed., pp. 67–95). New York: Raven Press.

Craig, K. D. (1992). The facial expression of pain: Better than a thousand words? *American Pain Society Journal, 1,* 153–162.

Craig, K. D. (1996). The back pain controversy—Reply. *Pain Research and Management, 1,* 183.

Craig, K. D., Hill, M. L., & McMurtry, B. (1999). Detecting deception and malingering. In A. R. Block, E. F., Kramer, & E. Fernandez (Eds.), *Handbook of chronic pain syndromes: Biopsychosocial perspectives* (pp. 41–58). Mahwah, NJ: Lawrence Erlbaum Associates.

Craig, K. D., Lilley, C., & Gilbert, D. (1996). Social barriers to optimal pain management infants and children. *Clinical Journal of Pain, 12,* 232–242.

Craig, K. D., & Pillai, R. R. (in press). Social influences, ethnicity, and culture. In G. A. Finley & P. J. McGrath (Eds.), *The contexts of pediatric pain: Biology, family, society, and culture.* Seattle, WA: IASP Press.

Craig, K. D., Prkachin, K. M., & Grunau, R. V. E. (2001). The facial expression of pain. In D. C. Turk & R. Melzack (Eds.), *Handbook of pain assessment* (pp. 153–169). New York: Guilford Press.

Derbyshire, S. W. G. (1996). Comment on editorial by Anand & Craig. *Pain, 67,* 210–211.

Derbyshire, S. W. G. (1999). Locating the beginnings of pain. *Bioethics, 13*(1), 1–31.

De Waal, F. (1988). Chimpanzee politics. In R. Byrne & A. Whiten (Eds.), *Machiavellian intelligence* (p. 123). Oxford, UK: Clarendon Press.

Engel, G. (1959). Psychogenic pain and the pain-prone patient. *American Journal of Medicine, 26,* 899–918.

Fernandez, E., & Turk, D. C. (1992). Sensory and affective components of pain: Separation and synthesis. *Psychological Bulletin, 112,* 205–217.

Fordyce, W. E. (1976). *Behavioral methods for chronic pain and illness.* St. Louis, MO: C. V. Mosby.

Fordyce, W. E. (1995). *Back pain in the workplace.* Seattle, WA: IASP Press.

Fordyce, W. E. (1996). Response to Thompson/Merskey/Teasell. *Pain, 65,* 112–114.

Fordyce, W. E., Fowler, R. S., Lehmann, J. F., & DeLateur, B. J. (1968). Some implications of learning on problems of chronic pain. *Journal of Chronic Diseases, 21,* 179–190.

Gagliese, L., & Katz, J. (2000). Medically unexplained pain is not caused by psychopathology. *Pain Research and Management, 5,* 251–257.

Gershoff, E. T. (2002). Corporal punishment by parents and associated child behaviors and experiences: A meta-analytic and theoretical review. *Psychological Bulletin, 128,* 539–579.

Giles, L. G., & Crawford, C. M. (1997). Shadows of truth in patients with spinal pain: A review. *Canadian Journal of Psychiatry, 42,* 44–48.

Glucklich, A. (2000). *Sacred pain.* Oxford: Oxford University Press.

Goodall, J. L. (1986). *The chimpanzees of Gombe: Patterns of behavior.* Cambridge, MA: Harvard University Press.

Grunau, R. V. E. (2001). Long-term consequences of pain in human neonates. In K. J. S. Anand (Ed.), *Pain in neonates* (2nd ed., pp. 55–76). Amsterdam: Elsevier.

Grunau, R. V., Whitfield, M. F., Petrie, J. H., & Fryer, E. L. (1994). Early pain experience, child and family factors as precursors of somatization: A prospective study of extremely premature and fullterm children. *Pain, 56,* 353–359.

Hadjistavropoulos, T. (1999). Chronic pain on trial: The influence of litigation and compensation on chronic pain syndromes. In A. R. Block, E. F. Kremer, & E. Fernandez (Eds.), *Handbook of pain syndromes* (pp. 59–76). Mahwah, NJ: Lawrence Erlbaum Associates.

Hadjistavropoulos, T., & Craig, K. D. (2002). A theoretical framework for understanding self-report and observational measures of pain: A communications model. *Behaviour Research and Therapy, 40,* 551–570.

Hadjistavropoulos, T., LaChapelle, D., MacLeod, F., Snider, B., & Craig, K. D. (2000). Measuring movement exacerbated pain in cognitively-impaired frail elders. *Clinical Journal of Pain, 16,* 53–63.

Hadjistavropoulos, T., von Baeyer, C., & Craig, K. D. (2001). Pain assessment in persons with a limited ability to communicate. In D. C. Turk & R. Melzack (Eds.), *Handbook of pain assessment* (pp. 134–152). New York: Guilford Press.

Harris, J. R. (1995). Where is the child's environment? A group socialization theory of development. *Psychological Review, 102,* 458–489.

Hendler, N. H., & Kozikowski, J. G. (1993). Overlooked physical diagnoses in chronic pain patients involved in litigation. *Psychosomatics, 34,* 494–501.

Hill, M., & Craig, K. D. (2002). Detecting deception in pain expressions: The structure of genuine and deceptive facial displays. *Pain, 98,* 135–144.

International Association for the Study of Pain, Subcommittee on Taxonomy. (1979). Pain terms: A list with definitions and notes on usage. *Pain, 6,* 147.

Jensen, M. P., & Karoly, P. (2001). Self-report scales and procedures for assessing pain in adults. In D. C. Turk & R. Melzack (Eds.), *Handbook of pain assessment* (pp. 153–169). New York: Guilford Press.

Keefe, F. J., & Lefebvre, J. C. (1999). Behavioural therapy. In P. D. Wall & R. Melzack (Eds.), *Textbook of pain* (4th ed., pp. 1445–1461). Edinburgh, UK: Churchill Livingstone.

Kouyanou, K., Pither, C. E., & Wessley, S. (1997). Iatrogenic factors and chronic pain. *Psychosomatic Medicine, 59,* 597–604.

Kroenke, K., & Mangelsdorff, D. (1989). Common symptoms in ambulatory care: Incidence, evaluation, therapy, and outcome. *American Journal of Medicine, 86,* 262–266.

LaChapelle, D., Hadjistavropoulos, T., & Craig, K. D. (1999). Pain measurement in persons with intellectual disabilities. *Clinical Journal of Pain, 15,* 13–23.

Leventhal, H., & Sherer, K. (1987). The relationship of emotion to cognition: A functional approach to a semantic controversy. *Cognition & Emotion, 1,* 3–28.

Loeser, J. D. (1996). The IASP report on back pain in the work place. *Pain Research and Management, 1,* 180.

Loeser, J. D., Butler, S. H., Chapman, C. R., & Turk, D. C. (2001). *Bonica's management of pain* (3rd ed.). Philadelphia: Lippincott, Williams & Wilkins.

McGrath, P. J. (1996). There is more to pain measurement in children than "ouch." *Canadian Psychology, 37,* 63–75.

McQuay, H., Moore, A., & Moore, R. A. (1998). *An evidence-based resource for pain relief.* Oxford, UK: Oxford University Press.

Meinhart, N., & McCaffery, M. (1983). *Pain: A nursing approach to assessment and analysis.* Norwalk, CT: Appleton-Century-Crofts.

Melzack, R. (1973). *The puzzle of pain.* New York: Basic Books.

Melzack, R. (1988). The tragedy of needless pain: a call for social action. In R. Dubner, G. F. Gebhart, & M. R. Bond (Eds.), *Proceedings of the Vth World Congress of Pain* (pp. 1–11). Amsterdam: Elsevier.

Melzack, R., & Casey, K. L. (1968). Sensory motivational and central controlled determinants of pain: A new conceptual model. In K. Shalod (Ed.), *The skin senses* (pp. 423–443). Springfield, IL: Charles C. Thomas.

Melzack, R., & Katz, J. (2001). The McGill Pain Questionnaire: Appraisal and current status. In D. C. Turk & R. Melzack (Eds.), *Handbook of pain assessment* (pp. 153–169). New York: Guilford Press.

Melzack, R., & Wall, P. D. (1965). Pain mechanisms: A new theory. *Science, 150,* 971–979.

Melzack, R., & Wall, P. D. (1996). *The challenge of pain* (2nd ed.). Toronto: Penguin Books.

Merskey, H. (1991). The definition of pain. *European Journal of Psychiatry, 6*, 153–159.

Merskey, H. (1996a). Re: Back pain in the work place (W. E. Fordyce, Ed.). *Pain, 65*, 111–112.

Merskey, H. (1996b). Back pain, psychology and money. *Pain Research and Management, 1*, 13.

Mosely, J. B., O'Malley, K., Petersen, N. J., Menke, T. J., Brody, B. A., Kuykendall, D. H., Hollingsworth, J. C., Ashton, C. M., & Wray, N. P. (2002). A controlled trial of arthroscopic surgery for osteoarthritis of the knee. *New England Journal of Medicine, 347*(2), 81–88.

Nader, R., Oberlander, T. F., Chambers, C. T., & Craig, K. D. (in press). Pain in children with autism. *Clinical Journal of Pain.*

Norton, P. J., Asmundson, G. J., Norton, G. R., & Craig, K. D. (1999). Growing pain: Ten-year research trends in the study of chronic pain and headache. *Pain, 79*, 59–65.

Oberlander, T. F., Gilbert, C. A., Chambers, C. T., O'Donnell, M. E., & Craig, K. D. (1999). Pain in children with significant neurological impairment. *Clinical Journal of Pain, 15*, 201–209.

Okifuji, A., Turk, D. C., & Kalauokalani, D. (1999). Clinical outcome and economic evaluation of multidisciplinary pain centers. In A. R. Block, E. F. Kremer, & E. Fernandez (Eds.), *Handbook of pain syndromes: Biopsychosocial perspectives* (pp. 77–97). Mahwah, NJ: Lawrence Erlbaum Associates.

Olden, A. J., Jordan, E. T., Sakima, N. T., & Grass, J. A. (1995). Patients' versus nurses' assessments of pain and sedation after ceasarean section. *Journal of Obstetric and Gynecological Neonatal Nursing, 24*, 137–141.

Pillai Riddell, R. R., & Craig, K. D. (2003). Time contingent schedules for post-operative analgesia: A review of the literature. *Journal of Pain, 4*, 169–175.

Porter, F. L., Grunau, R. E., & Anand, K. J. S. (1999). Long-term effects of pain infants. *Journal of Developmental and Behavioral Pediatrics, 20*, 253–261.

Preuss, T. M. (2001). The discovery of cerebral diversity: An unwelcome scientific revolution. In D. Falk & K. Gibson (Eds.), *Evolutionary anatomy of the primate cerebral cortex* (pp. 138–164). New York: Cambridge University Press.

Price, D. D. (2000). Psychological and neural mechanisms of the affective dimension of pain. *Science, 288*, 1769–1772.

Price, D. D. (2002). Pain in the electric chair. *APS Bulletin, 12*(3), 1–10.

Prkachin, K. M. (1997). Afterword: The consistency of facial expressions of pain. In P. Ekman & E. Rosenberg (Eds.), *What the face reveals* (pp. 198–200). Oxford: Oxford University Press.

Prkachin, K. M., & Craig, K. D. (1995). Expressing pain: The communication and interpretation of facial pain signals. *Journal of Nonverbal Behavior, 19*, 191–205.

Prkachin, K. M., Currie, N. A., & Craig, K. D. (1983). Judging nonverbal expressions of pain. *Canadian Journal of Behavioural Science, 15*, 409–421.

Rainville, P., Carrier, B., Hofbauer, R. K., Duncan, G. H., & Bushnell, M. C. (1999). Dissociation of sensory and affective dimensions of pain using hypnotic modulation. *Pain, 82*, 159–171.

Reesor, K. A., & Craig, K. D. (1988). Medically incongruent chronic back pain: Physical limitations, suffering, and ineffective coping. *Pain, 32*, 35–45.

Robertson, L., & Keeve, J. (1983). Worker injuries: The effects of workers compensation and OSHA inspections. *Journal of Health Politics Policy and Law, 8*, 581–597.

Rogers, R. (Ed.). (1997). *Clinical assessment of malingering and deception* (2nd ed.). New York: Guilford Press.

Romano, J. M., Turner, J. A., Jensen, M. P., Friedman, L. S., Bulcroft, R. A., Hops, H., & Wright, S. F. (2000). Chronic pain patient–spouse behavioral interactions predict patient disability. *Pain, 63*, 353–360.

Romsing, J., Moller-Sonnergaard, J., Hertel, S., & Rasmusses, M. (1996). Postoperative pain in children: Comparison between ratings of children and nurses. *Journal of Pain and Symptom Management, 11*, 42–46.

Scarry, E. (1985). *The body in pain.* New York: Oxford University Press.

Schwartz, L., Slater, M. A., & Birchler, G. R. (1996). The role of pain behaviors in the modulation of marital conflict in chronic pain couples. *Pain, 65*, 227–233.

Sternbach, R. A. (1968). *Pain: A psychophysiological analysis.* New York: Academic Press.

Summers, J. D., Rapoff, M. A., Varghese, G., Porter, K., & Palmer, R. E. (1991). Psychosocial factors in chronic spinal cord injury. *Pain, 47,* 183–189.

Sutherland, J. E., Wesley, R. M., Cole, P. M., Nesvacil, L. J., Daly, M. L., & Gepner, G. J. (1988). *Family Medicine, 20,* 343–346.

Taddio, A., Shah, V., Gilbert-MacLeod, C., & Katz, J. (2002). Conditioning and hyperalgesia in newborns exposed to repeated heel lances. *Journal of the American Medical Association, 288,* 857–861.

Tu, W. (1980). A religiophilosophical perspective on pain. In H. W. Kosterlitz & L. Y. Terenius (Eds.), *Pain and society* (pp. 63–78). Weinheim, Germany: Verlag Chemie GmbH.

Turk, D. C. (1996). Cognitive factors in chronic pain and disability. In K. S. Dobson & K. D. Craig (Eds.), *Advances in cognitive behavioural therapy* (pp. 83–115). Thousand Oaks, CA: Sage.

Turk, D. C. (1997). The role of demographic and psychosocial factors in the transition from acute to chronic pain. In T. S. Jensen, J. A. Turner, & Z. Wiesenfeld-Hallin (Eds.), *Proceedings of the 8th World Congress on Pain: Progress in pain research and management* (pp. 185–213). Seattle, WA: IASP Press.

Turk, D. C., & Melzack R. (2001). *Handbook of pain assessment.* New York: Guilford Press.

Turk, D. C., & Okifuji, A. (1999). A cognitive-behavioural approach to pain management. In P. D. Wall & R. Melzack (Eds.), *Textbook of pain* (4th ed., pp. 1431–1443). Edinburgh, UK: Churchill Livingstone.

Turk, D. C., & Okifuji, A. (2002). Psychological factors in chronic pain: Evolution and revolution. *Journal of Consulting and Clinical Psychology, 70,* 678–690.

Turner, J. A., Jensen, M. P., Warms, C. A., & Cardenas, D. D. (2002). Blinding effectiveness and association of pretreatment expectations with pain improvement in a double-blind randomized controlled trial. *Pain, 99,* 91–99.

Vertosick, F. T. (2000). *Why we hurt: The natural history of pain.* San Diego: Harcourt.

Waddell, G., Main, C. J., Morris, E. W., DiPaolo, M., & Gray, I. C. M. (1984). Chronic low back pain, psychological distress and illness behavior, *Spine, 9,* 209–213.

Waddell, G., Pilowsky, I., & Bond, M. R. (1989). Clinical assessment and interpretation of abnormal illness behaviour in low back pain. *Pain, 39,* 41–53.

Wall, P. D. (1999). *Pain: The science of suffering.* London: Weidenfeld & Nicolson.

Wall, P. D., & Melzack, R. (Eds.). (1999). *The textbook of pain* (4th ed.). Edinburgh, UK: Churchill Livingstone.

Walsh, N. E., & Dumitru, D. (1988). The influence of compensation on recovery from low back pain. *Occupational Medicine: State of the Art Reviews, 3,* 109–120.

Walters, E. T. (1994). Injury-related behavior and neuronal plasticity: An evolutionary perspective on sensitization, hyperalgesia, and analgesia. *International Review of Neurobiology, 36,* 325–427.

Williams, A. C. de C. (2003). Facial expression of pain: An evolutionary account. *Behavioral and Brain Sciences, 25,* 439–488.

Williamson, D., Robinson, M. E., & Melamed, B. (1997). Pain behavior, spouse responsiveness, and marital satisfaction in patients with rheumatoid arthritis. *Behavior Modification, 21,* 97–118.

Ethics for Psychologists Who Treat, Assess, and/or Study Pain

Thomas Hadjistavropoulos
Department of Psychology,
University of Regina

Most chapters in this volume primarily address the nature of pain and how pain problems can be alleviated. This chapter is more aspirational and outlines essential principles, values, and expectations that must be followed by professionals who study, assess, and treat pain. Maintaining high standards for the competent care and respectful treatment of clients and research participants, while staying in touch with important philosophical and moral traditions treasured in our society, is extremely important. Such traditions as well as codes of ethical conduct and guidelines should be taken into account at every step of our clinical and research endeavors.

The ethical issues that psychologists face in pain assessment, management, and research abound. Many of these concerns (e.g., limits to confidentiality, dual relationships) are not unique to work with pain patients and their thorough review is beyond the scope of this chapter. The interested reader is referred to comprehensive sources covering ethical issues for psychologists (e.g., Koocher & Keith-Spiegel, 1998). This chapter focuses on issues that are more particular to working with pain patients and on guidelines and standards that are especially relevant in this context.

Although psychologists are typically bound by codes of ethics that outline the importance of fundamental principles pertaining to respect for the dignity of persons, caring, integrity, responsibility to society, and the responsible care of animals (e.g., American Psychological Association [APA], 2002; Canadian Psychological Association [CPA], 2000), multidisciplinary organizations of pain researchers and clinicians have adopted

327

additional ethical standards that are more focused on the pain context (e.g., American Pain Society [APS], 1996–2001; Anand and the International Evidence-Based Group for Neonatal Pain, 2001; International Association for the Study of Pain [IASP], 1983, 1995). Moreover, clinicians and researchers do not practice in isolation, but instead are members of societies that have very rich philosophical, religious, and other values that influence our understanding of what is just and righteous (e.g., Pettifor, 1996). As such, it is important to recognize the values and ethical principles that underlie most of the standards adopted by professional organizations. It is for this reason that this discussion begins with a presentation of some of the dominant philosophical perspectives that affect ethical conduct and decision making. This analysis of philosophical perspectives is followed by their application to a specific case fraught with controversy and further discussion of specific ethical standards developed for practitioners and scientists addressing issues of pain.

ETHICS THEORY

Perhaps the most influential philosophical perspectives relating to ethics are *deontology* and *teleology*. The primary theme in deontological thought is the need to abide by principles. Transgression from such principles is considered unethical. Some deontological views are based on religion or divine doctrine (Brody, 1983) and others on intuition (i.e., intuitive deontology). *Intuitive deontology* refers to an individual's intuitive ability to reason ethically (Hadjistavropoulos & Malloy, 2000; Kant, 1788/1977; Ross, 1975). Although Immanuel Kant, whose name is most closely associated with deontological theory, spoke of the *categorical imperative* (i.e., the idea that moral and universal laws should guide all actions regardless of any situational constraints; e.g., according to the deontological principle of nonmaleficence one should not inflict unnecessary pain on others), other theorists (e.g., Ross, 1975) have argued that deontological rules can take into account situational constraints and demands.

In contrast to deontology, *teleology* emphasizes the consequences of one's actions (rather than the means of action). Within this perspective, *act utilitarianism* is focused solely on the ends of action, whereas *rule utilitarianism* advocates that the greatest good should be achieved by following prescribed rules (Sparks, 1991). As such, the minimization of pain (and maximization of happiness) would be an important goal of this approach. *Rule utilitarianism* differs from deontology because of its focus on consequences.

A third perspective on ethical behavior is the *ethics of care*. This perspective does not focus on the consequences or means of action but is primarily concerned with human relationships (e.g., Gilligan, 1982). Kluge (1999) stressed, for instance, the importance of acknowledging the functional embedding of all persons in their social contexts and attempting to reach resolutions on the basis of consensus and cooperation. Nonviolence is frequently emphasized within this perspective, and empathy (e.g., about pain and suffering) with other human beings is considered to be of vital importance. In other words, our actions must be guided by a sense of commitment to another person.

Although it has been argued that, ideally, codes of ethics should provide a balance of theoretical ethical orientations (e.g., between deontology and teleology) in their statements, most such codes are primarily deontological (Hadjistavropoulos, Malloy, Douad, & Smythe, 2002; Malloy, Hadjistavropoulos, Douad, & Smythe, 2002). That is, they tend to provide rules without conceptual justification or explanation. A more balanced approach would allow one to outline deontological expectations while at the same time providing a teleological rationale for ethical behavior. Such an approach would enhance the educational value of codes of ethics, which would be important because, although pain researchers and clinicians are knowledgeable in their fields, many do not have equivalent expertise in ethical philosophy.

The values behind good ethical conduct are outlined remarkably well in the code of ethics that has been adopted by the Canadian Psychological Association (CPA, 2000). Although many codes emphasize important ethical principles, the CPA code provides detailed and elaborate justifications for these. Specifically, the CPA code stresses the importance of dignity of persons, stating that each person must be treated primarily as a person or an end/in him or herself (as opposed to means to an end—e.g., as a means of obtaining an answer to a scientific question) because all persons have innate worth as appreciated human beings independent of their culture, background, or personal characteristics. The greatest responsibility is to those who are in a more vulnerable position (e.g., infants, children, persons with cognitive impairments). Despite this responsibility, evidence (e.g., Marzinski, 1991) suggests that pain among such individuals is undermanaged (this issue is discussed in detail later). Clinician and researcher obligations linked to consent, general respect/rights, nondiscrimination, and confidentiality/privacy all relate to the need to respect the dignity of persons. Similarly, *caring* is crucial because a basic ethical expectation of any discipline in our society is to do no harm. Consequently, it is important for scientists and professionals to show an active concern for human welfare. Special care should be taken when dealing with persons who are most vulnerable. Issues relating to competence and self/knowledge, the need to maximize benefit and minimize harm, and the need to care for the welfare of animals involved in scientific investigations are all underscored by the broad ethical principle of *caring*. Embedded in the principle of *integrity* in relationships is the recognition that relationships with clients/patients come with explicit and implicit mutual expectations that are vital to the advancement of scientific knowledge and the maintenance of public confidence in the health-care field. Issues relating to accuracy and honesty, straightforwardness and openness, minimization of biases and avoidance of conflicts of interest, all relate to the need for integrity. The ethical principles relating to *responsibility to the society* at large are based on the recognition that scientific and professional disciplines function in the context of human society. This comes with responsibilities and expectations. A very reasonable expectation of society is that professions that could not function without societal support will increase knowledge and conduct their affairs in a manner that will promote the welfare of all human beings. Freedom of inquiry and debate are exercised in a manner that is consistent with ethical requirements. Standards relating to respecting and benefiting society and developing knowledge are all based on such moral justifications.

Application of Ethical Theory

In order to demonstrate the manner in which ethical theory can inform ethical actions, one can consider the case of Tracy Latimer. This case has been the focus of much media attention in Canada over the last several years (McGrath, 1998). Tracy was a 12-year-old girl who suffered from severe cerebral palsy and who had very limited ability to communicate as a result of cognitive impairment. She suffered from severe pain caused by both the neuromuscular pathologies associated with the cerebral palsy and by the surgical interventions undertaken to release contractures. Although systematic pain assessment never took place, her father decided to end her life. He was subsequently convicted of murder, but his defense was that he chose to terminate Tracy's life in order to end her continuous and unremitting suffering. Canadian public opinion was largely divided, with Mr. Latimer's supporters arguing that unendurable, unremitting pain justifies active euthanasia whereas others were concerned about the implications of a potential acquittal for other disabled persons. They also raised concerns for vulnerable children and adults who cannot effectively express themselves. The Supreme Court of Canada heard the case and ruled that Mr. Latimer must spend at least 10 years in jail for killing his severely disabled daughter (*R. v. Latimer*).

It must be stressed that this analysis does not pass judgment on Mr. Latimer's character, as, by most accounts, he was a loving father who had the best interests of his daughter in mind. The analysis merely examines his action and implications from a variety of theoretical ethical perspectives.

One may apply ethical theory in conceptualizing this case. It is recognized that there are variations of deontological and teleological schools of thought (e.g., Ross's prima facie theory; Ross, 1975), but for the purposes of this illustration we focus on pure versions of teleology and deontology as well as on the ethics of care. In terms of deontological thought, Kant (1788/1977) spoke of the *categorical imperative* (i.e., moral and universal laws that should guide our actions). In other words, an individual should act in a way that his or her act could become a universal ethical law for all human beings. This implies that if it is ethical to terminate the life of a severely disabled child in pain, it follows that all parents of such children should do the same. Moreover, if such a universal law were to exist, it would logically follow that persons of disabled children (with severe and unremitting pain) who do not terminate their children's lives would be acting unethically. Such a conclusion would be untenable in our society. As such, it would be very difficult to justify the action to terminate Tracy's life from a deontological standpoint.

From a teleological standpoint, the focus of ethical decision making is on the consequences rather than the means of action. As such, one would have to take into account what results in the least amount of suffering (i.e., the greatest good) for the greatest number of people. Consequences that would have to be considered include the cost and burden to the family, society, groups of disabled persons, and, of course, Tracy. With respect to Tracy, one can consider the construct of *the injury of continued existence* (Engelhardt, 1999). This refers to a situation in which the continuation of life is construed as an "injury." But is it possible that Tracy would have grown to have a satisfying life? This is something that we cannot know. Some people consider death to be the ultimate form of harm. This may or may not be so, but something was certainly lost when Tracy died. Given the many unknowns involved in this situation, it could be possible to develop an argument in support of either position (i.e., either that the action to terminate Tracy's life was ethical or unethical). In other words, the many unknowns create subjectivity in the determination of what would constitute the greatest good for the greatest number.

In terms of the ethics of care, one could potentially argue that Mr. Latimer's action could be justified if he acted as a result of his empathy with his daughter's pain and his belief that he was acting in her best interest. Nonetheless, given that many ethics of care theorists would emphasize the importance of nonviolence, one might also have to make the case that the termination of Tracy's life (involving carbon monoxide inhalation) was nonviolent. It might be difficult to reach consensus on the nonviolence issue in this case.

If we, as a society, were ever prepared to argue that euthanasia to terminate unremitting pain is ethical, we would also have to ask the question as to who should make such decisions for people with severe cognitive impairments. Should it be parents and close relatives alone? We all know that parents and relatives often make mistakes. We also know that the extreme stress that can be associated with illness and disability in the family (e.g., Zarit, Orr, & Zarit, 1985) can affect judgment and take a toll on people. When it comes to the Latimer case, the truth is that we will never know exactly how much pain Tracy was in and what she would want. In various research projects that we conducted we demonstrated that biases (e.g., Hadjistavropoulos, McMurtry, & Craig, 1996; MacLeod, LaChapelle, Hadjistavropoulos, & Pfeifer, 2001) can often enter the process of assessing another person's pain and that people (depending on their background) can have tendencies to attribute relatively more or less pain. For instance, in one study we showed that trained health professionals observing videos of people undergoing a painful medical procedure attributed less pain to the patients than did untrained observers (Hadjistavropoulos et al., 1998). Any one individual making this decision for Tracy may have been influenced by factors that are not necessarily relevant to her pain experience.

Separate from the issue of euthanasia, there is a second ethical concern that relates to the Latimer case. This relates to the obligation of psychologists to help ensure that people with severe cognitive impairments have access to adequate pain assessment and management. This issue is less controversial than the ethical questions raised by Tracy's death because the perspectives of deontolology (e.g., "we have a duty to do good"), teleology (e.g., "we must do that which results in the greatest good"), and ethics of care (e.g., "it is important to care for other people") would all lead to similar conclusions. Nonetheless, as McGrath (1998) pointed out, our field as a whole has failed the Latimer family both in terms of our ability to systematically and accurately assess pain and in terms of our ability to manage it. Let us consider this case to be a wake-up call.

ETHICAL STANDARDS ADOPTED BY IASP AND APS

A basic background in ethics philosophy sets a foundation for pain clinicians and researchers who consult and study codes of ethics and standards. In addition to codes of ethics adopted by psychologists (e.g., APA, 2002; CPA, 2000), and standards adopted by various organizations (APS, 1996–2001; IASP, 1983, 1995), various other documents have been endorsed by groups of pain clinicians and researchers, such as the World Medical Association (WMA) Declaration of Helsinki, Recommendations Guiding Doctors in Clinical Research (World Medical Association, 1964/2000), the Declaration of Lisbon concerning the rights of the patient (World Medical Association, 1981), and the International Ethical Guidelines for Biomedical Research Involving Human Subjects (Council for International Organizations of Medical Sciences, 1993). Generally, such documents stress the importance of respect for dignity, caring, and the need for sound research designs where pain needs to be studied.

IASP Guidelines

The International Association for the Study of Pain (IASP, 1983, 1995) has published guidelines for pain research relating to the study of pain in both humans and animals. The IASP (1995) guidelines concerning humans stress that dignity, safety, and health are paramount in research and that the researcher always has the ultimate responsibility for maintaining high ethical standards. Moreover, IASP's guidelines stress the need for appropriate and thorough ethics review of research by a well-constituted ethics committee or board.

Consent should be informed, voluntary, and written (IASP, 1995). This implies that the elements of mental capacity and adequate information should also be present (Rozovsky, 1990). However, it is not always possible to clearly determine what constitutes "adequate information" in situations where consent is being sought. In making this determination it is important to know the type of information that potential research participants expect and want. Casarett, Karlawish, Sankar, Hirschman, and Asch (2001) set out to clarify this issue by presenting pain patients with vignettes describing various research studies and subsequently interviewing them about the type of information they would have liked to have had before enrolling. Participants stressed the need for information about study-related changes in medications, contingency plans, and assurances about how increased pain would be treated. They also raised concerns about addiction to opioids as a result of participation in the study (this is likely to arise when psychologists conduct research within the context of broader studies involving medical professionals). Most patients indicated that they would want to know how knowledge generated from their study might help them, as well as about burdens and inconveniences associated with study participation. Thirty-eight percent stated that they would like to know how study participation might give them improved access to a health care provider, 55% desired information about treatment availability following the completion of the study, 62% desired information about changes in medication and dose, 78% of patients described concerns about increased pain as a result of study participation, 70% said that they would want information about previous related studies of the treatment, and all patients indicated that they wanted information about potential treatment risks and side effects. Patients also wished to know whether they would have continued access to the treatment used in the study after the trial is over. Studies such as Casaret et al.

(2001), can be invaluable in assisting researchers in optimizing consent procedures for their research. Similar investigations focusing specifically on psychological studies of pain would be useful.

With respect to the IASP guidelines concerning the importance of written consent, we note that for some cultural groups in our society written consent may not be considered appropriate. In some instances, for example, it may be appropriate (for research ethics boards and institutional review committees) to approve consent by traditional native ceremony as long as this is fully voluntary and informed. Even in such instances, it would important to supply those consenting with all pertinent information about the study in writing.

According to the IASP (1995) document, special precautions should be taken with vulnerable populations. Pain studies with vulnerable persons (e.g., young children) should only be undertaken when it is essential given the goals of the project. Under such circumstances, consent should be obtained from those who have the legal responsibility for the patient's welfare. In all circumstances the intensity of any pain stimulus should be kept to the minimum necessary and should never exceed a participant's tolerance level. Effective forms of pain relief should be provided on request, even in sham and placebo studies, and the availability of alternative forms of pain relief should be made clear in the consent form and study instruction before the beginning of the investigation (IASP, 1995).

The IASP guidelines regarding the ethical use of animals in pain-related research (Zimmerman, 1983) are aimed at minimizing pain and avoiding unnecessary animal discomfort and distress. The following points are stressed: (a) the need for ethics review by appropriately constituted boards and/or committees and for a continuing justification of scientific research; (b) that the investigator should try the pain stimulus on himself or herself if possible (i.e., this applies to most noninvasive procedures); (c) the need to carefully examine the animal's deviation from normal behavior in order to closely assess for the presence of pain; (d) the need for assurances that the amount of pain to which the animal is exposed is the minimum necessary for the purposes of the study; (e) treating any animal presumed to experience chronic pain or allowing the animal to self-administer analgesic agents or procedures, provided that these will not interfere with the aim of the investigation; (f) not performing studies of pain in animals paralyzed with a neuromuscular blocking agent without a general anesthetic or an appropriate surgical procedure that eliminates sensory awareness; and (g) minimizing the duration of the experiment and keeping to a minimum the number of animals involved.

The IASP has also published a core curriculum for professional education in pain (Fields, 1995) and one that is more specific to psychology (IASP Ad Hoc Subcommittee for the Psychology Curriculum, 1997). These publications serve to guide both psychologists and educators about the necessary knowledge base for practice in this area. Discussion of ethical issues relating to research has been included in *Core Curriculum for Professional Education in Pain* (Fields, 1995). The volume stresses the importance of sound methodologies, and presents philosophical arguments against randomized controlled clinical trials (e.g., Gifford, 1994; Silverman, 1985) and against the use of placebo controls when effective forms of pain prevention or control are available. (It is noted that, in some instances, placebo treatments have been found to be as effective as widely used medical interventions [Moseley et al., 2002].) A strong recommendation is also made against the use of placebos in studies involving persons of diminished cognitive capacity, including infants, based on the argument that such individuals have no possibility of positive placebo effects. Nonetheless, the question of whether placebo effects can operate (under at least some circumstances) in these populations has not been investigated adequately. There is recognition that researchers should never exceed the research participant's tolerance limit in any type of investigation (whether it is of experimentally induced pain or pain that results from disease). Factors such as the need for ethics review, avoidance of conflict of interest, and knowledge of intricacies involved in both quantitative and qualitative research methodologies (e.g., Hadjistavropoulos & Smythe, 2001) are stressed. Sternbach (1983) suggested that attention needs to be paid to recruiting the smallest possible number of participants, using the least intense stimulation and the shortest possible pain duration. It is also important to advise participants of any and all risks involved in the study.

Although both Fields (1995) and the declaration of Helsinki (WMA, 1964/2000) raise strong objections to the use of placebos in the study of conditions for which alternative effective therapeutic methods are available, there may still be compelling scientific reasons to include placebos. For instance, a psychologist could make a valid scientific argument concerning the need to study the placebo response itself. Such a situation could raise very difficult issues for the researchers, research ethics boards, and organizations that adopt ethical guidelines concerning placebos. Nonetheless, the welfare, well-being, and dignity of the research participants should always be given the highest priority in decision making. The possible need to study the placebo response itself has not been directly addressed by the various ethical guidelines discussed here. Nonetheless, under ideal circumstances, researchers interested in studying the placebo response would do so within the context of larger studies that involve trials of new treatments for conditions for which effective interventions are not available.

Related to the IASP curriculum, one of the most fundamental ethical issues for psychologists working in the area of pain is that of competence. Competence is most directly linked to ethical principles relating to caring for others, as a lack of competence can have detrimental consequences for clients. The evaluation of a psychologist's comprehension of ethical issues should include the important determination of whether he or she is practicing within his or her area of competence. The expectations outlined in the IASP psychologists' curriculum include knowledge/understanding of nociceptive mechanisms, experimental and clinical pain measurement, psychological impact of different types of pain, psychological and behavioral assessments of individuals with pain, psychosocial impact of pain, pain syndromes particularly influenced by sex and gender, life span issues, health care seeking, economic and occupational impact of pain-associated disability, psychological and psychiatric treatment, pharmacological and invasive pain management procedures, interdisciplinary treatment programs, prevention and early intervention, treatment outcome and evaluation, and ethical standards and guidelines. In addition to familiarity with these topical areas, adequate supervised clinical and/or research experience is necessary to achieve an adequate level of competence. Finally, it is increasingly being suggested that psychologists should be utilizing empirically supported interventions (see Chambless & Hollon, 1998) when working with clients (e.g., Dobson & Craig, 1998; Hadjistavropoulos & Bieling, 2001).

APS Guidelines

The American Pain Society (APS) also adopted its own code of ethics (APS, 1996–2001). Its standards and principles address human and animal research as well as clinical practice. With respect to pain-related clinical research, the APS guidelines endorse the principles of a variety of organizations including the World Health Organization and the American Psychological Association. Much like the IASP document, the APS standards stress the need for thorough and impartial ethics review, informed consent (or consent from a proxy legally responsible for the research participant), not using in pain research persons who are incapable of providing consent (e.g., children, persons with cognitive impairments) unless it is essential for the purposes of the study, minimizing the intensity of noxious stimulation in pain studies, and allowing participants to terminate the painful stimulus at will, as well as ensuring that alternate treatments are available for patients who need them and who participate in placebo or sham treatment studies.

With respect to pain-related clinical practice, the APS document stresses that the principles of medical ethics published by the American Medical Association should apply to all clinical disciplines engaged in pain therapy and stress the importance of dedication to competent service with compassion and dignity, honesty, respect for the law, respect for the rights of others, continuation of research, application and dissemination of knowledge and consultation with other professionals. It also stresses that professionals can choose "whom to serve" except in emergencies, and recognizes the responsibility of participating in the activities of a free community. Many psychologists might criticize some of the standards put forth by the APS for pain-related clinical practice. For example, the APS document states, "A health care provider shall be dedicated to providing competent medical service with compassion, respect and dignity" (p. 3). Because psychologists provide psychological and not medical services, one could argue that the standard is not stated sufficiently broadly for their purposes. Moreover, an argument can be made that another standard ("A health care provider, in the provision of appropriate patient care, except in emergencies, shall be free to choose whom to serve, with whom to associate, and the environment in which to provide health-care services," p. 3) is also stated too broadly. That is, it can be argued that the standard can serve, in some people's minds, as justification for refusing treatment on grounds such as ethnicity and sexual orientation. Although such discrimination does not occur often in clinical settings, it would be important to emphasize within the standards that any refusal of service should be done only with adequate justification and in a manner that shows respect for the dignity of all persons. In terms of animal research, the APS endorses the IASP guidelines for research with animals aimed at minimizing pain and discomfort at all times as well as at avoiding unnecessary distress.

PRESSING ETHICAL ISSUES OF CONCERN TO PAIN CLINICIANS

A recent survey of the membership of the American Pain Society and the American Academy of Pain Medicine was conducted to determine beliefs about ethical dilemmas in pain management practice (Ferrell et al., 2001). The total sample of 1,105 respondents included 166 psychologists. The five issues that were found to raise the most frequent ethical concerns in the total sample (N = 1,105) were (in rank order): (a) management of pain at the end of life; (b) general undertreatment of pain; (c) undertreatment of pain in the elderly; (d) impact of managed care on pain treatment; and (e) undertreatment of pain in children. Among psychologists (N = 166), the top five issues of ethical concern were ranked as follows: (a) general undertreatment of pain; (b) management of pain at the end of life; (c) undertreatment of pain in the elderly; (d) undertreatment of pain in children; and (e) accepting patients' self-report of pain.

Scientific evidence shows that concerns about undertreatment of pain among specific populations have a factual basis. For example, Bauchner

(1991) conducted a study at a U.S. hospitals and concluded that although adults routinely received local analgesia for lumbar puncture, there was no evidence that any one of 252 children received it. Evidence for inadequate analgesia in children during and after surgery has also been obtained by other researchers (e.g., Eland & Anderson, 1977; Sutters & Miaskowski, 1997). Similarly, seniors with dementia also tend to be undertreated for pain problems. Despite the lack of evidence that dementia reduces pain-related suffering (e.g., Gibson, Voukelatos, Ames, Flicker, & Helme, 2001; Hadjistavropoulos, LaChapelle, MacLeod, Snider & Craig, 2000; Proctor & Hirdes, 2001), Kaasalainen et al. (1998) found that almost half of the cognitively intact patients were taking scheduled pain medications compared to only 25% of those with cognitive impairments. Marzinski (1991) found that although 26 of 60 inpatients with Alzheimer's disease had painful conditions, only three patients had orders for routinely scheduled analgesics. Seniors in general may also be undertreated for pain. Although psychosocial treatments for pain are available in many communities (e.g., LeFort, Gray-Donald, Rowat, & Jeans, 1998), these treatments are not geared toward the special concerns of seniors. Consequently, seniors are less likely to benefit from and participate in such treatment programs.

Cases of pain undertreatment may be taken to the legal arena. In North Carolina, for example, a health professional was found liable for failing to treat pain adequately (*Estate of Henry James v. Hillhaven Corp.*). Specifically, the jury deemed that Henry James' dying days were made intolerable by the decision of a nurse and her employer (a nursing home) to reduce or withhold medication ordered by the patient's physician.

Cassidy and Walco (1996) examined whether the undertreatment of pain can be construed as ethically justifiable from any one of three philosophical perspectives. The possible justifications were: (a) the revisionist justification (i.e., "pain is not bad"); (b) the pragmatic justification (i.e., "pain can produce a positive outcome"); and (c) the comparative justification (i.e., "the level of pain is not the worst"). Cassidy and Walco concluded that, given the lack of evidence for clinically significant reductions in pain sensitivity in undertreated populations and that the internal state of pain is not directly observable, the revisionist perspective is not tenable. The comparative justification is based on the view that the means of alleviating pain are sometimes more harmful than the pain itself. Although this can be true in rare instances, it would almost never apply to competently designed psychosocial interventions which are the focus of this volume. In terms of the pragmatic justification, pain can sometimes produce a positive outcome as it warns about injury or disease and alerts for the need for treatment. This does not apply to most instances of undertreatment of pain (e.g., most chronic diseases that are associated with aging, post-operative pain, diagnostic procedural pain). It can, therefore, be concluded that none of these justifications are typically applicable to populations that are neglected and undertreated and/or for whom effective psychosocial treatments can be developed or are available.

Hicks (2000) suggested that ethically sound pain management depends on professionals' understanding of themselves. That is, clinicians need to analyze and assess their own beliefs about what constitutes quality of life when it comes to specific patient groups (including patients with cognitive impairments). They also need to ask themselves how much they value quality of life for the patient. Second, clinicians should analyze their views and feelings about specific patient populations (e.g., What are clinicians' preconceived notions about older persons? Do they sometimes see nursing home residents not as persons, but as a commodity that is cared for in exchange for money?). Finally, Hicks (2000) suggested that clinicians should understand their views about clinical care and pain management. Is clinical care based on beneficence or nonmaleficence? Clinicians who believe primarily that their role is to *do no harm* may provide care that is quite different from those who believe that their primary role is to *do good*. According to Hicks, patient-focused care is most attainable when the clinician carefully analyzes his or her own views and beliefs about clinical management.

The area of pain assessment also raises a variety of concerns for clinicians (i.e., accepting the self-report of pain). After reviewing histopathological findings, Giles and Crawford (1997) showed that physical evidence of many legitimate soft-tissue injuries cannot be detected by conventional medical imaging procedures because of device limitations. The lack of such objective evidence has resulted in many conflicts and disagreements, especially in cases where pain patients make compensation and insurance disability claims. Experts are often asked by the parties concerned to provide or refute evidence in support of the legitimacy of such claims. Psychologists are frequently involved in these disputes partly because they possess expertise designed to identify malingering and deception, including symptom exaggeration (Craig, Hill, & McMurtry, 1999). Ethical issues abound in this context. Hadjistavropoulos (1999) raised some concerns given the divided loyalties that are often involved when psychologists conduct assessments of pain patients within the context of litigation and compensation/insurance claims. These divided loyalties tend to involve the claimant, the insurance company (or compensation board), and the legal system. Claimants may approach such assessments with suspicion and defensiveness, which could lead them to avoid genuine responses about factors such as job satisfaction and psychological concerns, fearing that their claim may be impacted in a negative fashion. The frequently adversarial nature of many such assessments can disrupt the trust and rapport that traditionally exist in the psychologist–client relationship. The best way to attempt to address such issues is by discussing and clarifying loyalties, limits to confidentiality, and all ethical obligations in advance of the assessment.

Although our ethics codes dictate that we must maintain impartiality when conducting independent assessments in adversarial and medico-legal contexts, an important concern is that third-party payers may be more likely to make referrals to professionals who tend to be least sympathetic to claimant concerns. Being motivated by such factors (i.e., the desire to secure additional insurance company business) when drawing conclusions concerning patient complaints would be unethical (Hadjistavropoulos, 1999).

Both self-report and behavioral observation play important roles in pain assessment. Hadjistavropoulos (1999) cautioned that unquestioningly accepting the claimant's self-report in the context of an independent third-party assessment (conducted largely in an effort to assess the genuineness of a client's complaints) could also raise serious ethical concerns (Hadjistavropoulos, 1999). Psychologists are sometimes overly concerned about the possibility of being complained against or sued by a disability claimant If they deem that the claimant is not disabled. Indeed, the risk for such action would be lower when the psychologist certifies that, in his or her professional opinion, the patient is disabled than when he or she certifies the opposite. Compromising the objectivity and integrity of one's conclusions in order to minimize the probability of a complaint is self-serving and unethical.

A related issue that needs to be considered in disability assessments (see Hadjistavropoulos, 1999) is the ethical obligation of the practitioner to provide feedback to the patient (e.g., concerning conclusions about the severity of a patient's condition). This ethical obligation is not typically diminished simply because a psychologist is retained by a third party (e.g., an insurance company). Releasing a copy of the report to the claimant's family physician is useful. The patient can be informed that he or she can go over the report with the general practitioner and that the psychologist will be available to provide clarifications. A feedback session with the patient is also useful. A concern is that insurance companies sometimes try to limit the feedback that the practitioner is to give to the claimant and do not permit the release of independent assessment reports without their permission. Consequently, practitioners sometimes ask claimants to waive their rights to a copy of the report. Nonetheless, withholding from claimants clinical information that pertains to them raises ethical concerns. It is imperative that practitioners who conduct third-party assessments educate such parties in order to facilitate the provision of adequate feedback to claimants.

CONCLUSIONS

Psychologists working in busy clinical settings and intensive research environments can become greatly preoccupied with managing large case loads and extensive research programs. As such, there is a risk of paying insufficient attention to important ethical issues and concerns that arise in such contexts. Familiarity with ethics codes and specific guidelines represents only the beginning of our ethical obligations to our clients, research participants, and society at large. Seeking the advice and assistance of experienced colleagues and mentors in resolving complex ethical problems is highly recommended. Maintaining a high level of competence, standards, and respect for clients and research participants, while staying in touch with important philosophical and moral traditions treasured in our society, is also vital. These traditions, as well as ethics codes and guidelines, should be considered in the resolution of complex ethical dilemmas.

ACKNOWLEDGMENTS

This chapter is not intended to provide legal advice nor to forecast adjudications by ethics committees. It merely raises possibilities. The author acknowledges the comments and advice of David Elliott and David Malloy concerning the brief analysis of the Latimer case. Portions of the Latimer case analysis were presented at the 2002 Annual Convention of the Canadian Pain Society, Winnipeg Manitoba. Preparation of this chapter was supported in part by a Canadian Institutes of Health Research Investigator Award.

REFERENCES

American Pain Society. (1996–2001). *Ethical principles of the American Pain Society*. Glenview, IL: Author. (retrieved from the World Wide Web on December 4, 2001, http://www.ampainsoc. org/about/ethics.htm)

American Psychological Association. (2002). *Ethical principles for psychologists and code of conduct*. Washington, DC: Author.

Anand, K. J. S., and the International Evidence-Based Group for Neonatal Pain. (2001). Consensus statement for the prevention and management of pain in the newborn. *Archives of Pediatric and Adolescent Medicine, 155*, 173–180.

Bauchner, H. (1991). Procedures, pain and parents. *Pediatrics, 87*, 563–565.

Brody, B. (1983). *Ethics and its applications*. New York: Harcourt Brace Jovanovich, Inc.

Canadian Psychological Association. (2000). *Canadian code of ethics for psychologists*. Ottawa, Ontario: Author.

Casarett, D., Karlawish, J. Sankar, P., Hirschman, K. B., & Asch, D. A. (2001). Obtaining informed consent for pain research: Patients' concerns and information needs. *Pain, 92,* 71–79.

Cassidy, R. C., & Walco, G. A. (1996). Pediatric pain: Ethical issues and ethical management. *Children's Health Care, 25,* 253–264.

Chambless, D. L., & Holon, S. D. (1998). Defining empirically supported therapies. *Journal of Consulting and Clinical Psychology, 66,* 7–18.

Council of International Organizations of Medical Sciences. (1993). *International ethical guidelines for biometical research involving human subjects.* Geneva: World Health Organization.

Craig, K. D., Hill, M. L., & McMurtry, B. (1999). Detecting deception and malingering. In A. R. Block, E. F. Kramer, & E. Fernandez (Eds.), *Handbook of chronic pain syndromes: Biopsychosocial perspectives* (pp. 41–58). Mahwah, NJ: Lawrence Erlbaum Associates.

Dobson, K. S., & Craig, K. D. (Eds.). (1998). *Best practice: Developing and promoting empirically validated interventions.* Thousand Oaks, CA: Sage.

Eland, J. M., & Anderson, J. E. (1977). The experience of pain in children. In A. Jacox (Ed.), *Pain: A sourcebook for nurses and other health professionals* (pp. 453–473). Boston: Little, Brown.

Engelhardt, H. T. (1999). Ethical issues in aiding the death of young children. In R. Munson (Ed.), *Intervention and reflection: Basic issues in medical ethics* (6th ed., pp. 158–163). Belmont, CA: Wadsworth/Thompson.

Estate of Henry James v. Hillhaven Corp., No. 89 CVS 64 (N.C. Sup. Ct. 1991).

Ferrell, B. R., Novy, D., Sullivan, M. D., Banja, J., Dubois, M. Y., Gitlin, M. C., Hamaty, D., Lebovich, A., Liman, A. G., Lippe, P. M., & Livovich, A. G. (2001). Ethical dilemmas in pain management. *Journal of Pain, 2,* 171–180.

Fields, H. (Ed.). (1995). *Core curriculum for professional education in pain* (2nd ed.). Seattle, WA: International Association for the Study of Pain Press.

Gibson, S. J., Voukelatos, X., Ames, D., Flicker, L., & Helme, R. D. (2001). An examination of pain perception and cerebral event-related potentials following carbon dioxide laser stimulation in patients with Alzheimer's disease and age-matched control volunteers. *Pain Research and Management, 6,* 126–132.

Gifford, F. (1994). The conflict between randomized clinical trials and the therapeutic obligation. In E. Erwin, S. Gendin, & L. Kleiman (Eds.), *Ethical issues in scientific research: An anthology* (pp. 179–200). New York: Garland.

Giles, L. G., & Crawford, C. M. (1997). Shadows of truth in patients with spinal pain: A review. *Canadian Journal of Psychiatry, 42,* 44–48.

Gilligan, C. (1982). *In a different voice.* Cambridge, MA: Harvard University Press.

Hadjistavropoulos, T. (1999). Chronic pain on trial: The influence of litigation and compensation on chronic pain syndromes. In A. R. Block, E. F. Kremer, & E. Fernandez (Eds.), *Handbook of pain syndromes* (pp. 59–76). Mahwah, NJ: Lawrence Erlbaum Associates.

Hadjistavropoulos, T., & Bieling, P. (2001). File review consultation in the adjudication of mental health and chronic pain disability claims. *Consulting Psychology Journal: Practice and Research, 53,* 52–63.

Hadjistavropoulos, T., & Craig, K. D. (2002). A theoretical framework for understanding self-report and observational measures of pain: A communications model. *Behaviour Research and Therapy, 40,* 551–570.

Hadjistavropoulos, T., LaChapelle, D., MacLeod, F., Hale, C., O'Rourke, N., & Craig, K. D. (1998). Cognitive functioning and pain reactions in hospitalized frail elders. *Pain Research and Management, 3,* 145–151.

Hadjistavropoulos, T., LaChapelle, D., MacLeod, F., Snider, B., & Craig, K. D. (2000). Measuring movement-exacerbated pain in cognitively impaired frail elders. *Clinical Journal of Pain, 16,* 54–63.

Hadjistavropoulos, T., & Malloy, D. C. (2000). Making ethical choices: A comprehensive decision-making model for Canadian psychologists. *Canadian Psychology, 41,* 104–115.

Hadjistavropoulos, T., Malloy, D. C., Douad, P., & Smythe, W. E. (2002). Functional linguistics, ethical orientation and the codes of ethics of the Canadian Medical Association and the Canadian Nurses Association. *Canadian Journal of Nursing Research, 34*, 35–52.

Hadjistavropoulos, T., McMurtry, B., & Craig, K. D. (1996). Beautiful faces in pain: Biases and accuracy in the perception of pain. *Psychology and Health, 11*, 411–420.

Hadjistavropoulos, T., & Smythe, W. E. (2001). Elements of risk in qualitative research. *Ethics & Behavior, 11*, 163–174.

Hicks, T. (2000). Ethical implications of pain management in a nursing home: A discussion. *Nursing Ethics, 7*, 392–398.

International Association for the Study of Pain. (1983). Ethical guidelines for investigations of experimental pain in conscious animals. *Pain, 16*, 109–110.

International Association for the Study of Pain. (1995). Ethical guidelines for pain research in humans. *Pain, 63*, 277–278.

International Association for the Study of Pain Ad Hoc Subcommittee for Psychology Curriculum. (1997). *Curriculum on pain for students in psychology*. Seattle, WA: International Association for the Study of Pain.

Kaasalainen, S., Middleton, J. Knezacek, S., Hartely, T., Stewart, N., Ife, C., & Robinson, L. (1998). Pain and cognitive status in the institutionalized elderly: Perceptions and interventions. *Journal of Gerontological Nursing, 24*, 24–31.

Kant, I. (1977). *Critique of practical reason* (L. W. Beck, Trans.). Indianapolis, IN: Bobbs-Merrill. (Original work published 1788)

Kluge, E. H. W. (1999). *Biomedical ethics: A Canadian focus*. Scarborough, ON: Prentice Hall Allyn.

Koocher, G. P., & Keith-Spiegel, P. (1998). *Ethics in psychology: Professional standards and cases*. New York: Oxford University Press.

LeFort, S. M., Gray-Donald, K., Rowat, K. M., & Jeans, M. E. (1998). Randomized control trial of a community-based psychoeducation program for the self-management of chronic pain. *Pain, 74*, 297–306.

MacLeod, F., LaChapelle, D., Hadjistavropoulos, T., & Pfeifer, J. (2001). The effect of disability claimants' coping styles on judgments of pain, disability and compensation. *Rehabilitation Psychology, 46*, 417–435.

Malloy, D. C., Hadjistavropoulos, T., Douad, P., & Smythe, W. E. (2002). The codes of ethics of the Canadian Psychological Association and the Canadian Medical Association: Ethical orientation and functional grammar analysis. *Canadian Psychology, 43*, 244–253.

Marzinski, L. R. (1991). The tragedy of dementia: Clinically assessing pain in the confused, nonverbal elderly. *Journal of Gerontological Nursing, 17*, 25–28.

McGrath, P. J. (1998). We failed the Latimers. *Journal of Pediatrics and Child Health, 3*, 153–154.

Moseley, J. B, O'Malley, K., Petersen, N. J., Menke, T. J., Brody, B. A., Kuykendall, D. H., Hollingsworth, J. C., Ashton, C. M., & Wray, N. P. (2002). A controlled trial of arthroscopic surgery for osteoarthritis of the knee. *New England Journal of Medicine, 347*, 81–88.

Pettifor, J. L. (1996). Ethics: Virtue and politics in the practice of psychology. *Canadian Psychology, 37*, 1–12.

Proctor, W., & Hirdes, J. (2001). Pain and cognitive status among nursing home residents in Canada. *Pain Research and Management, 6*, 113–125.

R. v. Latimer. 1 SCR 3 (2001).

Ross, W. D. (1975). The right and the good. In K. J. Struhl & P. R. Struhl (Eds.), *Ethics in perspective* (pp. 100–107). New York: Random House.

Rozovsky, F. A. (1990). *Consent to treatment: A practical guide* (2nd ed.). Boston: Little, Brown.

Silverman, W. A. (1985). *Human experimentation: A guided step into the unknown*. Oxford: Oxford University Press.

Sparks, A. W. (1991). *Talking philosophy*. New York: Routledge.

Sternbach, R. A. (1983). Ethical considerations in pain research in man. In R. Melzack (Ed.), *Pain measurement and assessment* (p. 259). New York: Raven Press.

Sutters, K. A., & Miaskowski, C. (1997). Inadequate pain management and associated morbidity in children after tonsillectomy. *Journal of Pediatric Nursing, 12,* 178–185.

World Medical Association. (1981). *Declaration of Lisbon: The rights of the patient.* Ferney-Voltaire Cedex, France: Author.

World Medical Association. (1964/2000). *Declaration of Helsinki: Recommendations for guiding doctors in clinical research* (rev. ed.). Edinburgh, UK: Author.

Zarit, S. H., Orr, N. K., & Zarit, J. M. (1985). *The hidden victims of Alzheimer's disease: Families under stress.* New York: New York University Press.

Zimmermann, M. (1983). Ethical guidelines for investigations of experimental pain in conscious animals. *Pain, 16,* 109–110.

Author Index

E

F

Subject Index